Mosby's First Responder

2nd edition

Richard L. Judd, Ph.D., EMSI, NREMT-A
Executive Dean and Professor, Emergency Medical Sciences,
Central Connecticut State University, New Britain;
Allied Health Staff, New Britain General Hospital;
New Britain, Connecticut

Dwight D. Ponsell, B.S., A.S., E.M.T.-P.
President, Scientific Paramedic Corporation
Formerly District Chief, Rescue Branch, Department of Public Safety;
Formerly Director, A.S. E.M.T. Program, Florida Junior College;
Jacksonville, Florida

with a foreword by **C. William Schwab, M.D., FACS**
with **495** *illustrations*

The C.V. Mosby Company
• St. Louis • Toronto • Washington, D.C. • 1988

Executive Editor: David T. Culverwell
Senior Editor: Richard A. Weimer
Editorial Project Manager: Lisa G. Cunninghis
Production/Manuscript Editor: A. Tony Melendez
Photography: Huntley S. Pierson
Art: Don Wittig
Index: A. Tony Melendez

Library of Congress Cataloging-in-Publication Data

Judd, Richard L.
    Mosby's first responder.

    Rev. ed. of: The first responder. 1982.
    Includes index.
    1. Medical emergencies. 2. First aid in illness and
injury. I. Ponsell, Dwight D. II. Judd, Richard L.
First responder. III. Title. [DNLM: 1. Allied Health
Personnel. 2. Emergency Medical Services—handbooks.
3. First Aid—handbooks. WX 39 J92m]
RC86.7.J83 1987   606.02'52   87-31450
ISBN 0-8016-2597-1

Printed in the United States of America

The C.V. Mosby Company
11830 Westline Industrial Drive
St. Louis, Missouri 63146

EG/VH/VH   9 8 7 6 5 4 3 2 1   01/D/075

To my family, Nancy, Sarah and Jonathan who support my goings and comings and abundantly enrich my life.

Richard L. Judd

Thanks to all those who have had a part in my development. The indulgence of my sweet wife cannot be overstated.

Thanks to all those who reviewed the manuscript; their helpful suggestions have dramitically improved this edition.

Dwight D. Ponsell

The emergency response to the critically ill and injured is based on a multitiered system that inter-links the site of the emergency and a receiving hospital. In most of these emergencies, after the person in distress is discovered, the first response comes from a group of "concerned" professionals–public safety, fire, or police–who with proper training can make the difference between life or death. Judd and Ponsell in their first text defined for us who these "first responders" are but more importantly, provided a text that enabled this group or any interested American to correctly learn what to do until the ambulance arrived. This widely accepted and masterfully presented textbook was the first of its kind and in just a few years has become the "standard" for initial emergency training.

Some may ask if educating firemen or policemen, especially those working within municipal or county wide EMS systems is beneficial. This is especially germane in an era of cost containment and restricted resource allocation to emergency medical systems. I believe the answer to the question is "yes," a resounding yes! Earlier this year the *New York Times* carried a dramatic picture story con-firming the impact the "First Responder" has on life. The picture was of the New York City firefighters bent over a small child and performing two-rescuer CPR. The story detailed that upon arrival at the burning home, they had found the child with no respirations or pulses. Following rapid evacuation to the street with simultaneous mouth-to-mouth resuscitation, a pulse was felt and as the EMS vehicle arrived, the child started to breathe spontaneously. An anecdotal story–yes, but in my experience a common occurrence and one that goes on daily throughout our land.

In this, the second edition of *Mosby's First Responder,* the authors have expanded and updated the entire first work. Environmental emergencies, abuse problems, including spousal and elderly, a special section on AIDS, and the topic of death and dying have been enhanced to provide a greater under-standing of these areas. Each chapter is presented in a well-designed, easy-to-read format with Key Concepts and Skills, and Key Words initially identified and consistently highlighted throughout the text. The common and expected medical emergencies are presented in an understandable fashion that is masterfully explained by concise anatomical and pathophysiologic explanations. Visual enhance-ment is afforded to each subject by the use of graphic illustrations and conceptual diagrams. The entire book flows so smoothly that one fails to realize they are actually reading a comprehensive field medi-cine manuscript. The authors accomplish this by the application of their own extensive field experi-ence to each of the subjects presented; that experience also enables them to authoritatively write about the knowledge and skills that any "First Responder" will need.

Though targeted to be an introductory medical text for public safety personnel, this textbook should be sought by anyone who may have to intervene in medical emergencies–coaches, office workers, all of us. In fact, any of us may become a "First Responder." This delightful but profound text provides the information that *will* make a difference in those first critical minutes.

C. William Schwab, M.D., FACS
Professor of Surgery
Chief, PENNSTAR
University of Pennsylvania

Preface to the second edition

First responders are perhaps the most important link in the emergency medical services system (EMSS) chain. The first responder is often the initial care provider on the scene of a medical or traumatic emergency. This care begins the systematic response to sudden illness and injury that often makes the difference between life and death. Without first responders trained in basic life support, no EMS system could be optimally effective. Simply, there are not enough EMS personnel available to be on the spot to render care when seconds and minutes count. The first responder in the tiered EMSS performs those life saving and stabilizing functions that reduce patient mortality and morbidity. They can and do make a difference.

The second edition of *Mosby's First Responder* reflects many changes that have come about since 1981 in prehospital emergency medical care. This edition, like its predecessor follows D.O.T. guidelines. The authors have added or strengthened subject material where they believed first responders were in need of additional information. The BLS-CPR chapters, updated to the 1986 AHA standards, describe the procedures involved in cardiac and respiratory arrest step by step, each step augmented with color figures. Two new appendices, one detailing oxygen administration and the other detailing communicable diseases, including AIDS, have been added.

The presentation of material has been simplified and emergency care procedures have been extensively complemented with 495 color figures. The figures provide easy to follow, step by step coverage of important emergency medical care skills. Key concepts, skills and words have been added to highlight important areas of emergency medical care. New sections have been included on pediatric trauma, spousal and elderly abuse, and death and dying.

A workbook and instructor's manual have also been added to enhance both the students' learning and retention, and instructors' methodologies.

The value of the first responder in the nation's emergency medical services system is a vital one, whether the first responder is a member of an organized public safety department, an employee of the U.S. Postal Service, a coach, a citizen, a public utility worker, teacher, or anyone coming to the aid of another person.

What makes the difference is the training that prepares one to act effectively, efficiently, and prudently when confronted with emergencies that threaten or reduce the quality of life of a person. Emergency medical care properly rendered by first responders truly does make a difference. This text is designed to meet the educational and training needs of the first link in a system of prehospital care that is truly a modern medical marvel!

Richard L. Judd

Dwight D. Ponsell

Acknowledgements

We express special thanks and appreciation to Mosby authors and artists for allowing us to use illustrations from their books that enriched this work substantially.

As all authors are aware, no work is fully that of the writers. Many persons share in the overall production process and in many supportive, technical and creative ways. This work is no exception and we are deeply grateful for the contributions of many persons and organizations. All of them, unfortunately, can not be listed, but several deserve our special thanks and recognition.

* Mildred Brayman and Eleanor Glennen who spent countless hours on manuscript production, telephone calls and other coordination activities.

* The team consisting of Huntley S. Pierson, Paul A. Ruel Jr., M.A., and Mark Wnuk, EMSI, who in addition to contractual obligations, expended many additional days in executing and coordinating the extensive photographic work, with special thanks to Sandra Wilson, EMT-I for her expertise in model make-up.

* The many persons associated with the New Britain Emergency Medical Services Foundation who provided equipment and technical assistance

* James A. Gosselin, EMSI and Paul Winfield Smith, workbook authors and colleagues, who offered many helpful suggestions throughout the manuscript production and for their continuing support

* The following persons who served as technical advisors during the photographic sessions expending many hours of their personal time:

James Lombardi, EMT-P
Glenn Bianchi, EMT-I
Joan Ruel, RN
Lynn Dizney, RN
Tom Ronalter, EMT-I
Glynis Skinner, EMT-A
David Mucci, MD

✳ The following departments, organizations and firms who provided personnel, equipment, space and other support services during manuscript production:

Central Connecticut State University Police Department
William McDonald, Chief

U.S. Postal Service, New Britain
Robert Paiva, Acting Postmaster

Southern New England Telephone Company
Daniel Fahey, Director of Public Relations

New Britain (CT) Police Department
Clifford J. Willis, Chief

New Britain (CT) Fire Department
Thomas J. Keough, Chief Engineer

Snowman's Oil Service
George A. Rothstein, President

Berlin (CT) Police Department
William Scalise, Chief

East Berlin (CT) Volunteer Fire Department
David Jorsey, Chief

Budney Industries, Newington, CT
Judith Budney, Vice President

Donald Sagarino Agency, New Britain, CT
Donald Sagarino, President

Empire Motors, New Britain, CT
John Curren, President

New Britain Transportation Company
Donald Agostini, President

Kensington Volunteer Fire Department
Vincent Lewandowski, Chief

New Britain Civil Preparedness
Domonic Colossale, Director

We also thank NancySue Hudson for her many helpful suggestions and the editorial staff of the C.V. Mosby Company, particularly Sue Lawson, Lisa Cunninghis and Rick Weimer for their assistance and support.

Richard L. Judd
Dwight D. Ponsell

Table of Contents

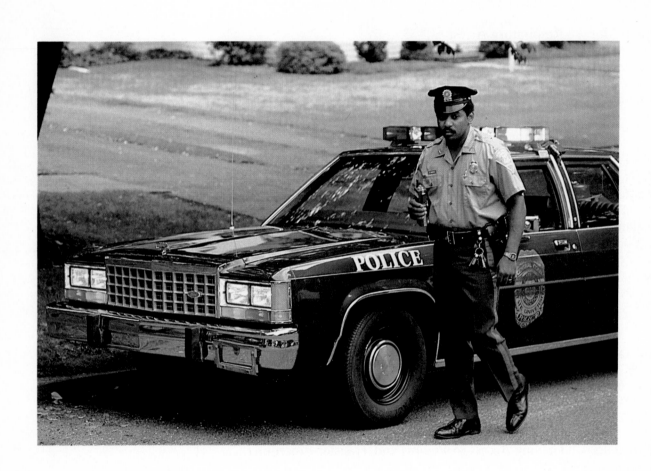

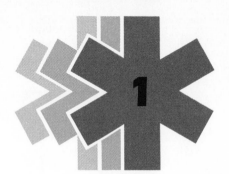

THE FIRST RESPONDER

KEY CONCEPTS AND SKILLS

By the end of this chapter, you will be able to:

❋ Identify key words associated with Emergency Medical Services (EMS)

❋ Define the need for a trained First Responder

❋ Describe the various roles of a First Responder

❋ Identify and describe the skills required to be a First Responder

❋ Describe the procedure necessary to stabilize a patient's condition at the scene of injury or illness until someone with greater medical knowledge can provide additional care.

KEY WORDS

Anaphylaxis – An acute, and sometimes fatal, reaction to a substance such as venom from a bee sting, drugs, chemicals or food. This may be characterized by a local rash, generalized itching, or, in more severe cases, collapse and shock.

Aura – An awareness of physical or mental factors that may precede an attack of migrane or epileptic seizure.

Cardiopulmonary Resuscitation (CPR) – A life-support procedure consisting of rescue breathing and manual, external massaging of the heart to restore circulation and breathing.

Emergency Medical Services System (EMSS) – A national network of services that provide medical assistance for traumatic or medical emergencies. EMSS is a tiered system linked by communications at the regional and local level.

First Responder – The first emergency care person to arrive at an accident scene. This person is trained to follow standards set up by the United States Department of Transportation (DOT).

Hazardous Materials – Substances that are lethal and harmful. These substances include chemicals, petroleum products and radioactive material.

Hazardous Material Incident – A dangerous situation such as a chemical spill or nuclear leak that can cause serious illness or injury.

Hemorrhage – A loss of a large amount of blood in a short period of time, either externally or internally.

Shock – A state of circulatory deficiency. A body's fast alarm to injury or allergic reactions.

Size-up – Scene assessment; starts the moment the "run" begins.

Stabilize – Firm and prepare a patient for transportation to an appropriate medical facility.

Trauma – An injury caused by violence or excessive physical force.

Unconscious – A state in which a person experiences no sensory impressions.

THE IMPORTANCE OF A FIRST RESPONDER

The First Responder, often called a Medical Response Technician, is a partner of the local Emergency Medical Services System (EMSS) (Figure 1-1 and Figure 1-2). A First Responder can be a police officer, a firefighter, a driver of an Emergency Medical Services (EMS) unit, a civil defense unit, or a private citizen.

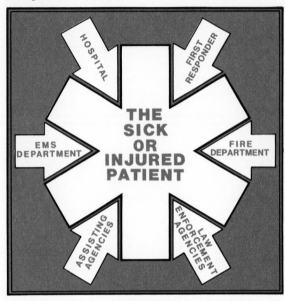

Figure 1-1. The EMS system.

The First Responder usually arrives at an emergency scene before other emergency medical care personnel, and plays a vital role in providing care that reduces or prevents further harm to a victim of trauma or sudden illness.

The actions of the First Responder may well be life saving. Proper handling and care in the first minutes following an accident or illness can lessen the patient's suffering, shorten the period of hospitalization, and reduce the period of recovery.

Although the patient's care becomes the responsibility of the EMS organization upon their arrival to the site, the First Responder should assist the ambulance team. The cooperation of partners in the

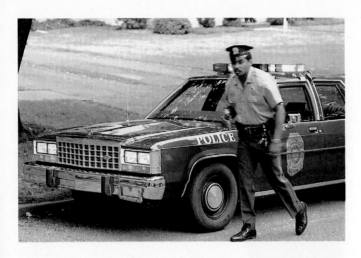

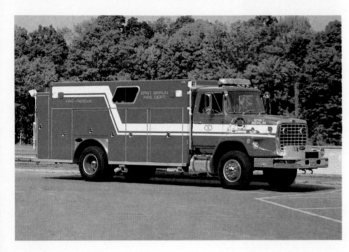

Figure 1-2. Parts of the EMS system.

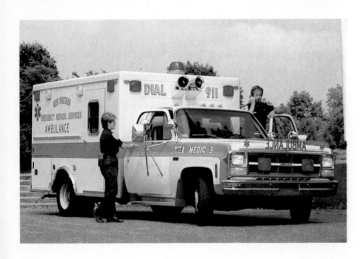

EMS delivery care system is of critical importance. Each responding unit must respect the qualifications, competencies, skills, and special resources provided by EMS, firefighters, police, utilities, and others (Figure 1-3).

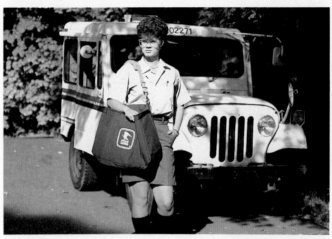

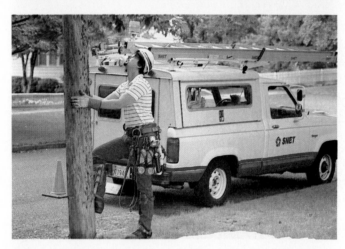

Figure 1-3. First responders.

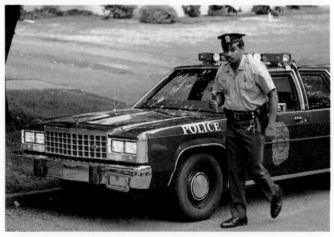

Many agencies participate in the provision of emergency medical services. They include the fire department, law enforcement, emergency medical services organizations, and other agencies such as Civil Preparedness and local utility companies. The First Responder may be a member of one of these agencies. If a sick or injured person is to be provided the best emergency medical care possible, all agencies must cooperate.

SCOPE OF RESPONSIBILITIES

In an emergency situation, the First Responder is required to make important decisions. The greatest responsibility is to the sick or injured person — doing what is necessary to stabilize the person's condition until someone with more advanced training and skills can take charge.

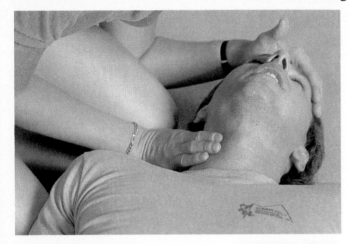

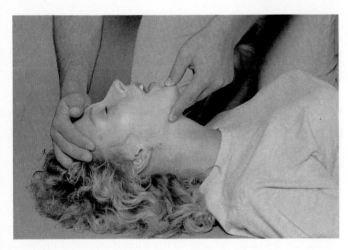

Figure 1-4. Basic life support functions.

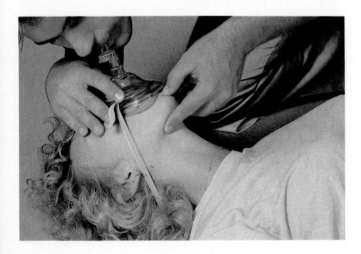

The greatest responsibility in rendering care is to be alert for life-threatening conditions (Figure 1-4) such as:

* Maintaining an airway with cervical spine protection
* Breathing for a person using artificial means (rescue breathing)
* Maintaining circulation with Cardiopulmonary Resuscitation - Basic Life Support (CPR-BLS)
* Controlling massive bleeding (hemorrhaging)
* Recognizing and caring for shock
* Activating the EMS system and notifying other necessary public safety and service departments
* Moving patients when absolutely necessary
* Directing traffic
* Controlling, directing, and asking bystanders for help
* Locating and stabilizing all patients
* Assessing all injured or ill patients
* Protecting the sick and injured from dangers at the scene such as traffic, energized power lines, or the presence of hazardous materials (HAZMAT) (Figure 1-5).

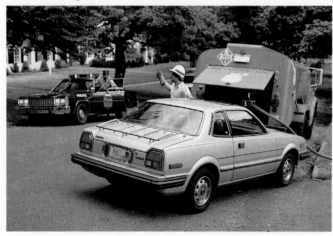

Figure 1-5. Accident scene.

While this list may not cover every situation, it is the responsibility of the First Responder to decide which actions must be taken. Prior planning is the key to good performance.

ASSESSING THE SCENE

Size-up, a quick evaluation of the emergency situation, is critical to protecting all persons at the scene. Size-up begins the moment you arrive at the scene of the incident. It may even begin when the dispatcher announces the emergency.

Emergency situations are seldom the same. Size-up helps you prepare and plan ahead by allowing you to consider the best route to the scene, route conditions (e.g., dry roads, dusk, traffic situations, rescue squad en route), type of emergency, and required equipment.

PERSONAL SAFETY

Your personal safety is of primary importance. Protecting and preserving life must include yourself, as well as those involved in the emergency. Never place your duty as a First Responder before your own personal safety. Duty does not mean being a hero.

As a First Responder, never:

* Enter a burning building unless properly equipped and trained as a firefighter

* Confront a mentally disturbed person who may be, or become, violent unless properly trained as a police officer in crisis intervention and are prepared to use appropriate force

* Enter the water and attempt to rescue a potential drowning victim unless properly trained in water-rescue techniques

* Attempt to remove an injured patient unless properly trained in difficult terrain rescue

* Enter a building where a bomb may be present unless properly equipped and trained for these situations

VEHICLE PLACEMENT

Vehicle placement depends on many factors (Figure 1-6):

* The nature of the emergency (e.g., a fire, gas leak, vehicle accident, aircraft crash, hazardous materials incident)

* Weather conditions such as fog, snow, or heavy rain

* Terrain, such as hills or curves in the road

* Services needed (e.g., firefighter, police, EMS, utilities, wrecker)

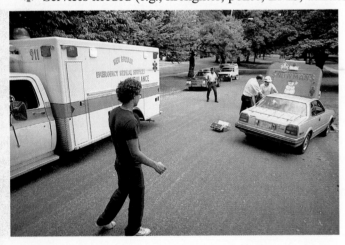

Figure 1-6. Vehicle placement at accident scene.

Since the First Responder is often the first person to arrive at the scene, park the response vehicle so that it is both accessible and out of the way of arriving vehicles. The First Responder arriving at the scene of a fire should park away from any fire hydrants.

Do not block the driveway to a residence or building if the services of an ambulance may be needed. After other emergency units have arrived, ask the person in charge of the scene if your vehicle should be moved. Always follow the directions of the individual in charge.

Do not stop at an emergency scene unless your services are needed. It is important for First Responders to provide care, but one should never become a spectator. If your services are no longer required, leave the scene. Your vehicle may be adding to the congestion.

NOTE: Many emergencies are potential crime scenes. Be careful when entering the area of a scene that may require the collection of evidence. Walking through such an area can disturb or destroy valuable evidence.

APPROACHING THE PATIENT

Initial contact with a patient is important (Figure 1-7). Your behavior, attitude, or words can communicate either trust or distrust, hope or lack of hope, caring or noncaring.

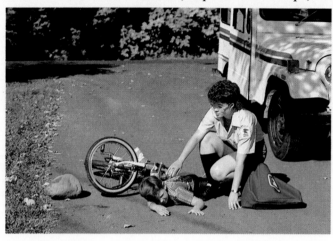

Figure 1-7. Patient approach.

As a First Responder, professional behavior is critical. Address all patients with respect. State clearly to the patient who you are and what you are trained to do. A positive and assertive attitude helps everyone.

Be careful what you say especially when treating unconscious or semiconscious persons. Such patients are often aware of much that is said. Information of a confidential, privileged nature may be revealed to the patient and can be harmful. Remarks such as, "Oh-oh," or "Oh-no, his leg is gone," do not help the patient and may needlessly frighten the victim. Put yourself in the place of the victim — what would you want to hear?

Do not treat children as miniature adults. Consider the child's age and maturity but do not underestimate the child. A child may be frightened of you or your uniform, be in pain, or simply be in an aura due to the emergency situation. An emergency is difficult for many adults to understand; for the child, it may be even more difficult. Careful explanation and attention to the child's needs will help.

Obtain consent from a patient or guardian to assist a minor. A parent or close adult should be with the child when emergency procedures are undertaken. If the parent or other adult interferes with what is going on, or is too upset to be of help, call the appropriate personnel (e.g., the police) to provide assistance. Life or death injuries can be stabilized without consent, but you should always seek out a responsible party if one is available.

SUMMARY

Early emergency care saves lives and reduces hospitalization. Trauma is the leading cause of death for persons between the ages of 1 and 37. This trauma occurs in homes, industrial settings, businesses, roadways, and playgrounds. The First Responder is often the first trained person to arrive at the scene where one is injured or ill.

The First Responder provides needed care until the EMS assumes responsibility for the sick or injured. Every member of the team is required if the patient is to be properly treated.

The First Responder must be able to survey the scene and provide the essential care to protect the patient from further harm.

Emergency care by the First Responder includes:

* Patient assessment
* Airway management
* Cardiopulmonary Resuscitation (CPR)
* Trauma care
* Bleeding control
* Fracture care
* Emergency childbirth
* Exposure to the environment
* Poisoning and drug control
* Mental health emergencies
* Hazardous materials assessment
* Victim access and transfer procedures

The First Responder must determine whether a patient is being handled effectively and may intervene accordingly.

POSTERIOR VIEW OF SKELETON
Axial skeleton is shown in blue. Appendicular system is
bone colored.

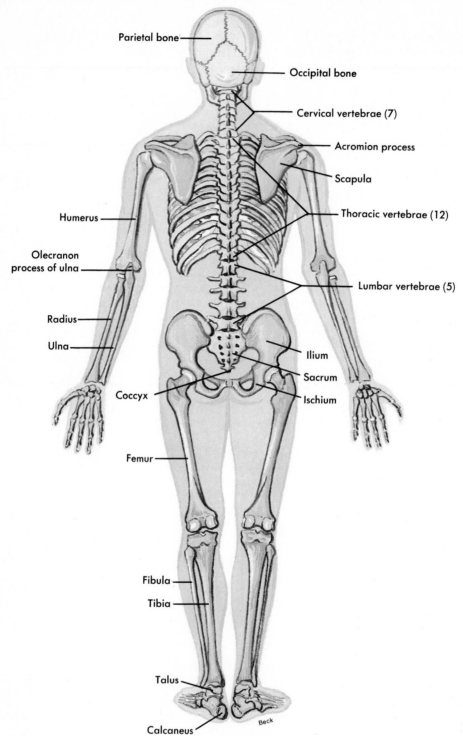

Parietal bone

Occipital bone

Cervical vertebrae (7)

Acromion process

Scapula

Humerus

Thoracic vertebrae (12)

Olecranon
process of ulna

Lumbar vertebrae (5)

Radius

Ulna

Ilium

Sacrum

Coccyx

Ischium

Femur

Fibula

Tibia

Talus

Calcaneus

Beck

ANATOMY OF THE HUMAN BODY

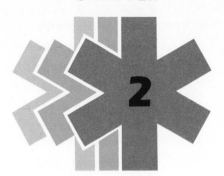

KEY CONCEPTS AND SKILLS

This chapter is an overview of the anatomy of the human body. As a First Responder, you will need to know the major body structures and their locations. It is not necessary that you know every detail of medicine or memorize a lot of medical terms. It is more important that you be able to identify and locate the major subdivisions of the body so that you can easily relate certain injuries or diseases to those parts of the body at an emergency scene.

Even though you are not expected to memorize a lot of medical terms, many of the medical names are in parentheses next to their common name or description in the text. This exposes you to terms that you may hear from more experienced medical personnel at an emergency scene.

By the end of this chapter, you will be able to:

✳ Identify various locations of the body and describe the directional relationship of two or more body parts.

✳ Identify and locate the five major cavities in the human body.

✳ Identify the function of each body system specified.

✳ Identify the location and function of major organs in the body.

KEY WORDS

Alveoli – Microscopic air cells (called sacs) that are found in the lungs. The exchange of oxygen and carbon dioxide takes place in these cells.

Appendix – An appendage attached to the large intestine. This sac-like tissue can become inflamed, resulting in appendicitis.

Anterior – Toward the front.

Artery – A large blood vessel that carries blood away from the heart.

Bronchi – The two main branches that lead away from the trachea to the lungs. The bronchi are the only passageways that allow air into the lungs.

Capillaries – Tiny blood vessels found between the veins and arteries.

Cartilage – A tough, fibrous tissue that is found in the joints, nose, ears, and the upper airway.

Colon – The portion of the large intestine that extends from the cecum to the rectum.

Diaphragm – A dome-shaped muscle that forms a wall separating the abdomen from the chest cavity. When the diaphragm shortens in size (contracts), it flattens downward, permitting the lungs to descend and fill with air.

Duodenum – The first part of the small intestine that connects at the stomach and extends to the second part of the small intestine (jejunum).

Epiglottis – A leaf-shaped tissue posterior to the tongue. This tissue covers the larynx during swallowing.

Epigastrium – The upper, central region of the stomach.

Esophagus – A muscular canal that connects the pharynx to the stomach. The esophagus starts in the neck and extends to the stomach.

Gallbladder – A pear-shaped sac organ that stores bile, located in the upper right quadrant of the abdomen.

Heart – A muscular, cone-shaped organ that pumps blood throughout the body.

Ileum – The third part of the small intestine that connects to the large intestine.

Jejunum – The second part of the small intestine that connects the duodenum to the ileum.

Kidney – One of a pair of bean-shaped organs located at the back of the abdominal cavity on each side of the spinal column. Its function is to filter blood and excrete urine.

Large Intestine – The last portion of the digestive tract. The large intestine is connected at the end of the small intestine by the ileum. The appendix is located next to the junction of the ileum and the large intestine.

Larynx – The voice structure that is part of the air passage connecting the pharynx with the trachea.

Liver – One of the larger organs in the body. The liver is found in the right upper portion of the abdominal cavity. The liver performs a variety of functions including the production of bile, which is stored in the gallbladder, and the distribution of glucose, proteins, vitamins, fats, and most other compounds used in the body.

Lungs – A pair of spongy organs that are located in the chest (thorax). The lungs are the main parts of the respiratory system.

Metabolism – A series of chemical changes that occur in the body resulting in growth, generation of energy, elimination of wastes, and other functions that relate to the distribution of nutrients in the blood after digestion.

Pancreas – A fish-shaped gland that stretches across both upper quadrants of the rear abdominal wall. The pancreas secretes digestive enzymes and insulin.

Pathogen – Any substance, microorganism or virus capable of producing diseases.

Peripheral – Of or pertaining to the outside, surface, or surrounding area of an organ or other structure.

Pharynx – The throat.

Plasma – Noncellular, fluid portion of the lymph and blood.

Posterior – Toward the back.

Pubic Bone – A portion of the pelvis.

Red Cells – Also called erythrocytes. Blood cells that contain hemoglobin, a substance that carries oxygen to the cells from the lungs.

Spleen – A sphere-shaped organ found between the stomach and the diaphragm. This organ is highly vascular.

Stomach – A major organ in the digestive system. The stomach is found in the upper right quadrant of the abdomen between the esophagus and the small intestine.

Trachea – The "windpipe." A cylindrical tube in the neck that extends from the larynx to the 5th thoracic vertebra where it then divides into 2 tubes (bronchi) to the lungs. The trachea provides the passageway for air to and from the lungs.

Ureters – A pair of tubes that carry urine from the kidney to the urinary bladder.

Urethra – A small, tubular canal that drains urine from the bladder.

Urinary Bladder – The muscular, membranous sac in the pelvis that stores urine before it is discharged through the urethra.

Vein – A vessel that carries unoxygenated blood back to the heart.

Vertabra – A spinal bone. There are 33 vertebra in the human spine.

White Cells – Also called leukocytes. These cells are found in the blood, They act as scavengers and fight infection.

Xiphoid Process – The lowest portion of the sternum. It has no ribs attached to it, but some of the abdominal muscles are attached to the xiphoid process.

DIRECTIONAL TERMS

Just as an atlas is divided by direction, (north, south, east, and west), so is the human body.

The following discussion describes the terms that are used to identify various locations of the body. When referring to the directional terms of the body, always assume the patient is facing you with hands open, fingers open, and palms facing forward.

The body is first divided down the middle. Think of an imaginary line running through the center of the body from head to toe. This imaginary line is called the midline. The midline establishes the patient's left and right. The front of the patient's body is called the anterior. The back of the patient's body is called the posterior.

There are other terms that describe the relative locations based on the midline. For example, any body part located toward the midline is referred to as medial. Any body part located away from the midline is called lateral. Body parts toward the head are called superior and any body parts toward the feet are called inferior. For example, the eyes are superior to the chest while the mouth is inferior to the nose but superior to the chin (Figure 2-1).

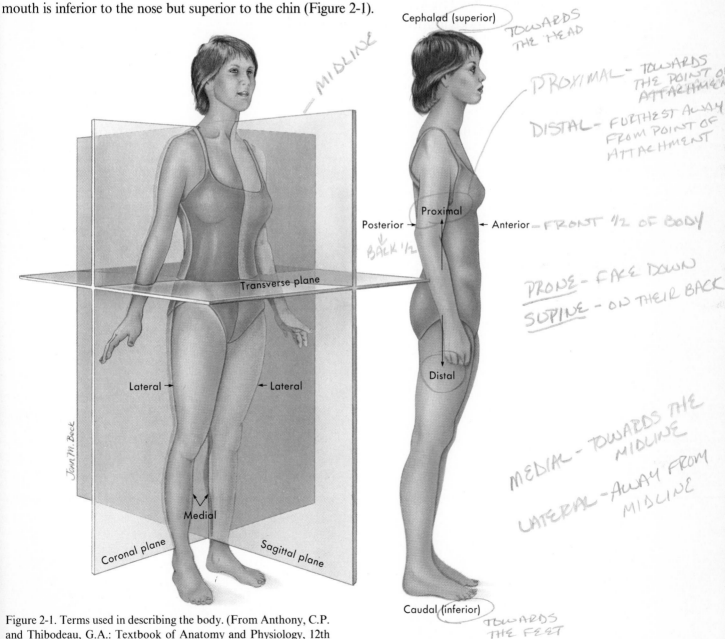

Figure 2-1. Terms used in describing the body. (From Anthony, C.P. and Thibodeau, G.A.: Textbook of Anatomy and Physiology, 12th edition, St. Louis, 1987, The C.V. Mosby Co.)

BODY REGIONS

After establishing direction, a map can be broken down into regions such as North America, South America, Asia and Europe. On a smaller scale, the regions can then be broken down into countries. The human body may also be divided into regions on much the same principle (Figure 2-2). From head to toe, these regions are:

✳ Head

  brain case (cranium)

  face

  jawbone (mandible)

✳ Neck

  spinal column

  airway tube (trachea)

  blood vessels (carotid arteries-jugular veins)

✳ Trunk

  spinal column

  chest (thorax)

  abdomen

  spinal column

  pelvis

✳ Upper Extremities

  shoulder

  upper arm

  elbow

  forearm

  wrist

  hand

✳ Lower Extremities

  thigh

  knee

  lower leg

  ankle

  foot

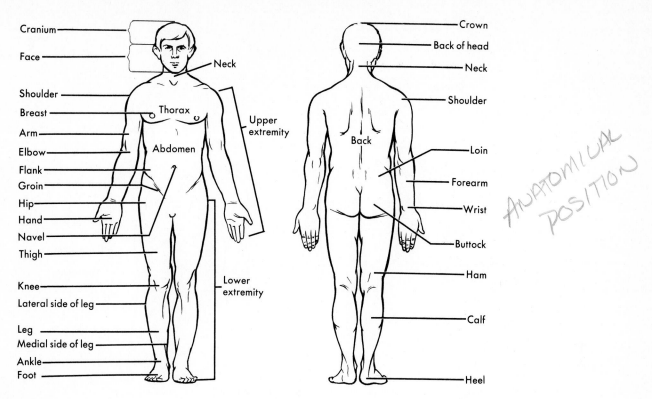

Figure 2-2. General descriptive areas of the body. (From McClintic,
J.R.: Human Anatomy, St. Louis, 1983, The C.V. Mosby Co.)

Study the basic geography of the human body. It is important the you be able to identify and locate these regions as you begin to learn more about the body and its functions.

BODY CAVITIES

There are five major body cavities that protect the major organs of the body (Figure 2-3).

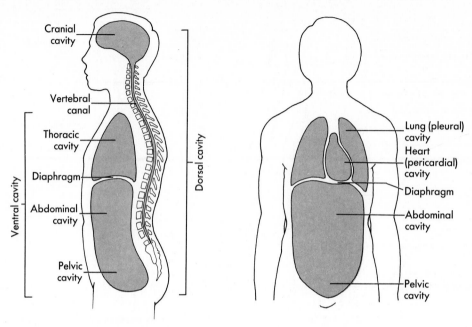

Figure 2-3. Major body cavities. (From McClintic, J.R.: Human Anatomy, St. Louis, 1983, The C.V. Mosby Co.)

1. *Cranial Cavity* – Protects the brain, eyes, and nasal airways.
2. *Spinal Cavity* - Protects the spinal cord, which is an extension of the brain.
3. *Chest Cavity* - Protects the heart, lungs, large blood vessels, part of the windpipe (the trachea) and a portion of the tube leading into the stomach (the esophagus). The lower portion of the chest cavity is a dome-shaped muscle called the diaphragm. The diaphragm separates the chest cavity from the abdominal cavity. The diaphragm aids in breathing.
4. *Abdominal Cavity* - Protects the stomach, liver, gallbladder, pancreas, spleen, small intestine, portions of the large intestine, the female reproductive organs, and the rectum. This cavity extends from below the ribs to the pelvis. The abdomen is a large body region. The only point of reference is the navel. Because so many organs are in the abdomen, it has been divided into the following 4 quadrants:

   ✽ Right Upper Quadrant (RUQ) - Containing most of the liver, the gallbladder, and part of the large intestine.

   ✽ Left Upper Quadrant (LUQ) - Containing most of the stomach, the spleen, and part of the large intestine.

   ✽ Right Lower Quadrant (RLQ) - Containing the appendix and part of the large intestine.

   ✽ Left Lower Quadrant (LLQ) - Containing part of the large intestine.

   Some organs and glands are located in more than one quadrant. The large intestine is found, in part, in the 4 quadrants. The same is true for the small intestine. Part of the stomach can be found in the right upper quadrant. Pelvic organs are included in these quadrants, with the urinary bladder being assigned to both lower quadrants.

5. *Pelvic Cavity* Protects the urinary bladder, part of the large intestine, and the female reproductive organs.

MAJOR BODY SYSTEMS

There are 10 major systems in the body. The following list briefly describes each system and its major functions. Figures 2-4 through 2-13 illustrate the locations of the various systems in the body. More detailed information for each system is found later in the text as it applies to specific emergency treatment, injuries, and diseases.

1. *Skeletal System* - Provides protection to the major organs through its intricate joint and bone structure. It allows for the movement of the body. The skeletal system is the supporting framework of the body (Figure 2-4).

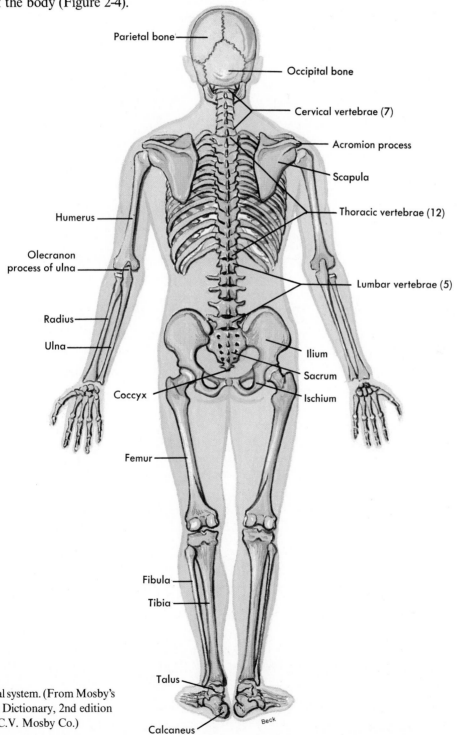

Figure 2-4. The skeletal system. (From Mosby's Medical and Nursing Dictionary, 2nd edition St. Louis, 1986, The C.V. Mosby Co.)

2. *Muscular System* - Muscles are a kind of tissue composed of fibers that are able to contract and relax, causing and allowing for the movement of the parts and organs of the body (Figure 2-5).

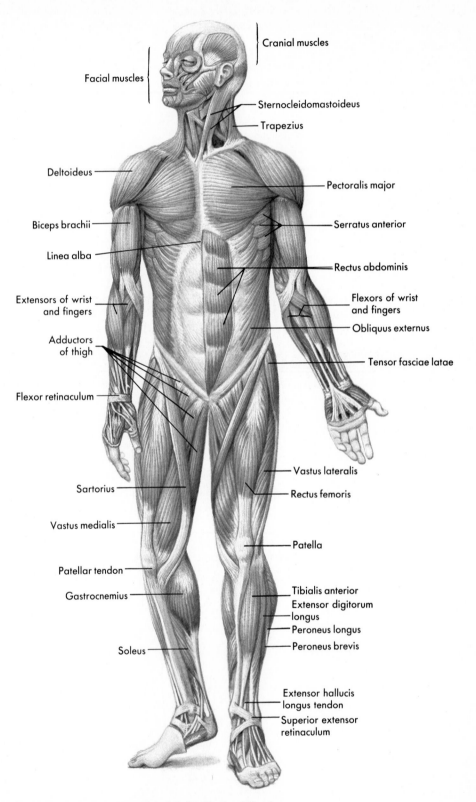

Cranial muscles

Facial muscles

Sternocleidomastoideus

Trapezius

Deltoideus

Pectoralis major

Biceps brachii

Serratus anterior

Linea alba

Rectus abdominis

Extensors of wrist and fingers

Flexors of wrist and fingers

Obliquus externus

Adductors of thigh

Tensor fasciae latae

Flexor retinaculum

Vastus lateralis

Sartorius

Rectus femoris

Vastus medialis

Patella

Patellar tendon

Gastrocnemius

Tibialis anterior

Extensor digitorum longus

Peroneus longus

Peroneus brevis

Soleus

Extensor hallucis longus tendon

Superior extensor retinaculum

Figure 2-5. The muscular system. (From Mosby's Medical and Nursing Dictionary, 2nd edition, St. Louis, 1986, The C.V. Mosby Co.)

3. *Circulatory System* - The heart and arteries transport oxygenated blood and nutrients through the body and remove wastes and carbon dioxide (Figure 2-6).

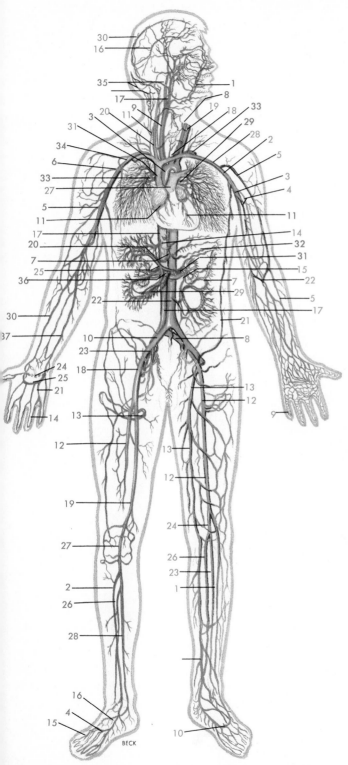

PRINCIPAL VEINS AND ARTERIES

Principal arteries

1 Angular
2 Anterior tibial
3 Aorta
4 Arcuate
5 Axillary
6 Brachial
7 Celiac
8 Common carotid, left
9 Common carotid, right
10 Common iliac, right
11 Coronary, left
12 Deep femoral
13 Deep medial
   circumflex femoral
14 Digital
15 Dorsal metatarsal
16 Dorsalis pedis
17 External carotid
18 External iliac
19 Femoral
20 Hepatic
21 Metacarpal
22 Inferior mesenteric
23 Internal iliac
   (hypogastric)
24 Palmar arch, deep
25 Palmar arch, superficial
26 Peroneal
27 Popliteal
28 Posterior tibial
29 Pulmonary
30 Radial
31 Renal
32 Splenic
33 Subclavian, left (cut)
34 Subclavian, right
35 Superficial temporal
36 Superior mesenteric
37 Ulnar

Principal veins

1 Anterior tibial
2 Axillary
3 Basilic
4 Brachial
5 Cephalic
6 Cervical plexus
7 Colic
8 Common iliac, left
9 Digital
10 Dorsal venous arch
11 External jugular
12 Femoral
13 Great saphenous
14 Hepatic
15 Inferior mesenteric
16 Inferior sagittal sinus
17 Inferior vena cava
18 Brachiocephalic, left
19 Internal jugular, left
20 Internal jugular, right
21 Lateral thoracic
22 Median cubital
23 Peroneal
24 Popliteal
25 Portal
26 Posterior tibial
27 Pulmonary
28 Subclavian, left
29 Superior mesenteric
30 Superior sagittal sinus
31 Superior vena cava

Figure 2-6. The circulatory system. (From Mosby's Medical and Nursing Dictionary, 2nd edition, St. Louis, 1986, The C.V. Mosby Co.)

4. *Endocrine System* - The glands that produce hormones that help regulate most bodily functions such as metabolism and growth (Figure 2-7).

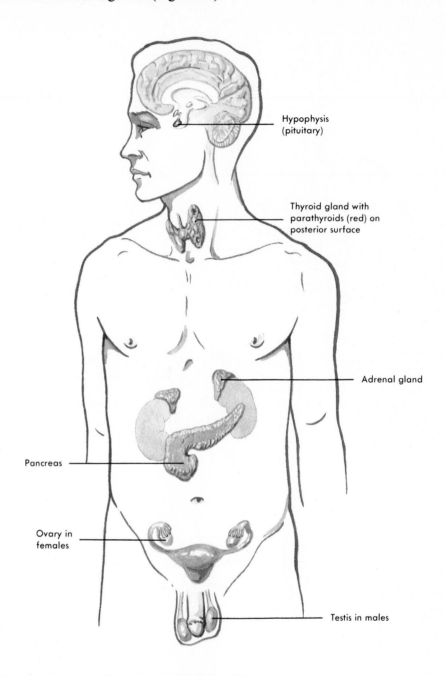

Figure 2-7. The endocrine system. (From Mosby's Medical and Nursing Dictionary, 2nd edition, St. Louis, 1986, The C.V. Mosby Co.)

5. *Lymphatic System* - Protects and maintains the internal fluid environment. The lymphatic system also carries fats, proteins, and other substances to the blood (Figure 2-8).

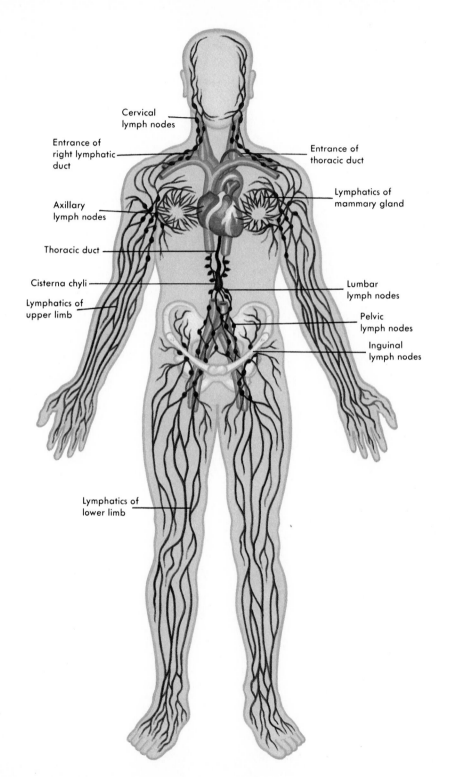

Figure 2-8. The lymphatic system. (From Mosby's Medical and Nursing Dictionary, 2nd edition, St. Louis, 1986, The C.V. Mosby Co.)

6. *Nervous System* - Consists of the brain, spinal cord, and a network of nerves that activate, coordinate, and control all bodily functions including the senses of light, smell, taste, touch, and hearing (Figure 2-9).

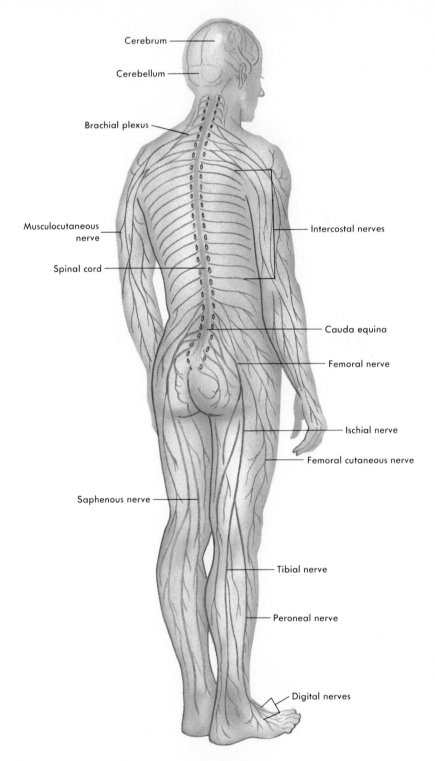

Figure 2-9. The nervous system. (From Mosby's Medical and Nursing Dictionary, 2nd edition, St. Louis, 1986, The C.V. Mosby Co.)

7. *Respiratory System* - Consists of the lungs and related organs that allow and provide for the exchange of oxygen and carbon dioxide to the blood stream, and assists in speech by providing air to the larynx and vocal cords (Figure 2-10).

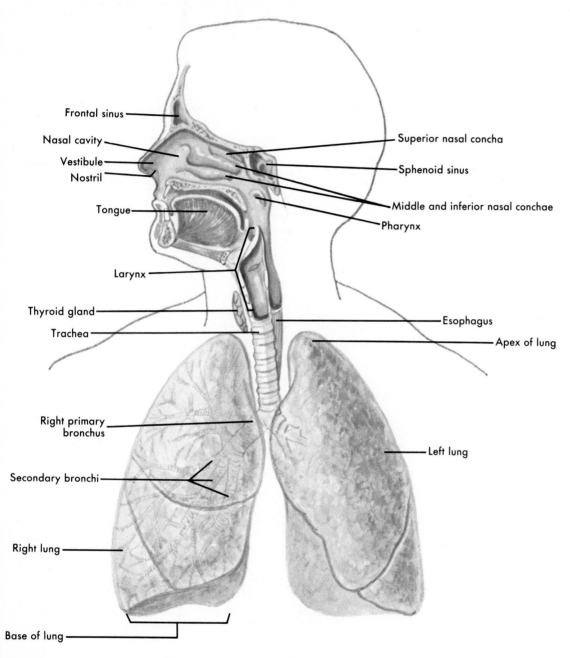

Frontal sinus

Nasal cavity

Vestibule

Nostril

Tongue

Larynx

Thyroid gland

Trachea

Right primary bronchus

Secondary bronchi

Right lung

Base of lung

Superior nasal concha

Sphenoid sinus

Middle and inferior nasal conchae

Pharynx

Esophagus

Apex of lung

Left lung

Figure 2-10. The respiratory system. (From Mosby's Medical and Nursing Dictionary, 2nd edition, St. Louis, 1986, The C.V. Mosby Co.)

8. *Digestive System* - Responsible for the digestion of foods and waste disposal (Figure 2-11).

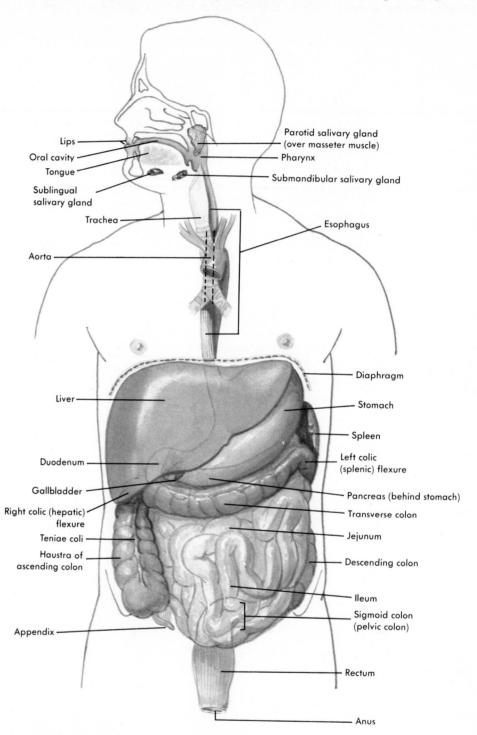

Figure 2-11. The digestive system. (From Mosby's Medical and Nursing Dictionary, 2nd edition, St. Louis, 1986, The C.V. Mosby Co.)

9. *Genitourinary System* - Controls the removal of fluid and wastes from the blood. This also includes the reproductive system (Figure 2-12).

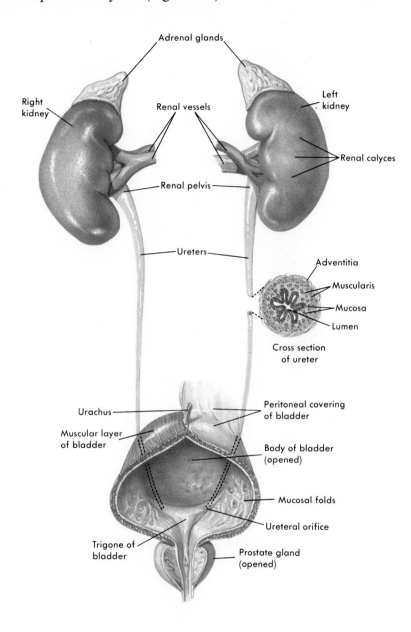

Figure 2-12a. The genitourinary system (male). (From Mosby's Medical and Nursing Dictionary, 2nd edition, St. Louis, 1986, The C.V. Mosby Co.)

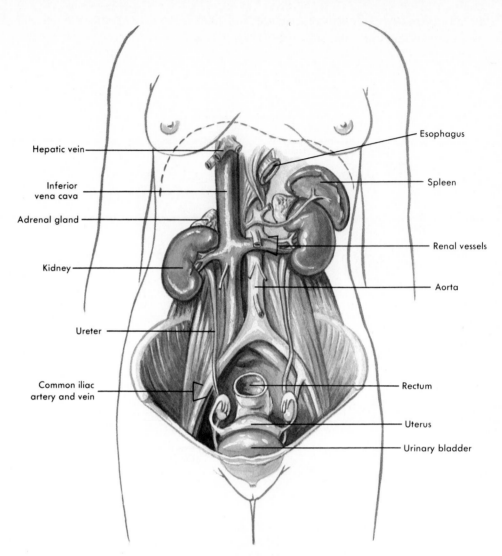

Hepatic vein

Inferior
vena cava

Adrenal gland

Kidney

Ureter

Common iliac
artery and vein

Esophagus

Spleen

Renal vessels

Aorta

Rectum

Uterus

Urinary bladder

URINARY SYSTEM AND SOME ASSOCIATED STRUCTURES

Fibure 2-12b. The genitourinary system (female). (From Mosby's
Medical and Nursing Dictionary, 2nd edition, St. Louis, 1986, The
C.V. Mosby Co.)

10. *Skin* - Layers of tissue that cover the entire surface of the body. The skin protects the body from disease-causing organisms, eliminates waste, and controls temperature. It is the largest organ of the body (Figure 2-13).

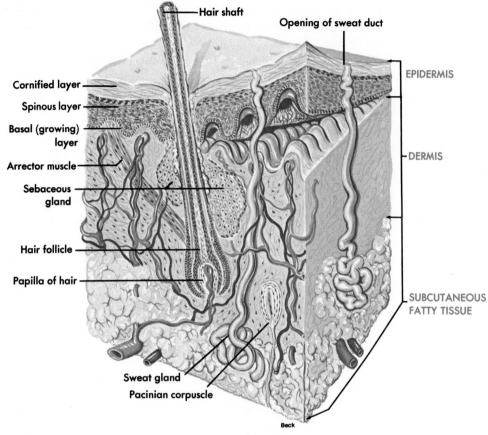

Figure 2-13. The skin. (From McClintic, J.R.: Human Anatomy, St. Louis, 1983, The C.V. Mosby Co.)

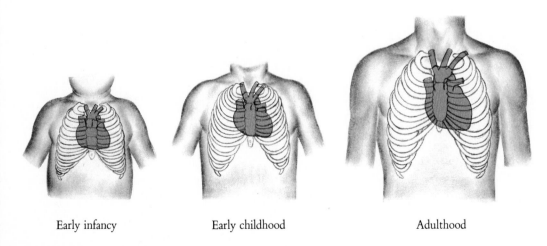

Early infancy   Early childhood   Adulthood

Figure 2-14. Location of the heart at various stages. (From Seidel, et al: Mosby's Guide to Physical Examination, St. Louis, 1987, The C.V. Mosby Co.)

MAJOR ORGANS

Now that you are familiar with directional terms, basic body regions, and the body's systems, you will more easily understand the major organs and related structures. As First Responder you must know the location and position of various structures in the body. Figures 2-14 through 2-16 illustrate the relative size and shape of the structures so that you can locate and relate the position of these organs to the exterior of the body.

The heart is one of the first organs you will locate (Figure 2-14). The heart is located in the chest. The ribs on the chest are divided by the breast bone (sternum). Use your finger to find the sternum, which is found in the middle of the chest cavity. The lowest part of the sternum is a small hard spot called the xiphoid (zi-foyd) process.

The lungs are also found in the chest cavity (Figure 2-15). The approximate center of the lungs is indicated by the nipples.

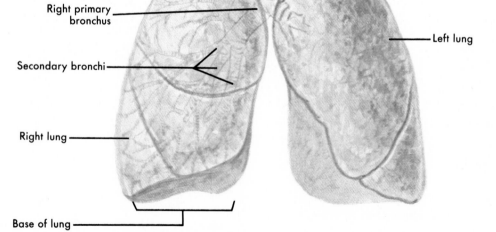

Figure 2-15. Organs of the respiratory system. (From McClintic, J.R.:
Human Anatomy, St. Louis, 1983, The C.V. Mosby Co.)

The stomach, liver, and first portion of the small intestine (the duodenum) are all found in the right upper quadrant of the abdominal cavity (Figure 2-16).

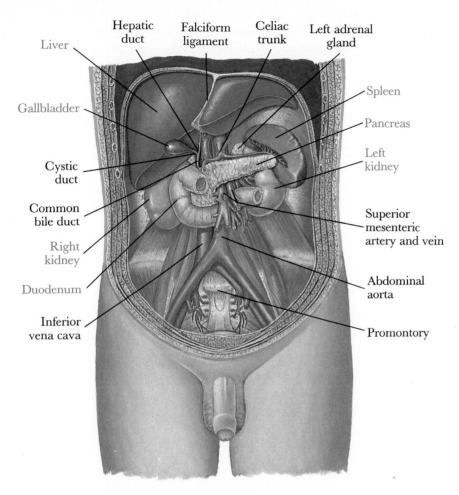

Figure 2-16. Organs of the abdominal cavity. (From Seidel, et al: Mosby's Guide to Physical Examination, St. Louis, 1987, The C.V. Mosby Co.)

The lower ribs protect the stomach and the liver. The location of the duodenum is important in emergency medical situations because this portion of the small intestine often receives severe blows during motor vehicle accidents (MVAs).

In relation to the stomach, liver, and duodenum, locate the gallbladder (behind the liver), the pancreas (behind the lower portion of the stomach), and the spleen (behind the left side of the stomach)(Figure 2-16).

The remainder of the small intestine (the ileum) takes up a large portion of the abdominal cavity. The large intestine surrounds the small intestine.

The kidneys are found behind the abdominal cavity . The bladder is in the pelvic cavity.

SUMMARY

As a First Responder, you need to know major body structures and their location. It is important for you to be able to locate and identify major organs. When you are at an emergency scene, you will need to communicate with other medical personnel. You will need to explain areas of pain by using directional terms in relation to various body regions such as the upper and lower extremities and the 4 quadrants of the abdomen.

You need to know various body cavities and which organs are contained within them. For example, the gallbladder is located in the right upper quadrant of the abdominal cavity. In addition, a First Responder should also be familiar with the 10 major body systems and their functions. The following quick reference list summarizes what you have learned in this chapter.

Directional Terms

* Midline - Center of the body from head to toe
* Left - Patient's left
* Right - Patient's right
* Anterior - Front of the patient's body
* Posterior - Back of the patient's body
* Medial - Toward the midline
* Lateral - Away from the midline
* Superior - Toward the head
* Inferior - Toward the feet

Body Regions

* Head
* Neck
* Trunk
* Upper Extremities
* Lower Extremities

Body Cavities

* Cranial
* Spinal
* Chest
* Abdominal
* Pelvic

Body Systems

* Skeletal
* Muscular
* Circulatory
* Endocrine
* Lymphatic
* Nervous (including special senses)
* Respiratory
* Digestive
* Genitourinary, including reproductive
* Skin

Major Organs

* Brain, spinal cord
* Heart
* Lungs
* Stomach
* Liver
* Gallbladder
* Pancreas
* Spleen
* Small and large intestines
* Kidneys
* Bladder
* Genitalia
* Skeleton

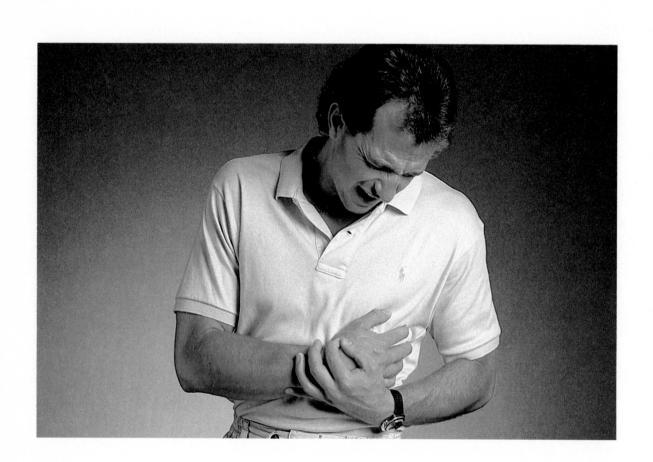

DIAGNOSTIC SIGNS AND PATIENT EVALUATION

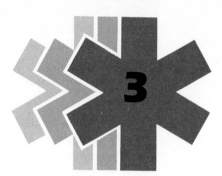

3

KEY CONCEPTS AND SKILLS

By the end of this chapter, you will be able to:

✳ Understand the concept of triage

✳ Identify the Medical Alert Symbol

✳ Describe and identify patient priority categories

✳ Describe vital signs and identify their normal ranges

✳ Describe various common symptoms of illness

✳ Perform the head-to-toe patient evaluation process for both trauma and medical illness.

✳ Describe and evaluate processes using the primary and secondary survey

KEY WORDS

AMPLE – An acronym for *A*llergies, *M*edications, *P*ast history, *L*ast meal, and *E*vents leading up to an emergency.

Antecubital – The area located anterior to the elbow; at the bend of the elbow; the location where palpation of the brachial artery occurs when taking a blood pressure.

Assessment – Determining the existence of life-threatening problems involving the airway (with cervical spine control), breathing, circulation, and massive hemorrhage. Also used to describe scene evaluation.

APVU – A method used to assess a patient's level of consciousness. The acronym stands for *A*lert, responds to *V*erbal commands, responds to *P*ain, or *U*nresponsive.

Blood Pressure – The pressure exerted by the blood on the walls of the arteries.

BP Cuff (Sphygmomanometer) – The instrument used to determine the pressure exerted on the arteries when the heart contracts and relaxes, always expressed in even numbers.

Brachial artery – The main artery of the upper arm. This artery is a continuation of the axillary artery on the inside of the arm.

Cardiac Arrest – Stoppage of effective heart action that can be detected by lack of central body pulses.

Carotid Artery – The main artery found anteriorly in the neck on either side of the larynx (voice box).

Cerebrovascular Accident (CVA) – (Stroke) An abnormal condition of blood vessels of the brain such as cerebral hemorrhaging resulting in decreased blood supply to an area of brain tissue, which may cause paralysis, weakness, a speech defect, or even death.

Cyanosis – Dark blue, gray, or dark purple discoloration of the skin, mucosa, or nail beds due to a decrease of oxygen in the blood.

Diastolic Pressure – Pressure exerted on the walls of the arteries during relaxation of the ventricles.

Dilate – Expand. For example, the pupil of an eye becomes larger if there is less light.

Distal – Farthest location from the center or median line; the opposite of proximal.

Dyspnea – A shortness of breath or difficult, labored breathing. May be caused by certain heart conditions, exercise, trauma, anxiety, or respiratory diseases.

Ectopic Pregnancy – An abnormal pregnancy in which the fertilized ovum implants outside the uterine cavity. There are different types of ectopic pregnancies.

Femoral Artery – The artery that begins in the same area as the external iliac and ends behind the knee as the popliteal artery on the inner side of the thigh.

Fracture – A break in a bone or cartilage.

Heat Exhaustion – Acute reaction to heat exposure; marked by weakness, dizziness, cool and clammy skin, dilated pupils, nausea, confusion, and chills.

Hypothermia – A condition in which the body temperature is below 94 °F (34.4 °C).

Laceration – A wound characterized by roughly jagged edges.

Mucosa – A mucous membrane composed of highly vascular tissue, which lines many structures of the body, e.g., the eyelids and mouth.

PERRLA – An acronym for *P*upils *E*qual, *R*ound, *R*eact to *L*ight. This is a method used to access eye response.

Primary Survey – The initial examination of a patient.

Priority Category – The earliest and most important emergency care to be carried out to support life.

Proximal – Closest location to the center of the median line, the opposite of distal.

Pubis – Pubic bone; the middle, front part of the pelvis.

Pulse – Rhythmic throbbing of an artery caused by the contraction of the heart.

Pulse Pressure – The numerical difference between systolic pressure and diastolic pressure.

Pupil – The opening at the center of the iris of the eye. It allows light to pass into the lens.

Radial Artery – An artery in the forearm that branches to the wrist and hand. Used to palpate a pulse on the thumb side of the wrist.

Respiration – The process of breathing.

Secondary Survey – A head-to-toe evaluation of the patient that is done when the primary survey and life-threatening emergencies have been treated.

Sign – Observable evidence or onset of an illness or trauma. Look, listen, and feel the patient for these signs.

Stethoscope – An instrument used to hear heart and lung sounds.

Symptom – Evidence of illness or injury related to the First Responder by the patient.

Systolic Pressure – Pressure exerted on the arteries during contraction of the ventricles of the heart.

Triage – A treatment or transport priority system to sort multiple ill or injured patients.

TRIAGE

In chapter 1, you learned the concept of size-up. Size-up is an assessment of the emergency scene. Until now the discussions assumed that only one patient is involved in an emergency situation. However, in many emergency situations there may be several injured or ill persons.

While size-up is an assessment of the emergency scene (environment), an assessment of the patient's state must be determined as well. As a First Responder, you must decide which patients require immediate emergency treatment or transport. The sorting and evaluating process is called triage (Figure 3-1). The decision to provide immediate emergency care should be based on the following criteria:

✳ The patient is not severely injured or critically ill

✳ Death could occur in minutes, or death could occur in hours

✳ The person is dead

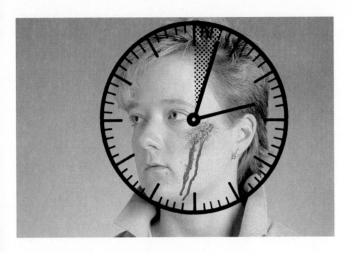

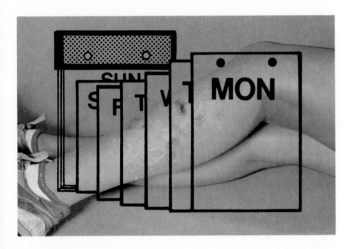

Figure 3-1. Time is important in triage.

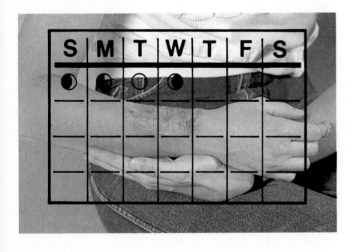

Each patient at the scene must be assessed and classified as either first, second, or third priority according to the seriousness of injury or illness.

First Priority - Those patients that have any of the following conditions. These patients require *immediate* emergency medical care and early transportation to a medical facility.

* Airway or breathing difficulty
* Cardiac arrest (if only one patient is present)
* Uncontrolled or suspected bleeding
* Open chest or abdominal trauma
* Severe laceration involving open fractures of major bones
* Severe burns of the face or upper respiratory tract
* Burns covering 40% of the body surface area
* Severe medical problems, such as poisoning or diabetic emergencies
* Severe head injuries
* Severe shock

Second Priority - Patients show the following conditions and should be transported to a medical facility as soon as possible:

* Rapidly correctable mechanical respiratory defects (obstructions)
* Controllable bleeding (hemorrhage) from an easily accessible area
* Severe crushing wounds of the extremities
* Burns involving 15-40% of body surface area
* Major multiple fractures
* Injuries to the spine
* Severe eye injuries

Third Priority - Patients show the following conditions and should be transported to a medical facility as soon as possible:

* Minor injuries
* Closed fractures (simple)
* Laceration without severe bleeding (hemorrhage)
* Burns that cover less than 15% of the body's surface (except of the respiratory tract)
* Emotionally distressed, but not severely injured
* Obviously dead

SIGNS VERSUS SYMPTOMS

As a First Responder, you should be able to identify certain signs or symptoms to help classify a patient's priority.

Signs are objective signals. They are obvious indications that you can see, hear, smell, or feel. For example, you can see obvious bleeding (hemorrhaging) or an object protruding from the chest. You can hear abnormal, loud breathing or verbal responses to pain. You can smell toxic odors or urine and you can feel abnormal body temperature.

Symptoms are more subjective signals. The patient may need to relate these signs to you. For example, a patient may state that he or she feels nauseous, or dizzy, feels pain, hears voices, or has blurred vision.

Vital Signs

Understanding vital signs and their evaluation in patient assessment is an important responsibility of the First Responder. When you arrive at an emergency scene, it is important to record a patient's vital signs and relate them to the appropriate medical personnel when they arrive at the scene. (For the sake of discussion, assume that proper size-up is complete and that there are no problems of traffic or access to the patient.) Vital signs are the level of consciousness, respiration, pulse and temperature of the patient.

It is important that you take a patient's vital signs immediately and then again at intervals during treatment. Changing vital signs can indicate rapid decline of the patient's status and the need for immediate transportation to a medical facility. For example, a patient may be hemorrhaging internally and show signs of complete consciousness but within 10 minutes or less, the patient may become dizzy and confused due to the loss of blood. These changes in vital signs help aid the diagnosis and proper emergency medical care of the patient.

There are different levels of consciousness. The normal person is alert and knows his or her name, location and date. However, following a trauma or medical emergency, a patient may be semiconscious, confused, in shock, or even unconscious.

The APVU method is an excellent way to determine a patient's level of consciousness. AVPU means:

* ❋ *A* - Alert and oriented to time and place (the patient is totally aware of his or her surroundings, e.g., time or date)
* ❋ *V* – Voice (the patient responds appropriately or inappropriately to voice commands)
* ❋ *P* - Pain (the patient responds appropriately or inappropriately to painful touch or pressure)
* ❋ *U* – Unresponsive (the patient does not respond to any stimulation)

Use the AVPU method for all patients. If there is no response to voice commands or light touch, gently squeeze the patient's arm. Rub the upper sternum or press an object such as a pen between the patient's fingers. If the patient moves away from the painful touch or pressure, the movement is purposeful. It is important to record the patient's reactions to the AVPU method.

Respiration

The normal rate of respiration for the adult ranges between 12-20 breaths/min. A child breathes somewhat faster than an adult. When evaluating the rate and depth of breathing, listen to the patient's chest or back with your ear or a stethoscope to determine whether air is reaching both lungs. (Figure 3-2A & B). Snoring and bubbling sounds are usually caused by upper airway obstructions involving the tongue. Wheezing and crackling usually occur in the lower airways and usually result from conditions such as chronic bronchitis, asthma, or smoking.

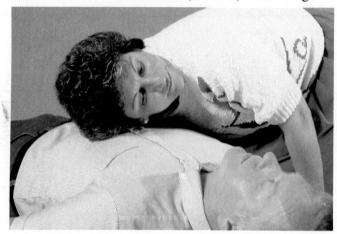

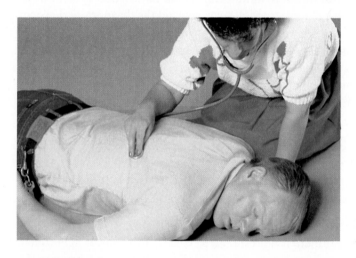

Figure 3-2. Listen to the patient's chest or back. **A,** Use your ear. **B,** Use a stethoscope.

To evaluate the patient's respiratory status, look, listen, and feel to determine whether the respirations are:

* Present or absent
* Fast or slow
* Deep or shallow
* Labored
* Noisy
* Regular or irregular

Record the respiratory state of the patient. Proper action procedures are discussed later in your training. For now you should just be aware of the various types of abnormal breathing.

Pulse

Pulses are palpated or felt at points where the arteries are located close to the surface of the skin. Always use the tips of two fingers when taking a pulse. Press the tips of the fingers lightly against the skin in any of the four common pulse areas as shown in Figure 3-3. The most common pulse areas are:

* Neck (Carotid) (Figure 3-3A)
* Groin (Femoral) (Figure 3-3B)
* Lower Arm (Radial) (Figure 3-3C)
* Upper Arm (Brachial artery) - particularly for infants (Figure 3-3D)

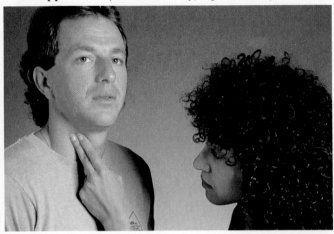

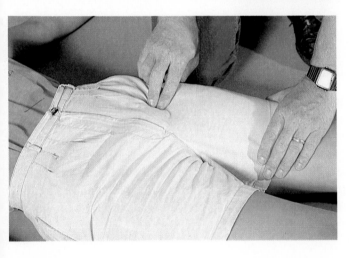

Figure 3-3. The most common pulse areas. **A,** Neck. **B,** Groin.

Evaluate the pulse for rate (beats per minute), rhythm (regular or irregular), and strength (strong, pounding, or weak).

The normal pulse rate for an adult is 60-100 beats/min at rest. The infant has a pulse of 100-120. A child's pulse ranges from 80-100 beats/min. Regularity and strength are as important as rate. Report any irregularity with the rate. The faster a pulse beats the weaker it feels because the filling time for the heart is reduced and less blood is being pumped.

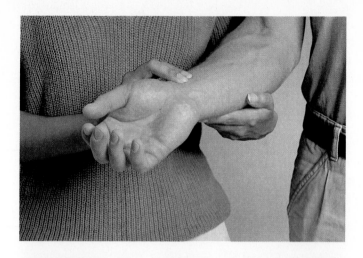

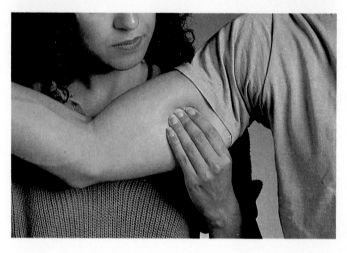

Figure 3-3. The most common pulse areas. **C,** Lower arm. **D,** Upper arm.

Many other pulses may be felt, but the four listed above are the commonly evaluated.

The most reliable pulse is found in the neck. You can assume that the patient's blood pressure is at least 60 mmHg if a carotid pulse is present. The femoral pulse is the next most reliable but is difficult to obtain on the clothed patient and should not be taken if a carotid pulse can be easily felt. The femoral pulse indicates that the patient's pressure is 70 mmHg or greater. The radial pulse is the least reliable but indicates a pressure of at least 80 mm Hg. If the patient is conscious, the radial pulse should be taken first. If the patient has a radial pulse, their systolic blood pressure is at least 80 mm Hg.

Temperature

The body may be cold and clammy, which could indicate shock, heat exhaustion, or warm and dry to indicate excessive temperature or heat stroke (hyperpyrexia). Skin that is cold and dry may indicate exposure to the cold (hypothermia). Hot, wet skin may suggest there is a fever.

Body Temperature

The body acquires heat through its metabolism, muscle activity, and external sources, e.g., hot foods, clothing, and environmental conditions.

Body temperature represents the balance between heat loss and heat gain.

The range of body temperature is 97.9-99.5°F (36.5-37.5° C) of a resting person when taken orally with a thermometer. Most people have an average oral temperature of 98.6°F (37°C). Most First Responders will not have oral thermometers available to them.

An alternate method, though not fully accurate, is to use the backs of your fingers to palpate a temperature.

Use the backs of your fingers to palpate for extremes in heat or cold. A person suffering from hyperthermia will feel very warm (105°F/40.6°C or higher); a person suffering from hypothermia (94°F/34.4°C or lower) will feel very cold.

You can roughly estimate the patient's body temperature against your own. After checking the patient's body surface with the backs of the fingers, with one hand, place them on the back of the fingers of the other hand. Any contrast should be apparent at once.

OTHER DIAGNOSTIC SIGNS

Other signs of diagnostic importance include skin color, dilation of the pupils, and blood pressure.

Skin Color and Temperature

Changes in skin color or temperature can be important signs of illness or injury. Skin color and temperature depend on blood circulation.

A patient may feel warm and wet, warm and dry, cool and dry, or cold and clammy. Changes in skin temperature can be important signs of illness or injury (Figure 3-4). The following list provides some examples of skin conditions and what they might indicate:

✳ Cool and clammy skin may indicate:

  Shock

  Heat exhaustion

✳ Cool and dry skin may indicate:

  Cold exposure, hypothermia

✳ Warm and wet skin indicate:

  Fever

✳ Hot and dry skin may indicate:

  Excessive temperature

  Heat stroke (hyperpyrexia)

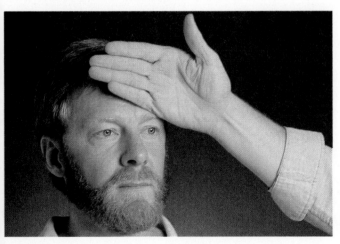

Figure 3-4. Hand to forehead for temperature evaluation.

Skin color can be a good diagnostic sign. The nail beds (Figure 3-5), the mucosa inside the mouth, or the palms of the hands are reliable indicators of color changes. These areas should always be reddish or pink in color. Abnormal skin color may indicate a variety of problems (Figure 3-6).

❋ Red skin is a good indication of:

High blood pressure

Burns

Heat stroke

Carbon monoxide poisoning in final stages

❋ Cyanotic skin is a good indication of:

Heart failure

Airway obstruction

Hypoventilation

Poisoning

❋ White, pale skin is a good indication of:

Insufficient circulation

Shock

Heart attack

Fright

Cold exposure

❋ Grayish skin is a good indication of:

Carbon monoxide poisoning (early)

Chronic obstructive pulmonary disease (COPD)

❋ Yellowish skin (jaundice) is a good indication of:

Gallbladder disease

Liver disease

Kidney disorders

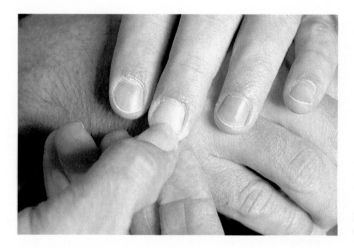

Figure 3-5. Use the capillary blanch test to evaluate the nail beds.

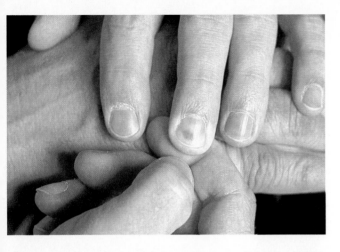

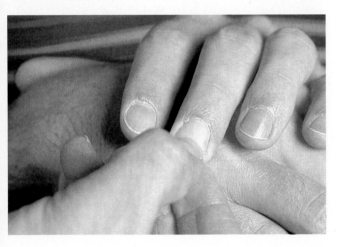

Figure 3-5 (cont.). Use the capillary blanch test to evaluate the nail beds.

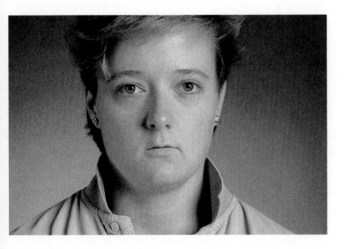

Figure 3-6. Abnormal skin color.

Pupils

The pupils of the eyes are the windows of the brain, since they can quickly reflect the status of the central nervous system. The pupils in both eyes should always be of equal size. Pupils become smaller, or constrict, in bright light. In darkness, the pupils become larger, or dilate. Even if you shine a light in one eye, both pupils should constrict (Figure 3-7 and 3-8).

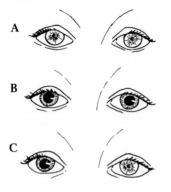

A

B

C

Figure 3-7. Pupil size may vary. **A,** Normal pupils, **B,** Dilated pupils, **C,** Irregular pupils. (From Arnheim, D.D.: Modern Principles of Athletic Training, St. Louis, 1985, The C.V. Mosby Co.)

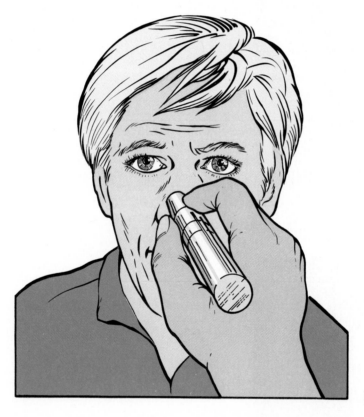

Figure 3-8. The corneal light reflex.

If one pupil is larger than the other, it usually means that there is a possible head injury. Abnormal pupil sizes may be a sign of the following:

✱ Constricted pupils

Bright light

Stroke

Use of amphetamines, heroin, or cocaine

Use of narcotics

✱ Dilated pupils

Darkness

Unconsciousness

Cardiac arrest

Head injury

✱ Unequal pupils

Head injury

Stroke (cerebrovascular accident)

Artificial eye

If a patient is dead, pupils are dilated and do not respond to light. If the patient is alive and pupils do not respond to light, record the information and evaluate other vital signs as you initiate proper care.

Blood Pressure

To assess blood pressure (abbreviated BP), use a BP cuff (Figure 3-9). Do not take a patient's blood pressure until you have taken care of the patient's life-threatening needs. Obtaining a blood pressure is not part of the initial patient survey; you may, however, be required to take blood pressures as part of your job. A pulse reading is sufficient for the initial assessment. It is discussed here, however, because you may be requested by other medical personnel to report the blood pressure during triage.

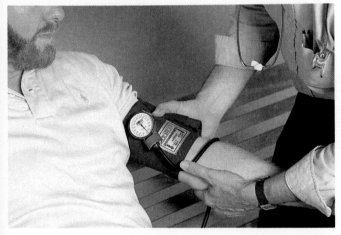

Figure 3-9. A blood pressure cuff or sphygmomanometer is merely a rubber bladder to be wrapped around the patient's arm.

Blood pressure is the pressure exerted on the walls of the arteries as blood is forced through them by the pumping action of the heart (Figure 3-10). Extremely high blood pressure can damage weak blood vessels in the body. Low blood pressure can be one of the later signs of shock.

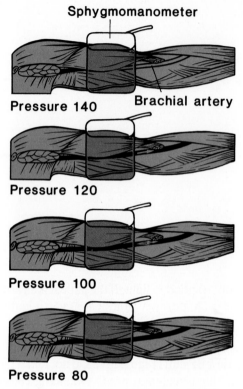

Figure 3-10. Blood pressure. This patient's pressure is 120/80.
NOTE: Blood must flow beneath the bladder of the cuff for sounds to be heard. After the bladder is relaxed to the same pressure as the arterial residual (diastolic) pressure, the sounds of blood moving disappear.

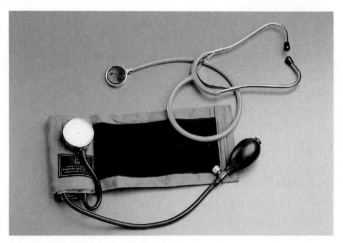

Figure 3-11. A stethoscope.

You must compare blood pressure with other signs and symptoms of the patient. Do not base a diagnosis on a blood pressure reading as fear or nervousness can cause a patient's blood pressure to rise.

To take a blood pressure reading you need a blood pressure cuff (also known as a sphygmomanometer), and a stethoscope (Figure 3-11). Follow this procedure to use a blood pressure cuff:

❋ Center the bladder of the cuff over the brachial artery and attach the cuff firmly to the patient's arm (Figure 3-12A).

❋ Place the stethoscope in your ears with the bell of the stethoscope on the artery at the antecubital area (Figures 3-12B-C).

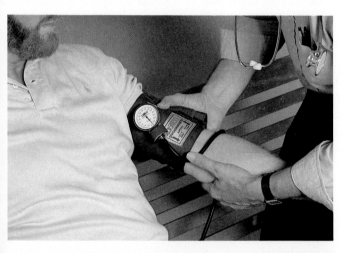

Figure 3-12A. Center the cuff over the brachial artery.

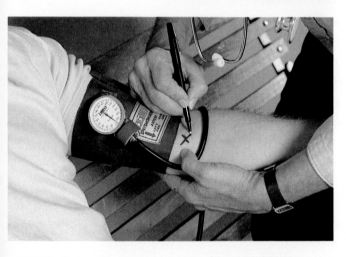

Figure 3-12B. Locate the brachial artery.

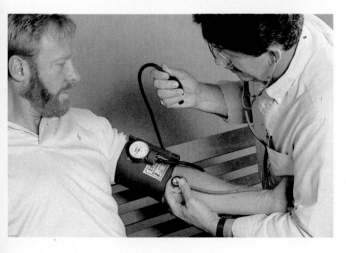

Figure 3-12C. Placement of the stethoscope.

✳ Pump the bladder up to approximately 200 mmHg. Listen for the sound of the pulse. If you can hear the pulse, the pressure on the cuff must be increased until no sounds are heard. When no pulse is heard, open the valve slowly, allowing the needle in the gauge to drop very slowly.

✳ The first sound heard is the systolic pressure. The systolic pressure is the pumping of the heart. The last, or diminished, sound heard is the diastolic pressure; it is the residual pressure in the arterial system. The diastolic pressure occurs when the blood presses against the walls of the arteries and in the ventricles of the heart during relaxation.

✳ Record the corresponding numbers once you have heard each sound.

The average pressure for the adult is 120/80. A useful rule of thumb is 100 plus the patient's age for systolic pressure up to 150 mmHg. Normal diastolic pressure should range from 60-90 mmHg in men with women ranging from 10-15 mmHg lower. A small woman may have a normal pressure of 90/60. A newborn child's BP averages 50/30. Pressure increases with growth until about age 14, when adult ranges are achieved.

The difference between systolic pressure and diastolic pressure is called pulse pressure. Pulse pressure is normally 30-40 mmHg but may vary with specific injury or illness. Remember, blood pressure is always recorded in even numbers.

SYMPTOMS

To evaluate pain, check for the following symptoms:

✳ *Quality* - Is the pain sharp, dull, heavy, smothering, or squeezing? Is there an increase in pain when you apply pressure to the area that hurts?

✳ *Quantity* - Is the pain consistent, does it come and go, is it prolonged and did the pain increase in intensity from the onset?

✳ *Location* - Have the patient point to the area that hurts.

✳ *Radiation* - From the point of location, where does the pain spread to?

✳ *Duration* - When did the pain begin?

✳ *Alleviate or relieve pain* - What makes or decreases the pain (e.g., having the patient sit up or stay in a particular position)?

✳ *Associated symptoms* - Is the pain accompanied by other symptoms, e.g., nausea, vomiting, coughs, or a lack of sensation?

Other signs include the following:

✳ The abdomen - Does the patient have cramps, make gurgling sounds, feel bloated or gaseous, or have a bubbling feeling in the abdomen?

✳ The back - Does the patient feel numbness in the back, legs or arms?

✳ Sight - Can the patient see? Is his or her vision blurred or fuzzy?

✳ Taste - Does the patient have a sour, sweet, metallic, foul, or salty taste in his or her mouth?

✳ Smell - Can you detect any foul, fragrant, or unusual odor to the patient?

✳ Touch - Does the patient feel numbness, tingling, referred sensation, burning, tenderness, or response to hot and cold?

✳ Hearing - Can the patient hear or is there a ringing or buzzing in the ears?

✳ Gait - Is the patient dizzy, staggering, weak, swaying, listing, or immobile?

✳ Is the patient choking?

✳ Urine – Is the patient's urine absent, dark, have an ammonia smell to it, or does it hurt the patient to urinate?

EVALUATING THE PATIENT

It is important that you are able to understand and identify the vital signs previously discussed. These signs are critical when assessing a patient during triage. There are two types of assessments or surveys that must be performed on each patient at the scene, the primary survey and the secondary survey.

For the sake of discussion, assume that there are no problems at the scene and that all size-up has been performed. You have identified yourself to the patient and there are no problems such as traffic or equipment needs. The focus is on the patient.

Primary Survey

When you reach the patient, conduct a primary survey. The primary survey consists of determining if there are any life-threatening conditions. This includes classifying the patient's level of priority in the following manner:

* Determine the patient's level of consciousness using the AVPU method.

* Assessment including airway maintenance with cervical spine control (described in Chapter 4).

* Breathing (adequate air exchange; refer to Chapter 4).

* Circulation with bleeding (hemorrhage) control (refer to Chapter 6).

* Determine whether the patient is bleeding and if so, is it under control or is the patient hemorrhaging?

* Check the patient's pupils for dilation or constriction.

* Observe the patient's skin color and temperature.

* Repeat the primary survey immediately if there is a change in the patient's respiration or pulse.

Secondary Survey

When all primary vital signs have been assessed and recorded, evaluate the patient's wounds or illness. These may not be obvious at first. Start at the patient's head and work toward the patient's toes. Record all presenting signs and symptoms. Using your senses, look, listen, smell, and feel for any objective signs and subjective symptoms.

Assessing the Patient for Trauma

When you assess a patient for trauma, consider the accident site and mechanism of injury. For example, consider a motor vehicle accident. In Chapter 2 you learned that the first portion of the small intestine is often injured due to blunt trauma.

The Head - Begin assessing the patient at the head. Always keep the head in a neutral position and protect the neck. One out of every four patients with major head injuries has some type of neck injury as well. Evaluate the head for:

* Bleeding and pain – Look and feel for bleeding.

* Deformity – look and gently feel for any deformity to the neck or skull.

* Level of consciousness – Use the APVU method to check for consciousness.

* Tenderness – Gently feel for any tender areas.

* Pupils – Check for eye movement and size of pupils using the PERRL method (Pupils Equal, Round, Reactive to Light).

* Fluids – Check if fluids are coming from the ears or nose.

* Bruises – Examine around the eyes and behind the ears for bruising; (This is an excellent time to evaluate the skin for temperature and color.)

* Check the inside of the mouth for injury or foreign materials.

Talk with the patient as you feel the head. While defining any points of injury or pain, determine if the patient is oriented to time, place, and person.

The Neck - Do not ask the patient to move if you suspect a neck injury. A patient can become paralyzed during the secondary examination. A patient with an intact cervical spine could possibly sever the nerve supply while shaking the head yes or no to your questions.

Evaluate the neck for the presence or absence of:

❋ Pain – Ask the patient if any part of the neck hurts.

❋ Deformity – Look and gently feel for any deformities in the neck and bones of the face.

❋ Bleeding – Look and gently feel for any bleeding.

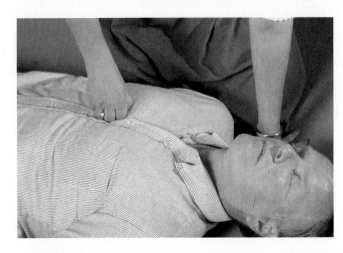

Figure 3-13. Applying pressure to the sternum.

Chest - Evaluate the chest for:

❋ Pain – Pain can be elicited by applying pressure to the sternum (Figure 3-13) or by asking the patient to cough. If the ribs are fractured, the patient will complain of pain in a specific area.

❋ Deformity – Examine the movement of the chest as the patient breaths. If one segment of the chest moves in as the remainder of the chest moves out, it may indicate that the patient is breathing air from one lung to the other rather than from the atmosphere. This condition is called flailed section and can cause death in minutes.

❋ Shortness of breath – A conscious patient can relate any sensation of breathing difficulty (dyspnea — pronounced disp-knee-a). Observe and listen for any abnormal breathing in the unconscious patient.

❋ Open wounds – Bubbly, bright red blood from the patient's nose or mouth indicates damage to lung tissue. Open chest wounds may produce a sucking sound when the patient inhales. This is a life-threatening injury and must be treated immediately.

Abdomen - The solid organs of the abdomen may bleed when damaged, and the hollow organs may spill contents and contaminate the abdominal cavity. Use great care when gently applying pressure to the abdomen.

Evaluate the abdomen for:

❋ Pain – Ask the patient if any area hurts.

❋ Tenderness, Rigidity – Gently feel the patient's abdomen for tenderness or rigidity.

❋ Bruising – Look for bruises. Bruising is often a sign of internal bleeding.

❋ Open wounds or distention.

Remember! Be gentle!

Assessing the Patient's Illness

It is important that you understand and can identify the signs and symptoms discussed earlier in this chapter. Good patient assessment takes practice. Symptoms of an illness are subjective. Much depends on the patient's level of consciousness and how well the patient can relate the information to you. When assessing an illness, begin at the patient's head and work toward the feet.

Use the AMPLE method to gather important information about a patient's illness or injury. AMPLE stands for:

A - Allergic (Check whether the patient is allergic to any substance, e.g., bee stings, food, or medications.)

M - Medication (Check whether the patient is currently taking medication.)

P - Past medical history (Check whether the patient has any history of serious illness. For example, heart disorders, known respiratory diseases, diabetes, etc.)

L - Last meal (When was the patient's last meal?)

E - Events (What events took place that may have led to the problem?)

Record the information and report it to the appropriate medical personnel as soon as the are available.

Before you begin the head-to-toe evaluation, check for various signs. If the patient is conscious, speak clearly and to the point. Ask only pertinent questions and treat the patient with respect. Check for the following:

❋ Level of consciousness AVPU

❋ Skin color and temperature

❋ Dilation of pupils

❋ Breathing and pulse

MEDIC ALERT®

Always check the patient's neck, wrists, ankles, and wallet for a Medic Alert® tag (Figure 3-14) or card. If it is necessary to look in a wallet or pocketbook, have someone assist you. Document all valuable items present. These informative tags may supply you with data that may be otherwise unobtainable from a disoriented or unconscious patient. The toll-free Medic Alert number is 1-800-344-3226. More information about Medic Alert can be obtained by contacting the Medic Alert Foundation, Turlock, California.

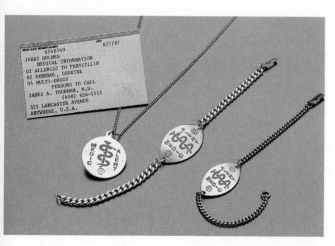

Figure 3-14. Medic Alert® tag.

SUMMARY

As a First Responder, you will be required to make decisions regarding which patients require immediate care. These decisions should be based on the patient's need for care. For example, highest priority care should be given to the most seriously injured or ill person who can be quickly stabilized and transported. Urgent care should be initiated as soon as possible.

The walking wounded or those with minor injuries can be cared for in a slower, more deliberate manner after the higher priority care is completed or a sufficient number of responders are present to provide delayed care.

Lowest priority patients are those that are either dead or who are going to die no matter what care they are given. Many times the level of priority will not be as clear to you as described in this chapter.

Making decisions requires a knowledge of evaluating vital signs and symptoms. They include level of consciousness, breathing, pulse rate, and temperature. Diagnostic signs are also discussed in this chapter. These signs include all the other methods used to evaluate the severity of illness or injury. Normal vital signs are:

* Level of consciousness - Alert
* Respiratory rate (12-20 breaths/min with a sufficient volume of air moving with each breath).
* Pulse rate (60-120 beats/min).
* Temperature (between 98 and 100°F (36.7°C and 37.8°C).

A head-to-toe survey should be conducted on all injured or ill persons. You should look, listen, smell, and feel when performing a complete survey.

Always be aware of the methods used to note medical information that a person may wear or carry with them. Check a person's neck, wrist, ankles, wallet, and purse for information that will alert you to any medical abnormalities such as disease or allergies. It is best to have a responsible witness when searching through a person's belongings.

As a First Responder, you are a very important link in a chain to obtain information concerning a sick or injured patient. Take appropriate care to ensure that all information is passed on to the physician. Care must be quickly instituted when injury or illness is recognized.

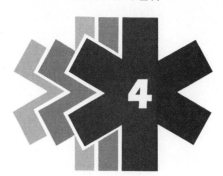
RESPIRATORY ARREST

KEY CONCEPTS AND SKILLS

By the end of this chapter, you will be able to:

* State the amount of time the brain is able to live without oxygen.
* Identify the control center for breathing.
* Identify and describe each of the components of the respiratory system.
* Describe how air travels through the respiratory system to exchange oxygen and wastes.
* Describe the difference between a total and partial neck breather; identify the patient with a stoma.
* Describe the signs of adequate and inadequate breathing.
* Demonstrate on a manikin, two methods of opening an airway.
* Perform, on a manikin, mouth-to-mouth and mouth-to-nose rescue breathing.
* Perform rescue breathing on an adult, infant, and child manikin.
* Perform the appropriate procedures used to clear an obstructed airway for the conscious and unconscious adult, child, and infant.
* Describe airway care and rescue breathing for the partial and total neck breather.
* Describe airway care for the near-drowning victim.

KEY WORDS

Abdominal Thrust – Heimlich maneuver - The procedure used when attempting to relieve a complete airway obstruction. To push or drive with force in the epigastric region of the airway.

Airway Obstruction – Clogged or blocked airway passage.

Artificial Ventilation – Rescue-breathing procedures.

Aspiration – Sucking or drawing in; foreign bodies may be sucked into the nose, throat, or lungs. This often occurs in drowning victims.

Cardiopulmonary Resuscitation – Artificial restoration of breathing (rescue breathing) and circulation.

Child – A person between the ages of 1 and 8 years.

Cyanosis – Blue coloration of the nail beds, area around the mouth, face, ears, and sometimes other parts of the body due to decreased oxygen in the blood.

Epiglottis – Leaf-shaped tissue that covers the larynx during swallowing.

Gastric Distention – Swelling of the stomach due to air, fluid, or food.

Hyperventilation – Rapid, increased rate of breathing.

Hypoventilation – Slow, reduced rate of breathing.

Hypoxemia – Insufficient oxygenation of the blood.

Hypoxia – Reduced amount of oxygen in the body.

Infant – A child under the age of 1.

Laryngectomee – A person who has undergone a laryngectomy (partial or full removal of the larynx).

Partial Neck Breather – Person who partially exchanges air through both the stoma and upper airway passages.

Rescue Breathing – Method used to provide air for the nonbreathing (or breathing impaired) patient by artificial means.

Respiratory Rate – The rate at which a person breathes. The normal adult rate ranges between 12-20 respirations per minute.

Total Neck Breather – A person who has undergone a total laryngectomy and breathes through the stoma.

Vomitus – Material ejected from the stomach through the mouth.

THE RESPIRATORY SYSTEM

The respiratory system provides the means to exchange oxygen and carbon dioxide. Air from the atmosphere contains oxygen, carbon dioxide, and other gases. The respiratory system delivers the oxygen to the cells of the body and disposes of the carbon dioxide. The respiratory system (Figure 4-1) consists of:

* Nose
* Mouth
* Pharynx
* Trachea
* Epiglottis
* Larynx
* Bronchi
* Lungs (including the alveoli)
* Diaphragm
* Rib muscles

The nose is the primary organ of breathing. As air passes through the nose, it is filtered, heated, cooled, moistened, or dried, depending on the temperature and humidity of the atmosphere.

The mouth is the secondary external organ for accepting air. It does not have the purifying or cleansing characteristics of the nose.

The pharnyx (throat) extends from the area in the back of the mouth between the lower palate of the nostrils in the roof of the mouth and the opening to the trachea. Air enters the nose and travels through the pharynx to the trachea, epiglottis, and larynx.

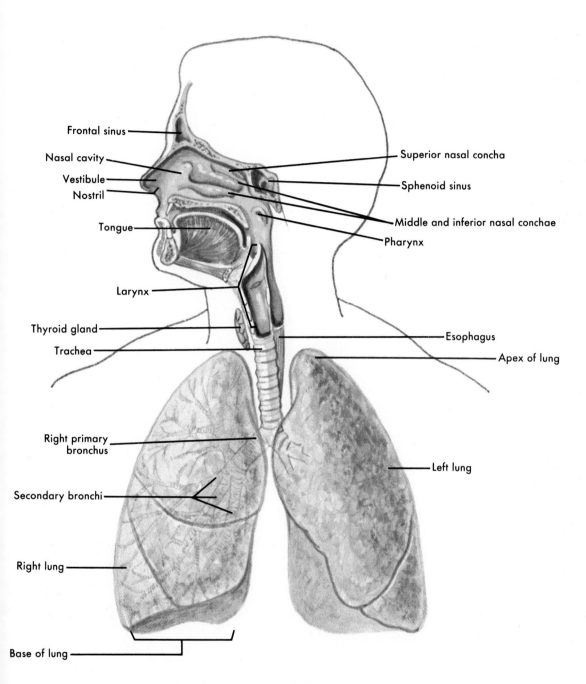

Frontal sinus

Nasal cavity

Vestibule

Nostril

Tongue

Larynx

Thyroid gland

Trachea

Superior nasal concha

Sphenoid sinus

Middle and inferior nasal conchae

Pharynx

Esophagus

Apex of lung

Right primary bronchus

Secondary bronchi

Right lung

Left lung

Base of lung

Figure 4-1. The respiratory system. (From Mosby's Medical and Nursing Directory, 2nd edition, St. Louis, 1986, The C.V. Mosby Co.)

The chest is an enclosed area with only one opening, the trachea. The trachea begins at the lower border of the cricoid cartilege and extends 6 inches and then divides into the bronchi (Figure 4-2). The trachea is called the windpipe.

The epiglottis is a flap of tissue that covers the trachea when swallowing to keep food particles out of the airway. When breathing, the epiglottis is open.

The larynx, also called the voice box, is attached to the uppermost portion of the trachea. The larynx contains the vocal cords. You can locate the larynx by feeling for a patient's Adam's apple.

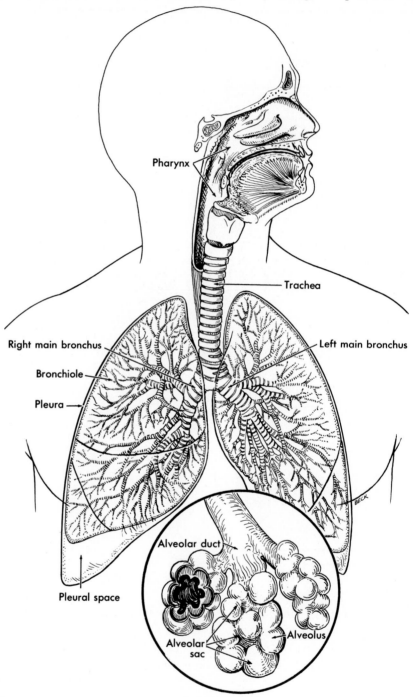

Figure 4-2. The lower respiratory tract. (From Anthony, C.P. and Thibodeau, G.A.: Textbook of Anatomy and Physiology, 12th edition, St. Louis, 1987, The C.V. Mosby Co.)

The diaphragm is a bell-shaped muscular structure that separates the abdominal and chest (thoracic) cavities (Figure 4-3). When this muscle contracts, the patient breathes. Muscles between the ribs contract causing the chest cavity to increase in size as the diaphragm contracts. This increase in size allows air to rush in because of the reduced pressure within the enclosed area. When the muscles relax and the pressure in the chest cavity increases, air passes out of the body.

The bronchi are the two tubes that enter the lungs from where the trachea divides. The bronchi continue to divide into small branches called the bronchioles. The bronchi feed the air sacs (alveoli) in the lungs.

The lungs are where the actual exchange of oxygen and carbon dioxide occurs.

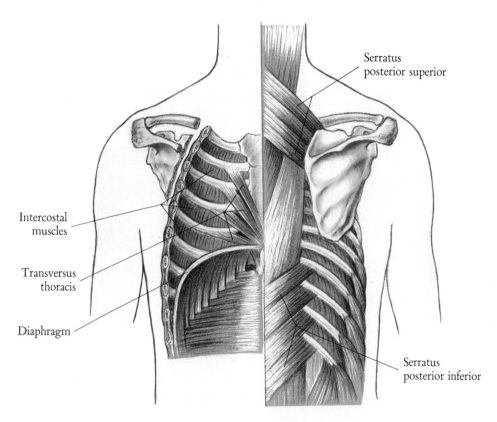

Figure 4-3. The diaphragm and muscles of ventilation. (From Seidel, H.M., et al: Mosby's Guide to Physical Examination, St. Louis, 1987, The C.V. Mosby Co.)

BREATHING CONTROL

There are two distinct phases of breathing, external and internal. External breathing involves movement of air from the atmosphere into the minute air sacs in the lungs (alveoli) and the exhalation of waste gases. Internal breathing involves the exchange of gases that occur in the alveoli of the lungs and in the capillaries between the arteries and veins.

The body has specific receptors that measure oxygen and carbon dioxide in the bloodstream. These receptors send information to the brain where absolute breathing control occurs.

Normal breathing is regulated by the carbon dioxide content in the blood stream. Oxygen must be available to cells for food to be converted into energy. Air from the atmosphere containing oxygen is delivered to the cells. Although some cells can live for extended periods without oxygen, the brain begins to die within 4-6 minutes. When a sufficient number of brain cells die, a person cannot live.

ASSESSING AND CORRECTING BREATHING DIFFICULTIES

Breathing is the body's vital function. If the breathing process becomes obstructed or stops, the heart will soon stop. Cells in the brain begin to die and signals from the nervous system to the brain are cut off. Once brain cells die, they cannot carry out their normal functions and will never do so again. If enough cells die, the person dies.

There are two forms of death, clinical death, and biological death. As a First Responder, it is important that you understand the differences.

Clinical death occurs the moment the patient stops breathing and the heart stops. However, the patient usually has 4-6 minutes before the brain stops functioning. This means that clinical death can be reversed and treated in time.

Biological death occurs when a person is not receiving oxygen and brain cells are dead. Biological death is irreversible.

As a First Responder, you will be trained to provide Basic Life Support - Cardio Pulmonary Resuscitation (BLS-CPR) services to patients that are clinically dead.

The first steps in Basic Life Support are to determine if there is responsiveness, breathlessness, an open airway, or pulselessness.

Adequacy of breathing can be determined by:

* Watching the chest and abdomen rise and fall
* Listening for the air moving out of the nose and mouth
* Feeling the air coming from the nose and mouth
* Observing the color of the patient's skin and mucosa

As discussed in Chapter 3, the normal adult respiratory rate ranges from 12-20 breaths/min. During each breath an adult at rest moves an average of 1 pint of air; for a child or infant, the respiratory rate exceeds 20 breaths/min., and the volume of air exchanged is lower.

You can identify inadequate breathing if:

* No air is heard or felt at the nose or mouth
* The patient is obviously having difficulty breathing
* The chest and stomach are moving but there is no exchange of air (usually indicates complete airway obstruction)
* The breathing rate is over 20 breaths/min (hyperventilation) or less than 12 breaths/min (hypoventilation)
* Bubbling, snoring, or other noisy respirations are present (indicates partial airway obstruction)
* The nail beds, areas around the mouth, face, or ears have a blue coloration (cyanosis).
* Nasal flaring, sternal retraction are present

Irregular breathing patterns may indicate head injury or stroke. The most severe problem is the patient who is not breathing.

OPENING THE AIRWAY

The initial step to ensure adequate respiration is to open the patient's airway. The tongue is the most common cause of airway obstruction in the unconscious patient (Figure 4-4). This occurs when the relaxed tongue presses down on the epiglottis and seals off the upper airway. Because the tongue is attached to the lower jaw, moving the lower jaw forward often lifts the tongue away from the back of the throat and opens the airway.

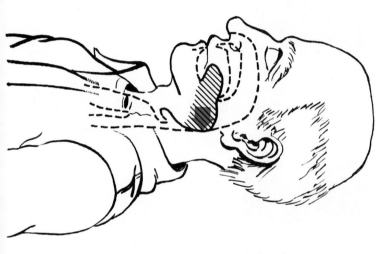

Figure 4-4. The tongue obstructing the airway.

NOTE: If the patient has a head injury, is unconscious, or shows any signs of a possible neck injury, stabilize the patient's neck.

There are two techniques used to open the airway, the head-tilt/chin-lift and modified jaw thrust maneuvers.

CAUTION: Do not use the head-tilt/chin-lift technique if the patient has possible spinal injuries.

The patient may try to breathe but air may not exchange because of an obstruction. If the patient is not breathing or if air exchange is inadequate, begin rescue breathing at once.

The Head-Tilt/Chin-Lift Maneuver

The head-tilt/chin-lift maneuver (Figure 4-5) has shown to be the most effective method. It is the recommended method to open the airway for the nontrauma patient.

The following 4 steps outline the procedure to perform the head-tilt/chin-lift maneuver.

1. Place one hand on the patient's forehead and apply firm, backward pressure with the palm to tilt the head back (Figure 4-5a).

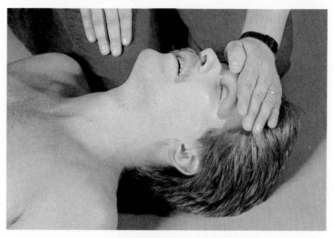

Figure 4-5a. Apply firm backward pressure.

2. Place the tips of the fingers of one hand under the bony part of the patient's lower jaw near the chin (Figure 4-5b). Do not compress the soft tissues under the chin with your fingers (Figure 4-5c). This could obstruct the airway.

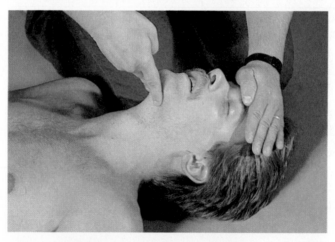

Figure 4-5b. Place the tips of your fingers under the patient's lower jaw.

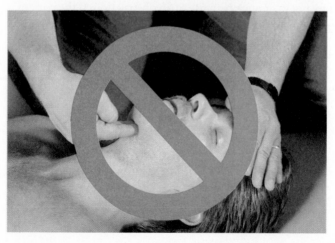

Figure 4-5c. Do not compress the soft tissues under the chin.

3. Lift the chin forward (Figure 4-5d). Continue to press on the patient's forehead with your other hand to tilt the head back.

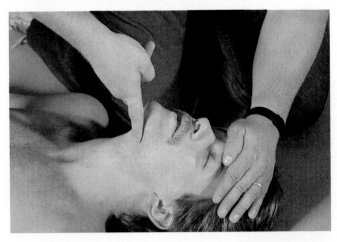

Figure 4-5d. Lift the chin forward.

4. Lift the chin so that the teeth are nearly together but the mouth is not closed completely (Figure 4-5e).

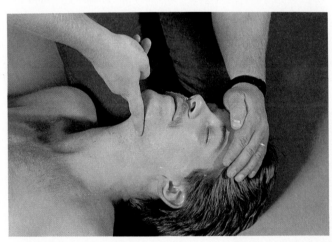

Figure 4-5e. Lift the chin.

NOTE: Dentures are usually left in place because achieving the mouth-to-mouth seal is easier. However, if the dentures are loose or interfere with maintaining the seal when performing mouth-to-mouth resuscitation, remove them.

The Modified Jaw Thrust Maneuver

This technique is the safest first approach in opening the airway of a patient of a suspected cervical spine injury. The following 4 steps outline the procedure to perform the modified jaw thrust maneuver:

1. Rest your elbows on the surface on which the patient is lying (Figure 4-6a).

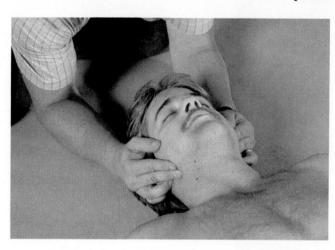

Figure 4-6a. Rest your elbows on the surface on which the patient is lying.

2. Support the patient's head carefully without tilting it backward or turning it from side to side (Figure 4-6b).

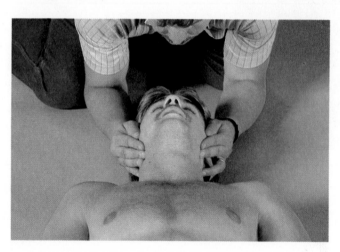

Figure 4-6b. Carefully support the patient's head.

3. Place one hand on each side of the patient's head and grasp the angles of the patient's lower jaw (mandible) (Figure 4-6c).

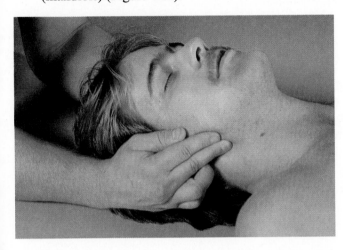

Figure 4-6c. Grasp the angles of the patient's lower jaw.

4. Gently pull up the patient's lower jaw with both hands, one on either side. This should move the mandible forward without tilting the head backward (Figure 4-6d).

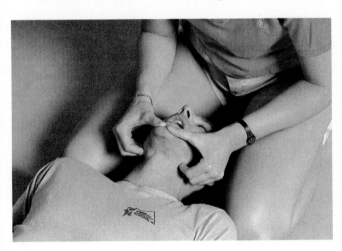

Figure 4-6d. Gently pull the patient's lower jaw with both hands.

RESCUE BREATHING

There are three kinds of rescue breathing techniques:

❋ Mouth-to-Mouth

❋ Mouth-to-Nose

❋ Mouth-to-Stoma

Mouth-to-mouth rescue breathing is the most common technique. The mouth-to-nose technique is used if it is impossible to open a patient's mouth or seal the mouth fully, or if there is a serious injury near the mouth. The mouth-to-stoma technique is used on patients who have a full or partial removal of the larynx. Ventilation is required in this surgical opening of the trachea.

> **NOTE:** In infants and some small children, both the mouth and the nose must be covered in order to make a seal. If the child's mouth is too large for you to make a tight seal over both the nose and mouth, pinch the nose as in the technique for adults and breathe through the child's mouth.

The procedures for each technique are outlined in the following paragraphs:

Mouth-to-Mouth Rescue Breathing

1. Place one hand on the patient's forehead and the other hand under the chin to stabilize the head (Figure 4-7a).

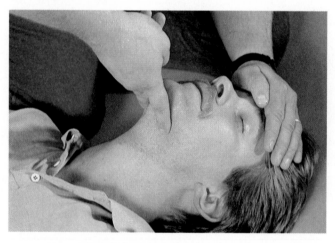

Figure 4-7a. Placement of hands.

2. Using the thumb and index finger of the hand on the forehead, gently pinch the nostrils closed to prevent the escape of air (Figure 4-7b).

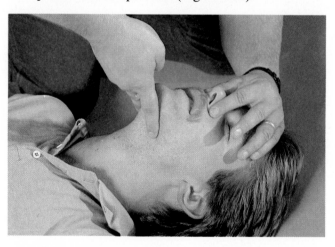

Figure 4-7b. Gently pinch the nostrils closed.

3. Open your mouth wide and take a deep breath (Figure 4-7c).

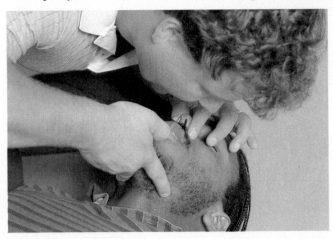

Figure 4-7c. Take a deep breath (no mask used).

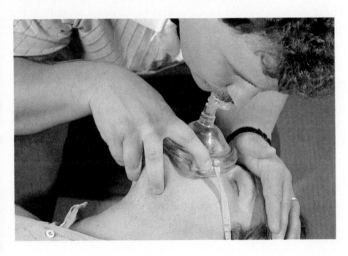

Figure 4-7c. Take a deep breath (mask used).

4. Seal the patient's mouth by placing your mouth around the outside of the patient's mouth (Figure 4-7d).

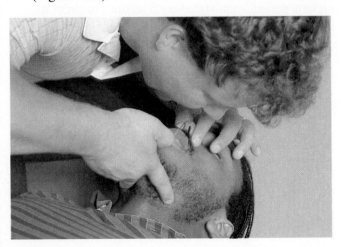

Figure 4-7d. Seal the patient's mouth (no mask used).

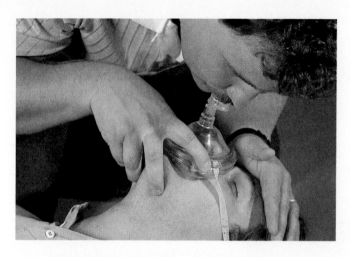

Figure 4-7d (cont.). Seal the patient's mouth (mask used).

5. To begin rescue breathing, give two full breaths of 1-1½ seconds/breath allowing the patient's lungs to deflate between breaths. These breaths should be slow and purposeful to reduce the probability of gastric distention, which may interfere with rescue breathing and cause vomiting. (Gastric distention is described in more detail later in this chapter.)

6. Forcefully exhale the air from your lungs into the patient's mouth (Figure 4-7e).

   NOTE: The average exhalation from the lungs during nonstrenuous activity is about 1 pint of air. In order to inflate the lungs of a nonbreathing person, it may take 1½ pints of air to break the resistance and back pressure of the patient's lungs.

7. Watch the patient's chest (Figure 4-7f) to see if:
   * The chest is rising and falling
   * Resistance is felt
   * The patient's lungs are compliant
   * You can hear and feel air escaping during exhalation

If all of these are true, then adequate ventilation has been accomplished.

   NOTE: In the nonbreathing, unconscious patient, ventilate every 5 seconds in order to achieve 12 ventilations/min. Use the following count, one one-thousand, two one-thousand, three one-thousand, four one-thousand, five one-thousand, breathe.
   For infants, inflate the lungs once every 3 seconds using the one one-thousand count method.
   For children, inflate the lungs every 4 seconds using the one one-thousand count method.

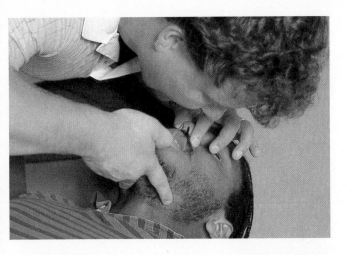

Figure 4-7e. Forcefully exhale air into the patient's mouth (no mask used).

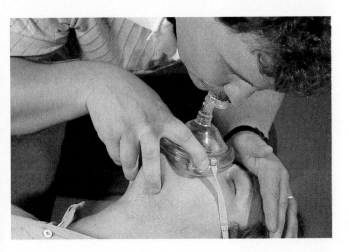

Figure 4-7e. Forcefully exhale air into the patient's mouth (mask used).

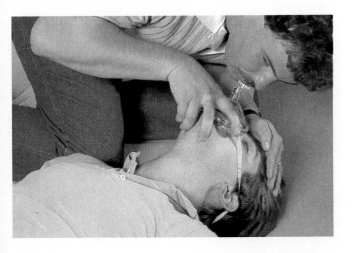

Figure 4-7f. Watch the patient's chest.

Mouth-to-Nose Rescue Breathing

1. Maintain the head-tilt/chin-lift position with one hand (Figure 4-8a).

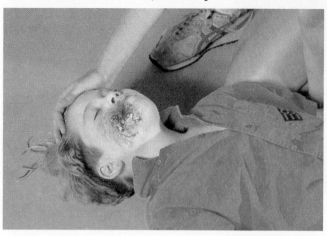

Figure 4-8a. Maintain head-tilt/chin-lift position.

2. Lift the patient's lower jaw and close the mouth with the other hand (Figure 4-8b).

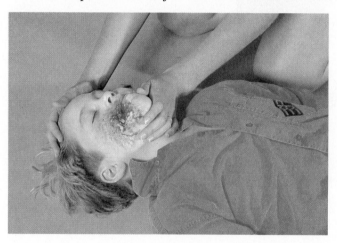

Figure 4-8b. Lift patient's lower jaw and close the mouth.

3. Take a deep breath, seal your lips around the patient's nose, and give two full breaths of 1-1½ seconds each until compliance is felt (Figure 4-8c).

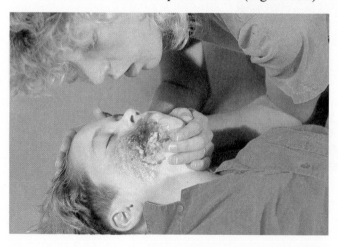

Figure 4-8c. Seal the patient's nose.

NOTE: In the nonbreathing, unconscious patient ventilate every 5 seconds in order to achieve 12 ventilations/min. Use the count, one one-thousand, two one-thousand, three one-thousand, four one-thousand, five one-thousand; breathe.

For infants, inflate the lungs once every 3 seconds using the one one-thousand count method.

For children, inflate the lungs every 4 seconds using the one one-thousand count method.

4. Remove your mouth to allow the patient to exhale and watch the chest fall (Figure 4-8d).

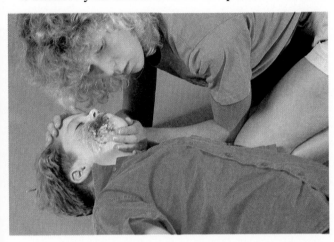

Figure 4-8d. Remove your mouth to allow patient to exhale.

NOTE: If passive exhalation is not observed, it may be necessary to open the mouth to allow the escape of air (Figure 4-8e). This may occur because of a valve-like obstruction caused by the soft palate.

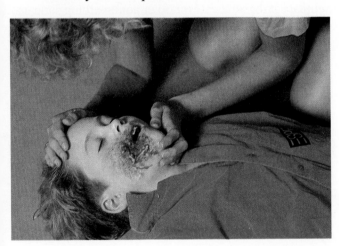

Figure 4-8e. It may be necessary to open the mouth to allow the escape of air.

Mouth-to-Stoma Rescue Breathing

CAUTION: Do not remove any appliances from the stoma. Doing so may cause collapse of the tissues around the stoma and may completely prevent breathing.

1. Clear the stoma of any obstructions (Figure 4-9a). If a mucous plug or other obstruction is in the appliance, remove it with either suctioning equipment or by fully opening a 4 x 4 inch gauze pad of the stoma and doing the suctioning by inhaling through the pad.

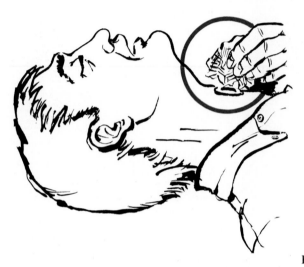

Figure 4-9a. Clear the stoma of any obstruction.

2. Seal your mouth over the stoma and ventilate at the same rate for other nonbreathing patients (1 breath of 1-1½ seconds every 5 seconds) into the stoma (Figure 4-9b).

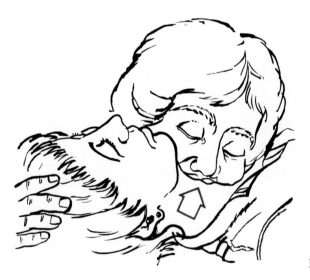

Figure 4-9b. Seal your mouth over the stoma.

NOTE: If the patient has had a partial laryngectomy or has a tracheostomy tube, you will have to seal both the mouth and nose with your hand to prevent the air you are exhaling into the stoma from escaping via the upper airway (Figure 4-9c).

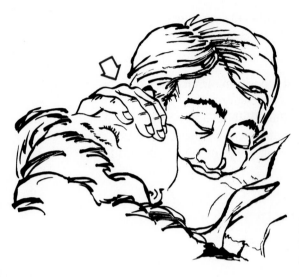

Figure 4-9c. If the patient has a partial laryngectomy or tracheostomy tube, you will need to seal both the mouth and nose.

Gastric Distention

During the process of rescue breathing, the stomach often swells because of excessive pressure being used to inflate the lungs, or it can result when the airway is partially or fully obstructed. Gastric distention is more common in children but occurs in adults as well. It can be minimized by slow, purposeful ventilation every 1-1½ seconds.

As distention increases, the patient may vomit and possibly aspirate the vomitus. In addition, as the diaphragm is elevated in the abdominal cavity, lung volume is reduced.

Relieving Gastric Distention

If the stomach becomes distended, recheck and reposition the airway. Continue checking for the rise and fall of the chest and avoid excessive airway pressure.

Relieving distention almost always causes vomiting. Without appropriate suctioning equipment, it is difficult (if not impossible), to remove vomitus from airway passages. Distention should be relieved only if it fully inhibits ventilatory efforts. The following 4 steps outline the procedure to relieve distention:

1. Turn the patient on his or her side (Figure 4-10a)

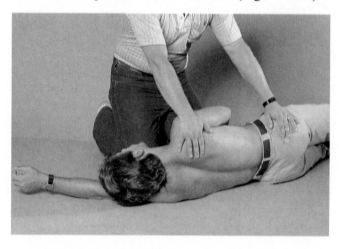

Figure 4-10a. Turn the patient on his side.

2. Gently depress the abdomen just below the sternum with one hand as shown in Figure 4-10b (the patient may vomit).

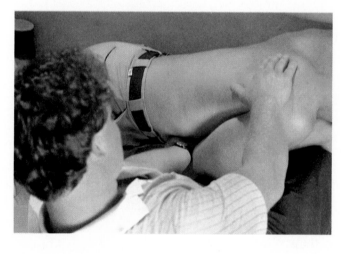

Figure 4-10b. Gently depress the abdomen.

3. Clear the patient's mouth of vomitus (Figure 4-10c).

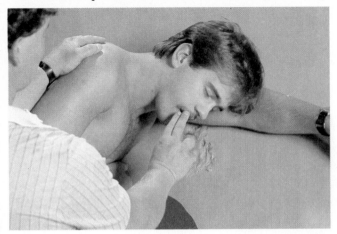

Figure 4-10c. Clear the patient's mouth of vomitus.

4. Continue Basic Life Support.

AIRWAY OBSTRUCTION

Airway obstruction is caused by a variety of factors including the tongue, foreign bodies such as loosened teeth, trauma to the respiratory system, inhalation burns, severe allergic reaction, strangulation and drowning. The classic signal for choking is illustrated in Figure 4-11.

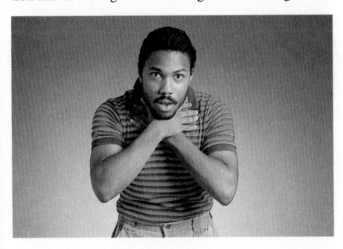

Figure 4-11. The classic signal for choking.

Airway obstruction may be either partial or complete. In partial obstruction, the air exhange can be good or poor although the patient is wheezing or coughing.

If the patient is getting good air exchange, assistance should not be rendered. However, continue to observe the patient. Encourage the patient's attempts to clear the airway by coughing.

If air exchange is poor and coughing becomes weak, attempt to clear the airway obstruction using the techniques described in the following paragraphs.

> **NOTE:** Procedures for correcting airway obstructions differ between adults and small children and infants. If the patient is an infant or small child, refer to the "Modified Correction of Airway Obstruction for Infants and Children" section.
> For patients that are obese or women in the late stages of pregnancy, refer to the "Chest Thrusts" sections. Use this technique when you are unable to reach around the patient's abdominal area.

Correcting the Obstructed Airway

To correct the obstructed airway of the conscious adult that is standing or sitting:

✱ Ask the person if they are choking. Observe for cyanosis and exaggerated breathing efforts.

✱ If the person is not exchanging air, apply abdominal or chest thrusts (called the Heimlich maneuver) as described in the following procedure:

1. Stand behind the patient as shown in Figure 4-12a

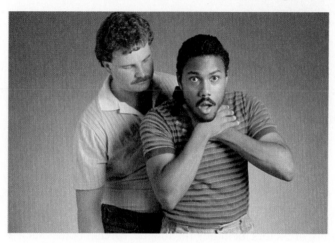

Figure 4-12a. Stand behind the patient.

2. Wrap your arms around the patient's waist (Figure 4-12b).

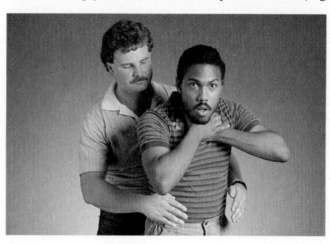

Figure 4-12b. Wrap your arms around the patient's waist.

3. Place the thumb side of your fist against the patient's abdomen between the waist and the rib cage and grasp your fist with the other hand (Figure 4-12c).

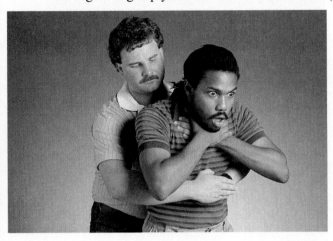

Figure 4-12c. Place the thumb side of your fist against the patient's abdomen between the waist and the rib cage. Grasp your fist with the other hand.

CAUTION: Never place your hands on the xiphoid process or the lower margins of the rib cage. The position of your hands is important to prevent possible damage to internal organs when applying chest thrusts. Vomiting may occur as a result of chest or abdominal thrusts.

4. Press your fist, using a quick inward and upward thrust into the patient's abdomen (Figure 4-12d). Each thrust should be distinct and delivered with enough force to relieve the obstruction.

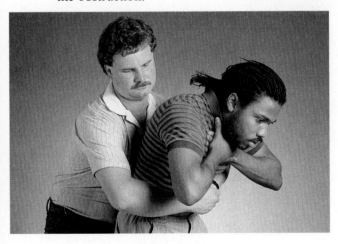

Figure 4-12d. Use a quick inward and upward thrust.

5. Repeat manual thrusts until they are effective or until the patient becomes unconscious.

To correct the obstructed airway of the unconscious adult:

1. Place the patient horizontally on their back (in a supine position) with his or her head in the normal anatomical position as shown in Figure 4-13a).

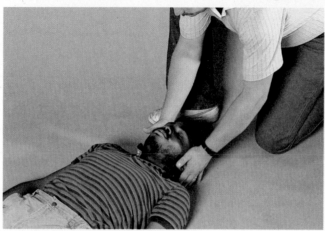

Figure 4-13a. Place the patient horizontally on their back.

2. Call for help.

3. Perform a finger sweep using the tongue-jaw lift to check for foreign objects (Figure 4-13b).

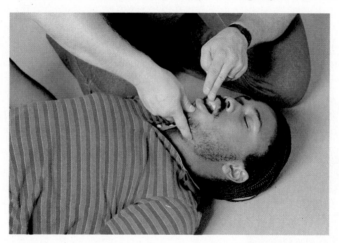

Figure 4-13b. Use the tongue-jaw lift to check for foreign objects.

Here is the tongue-jaw lift procedure:

NOTE: Never insert your finger into the mouth of a conscious or semiconscious person.

✳ Place the patient's head in its normal anatomical position.

✳ Using your thumb and fingers, open the mouth. Grasp the tongue and lower jaw and lift. This may partially relieve the obstruction (Figure 4-13c).

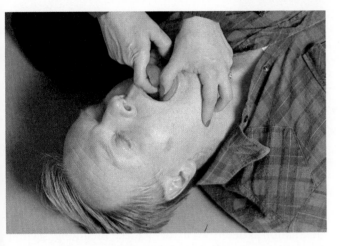

Figure 4-13c. Using your thumb and fingers, open the mouth.

✳ Insert the index finger of your other hand along the inside of the cheek and deeply into the throat to the base of the tongue and across to the other cheek (Figure 4-13d).

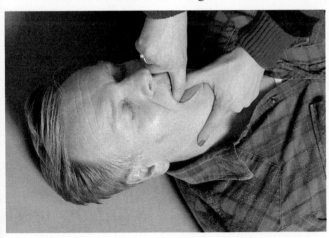

Figure 4-13d. Insert index finger of other hand along the inside of the cheek deeply into the throat.

✳ Using a hooking motion, try to dislodge the foreign body into the mouth to remove it (Figure 4-13e).

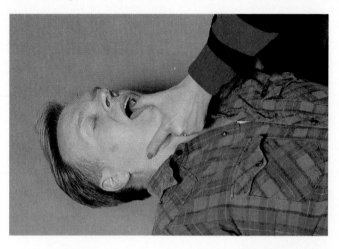

Figure 4-13e. Use a hooking motion to dislodge the foreign body.

CAUTION: Do not force foreign objects deeper into the airway.

4. Open the airway using the head-tilt/chin-lift method described earlier in this chapter.
5. Seal the mouth and nose and attempt ventilation as described in the "Rescue Breathing" section.
6. Sit astride the patient or straddle one leg (Figure 4-13f).

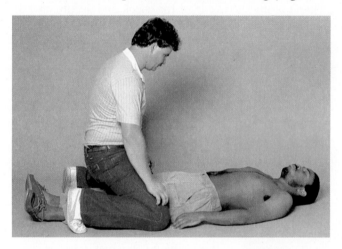

Figure 4-13f. Sit astride the patient.

CAUTION: Do not thrust from the side of the patient. Damage can occur to internal organs. Perform thrusts astride the patient.

7. Place the heel of one hand against the patient's abdomen between the navel and the xiphoid process. Put one hand on top of the other (Figure 4-13g). Your hands should be directly over the middle of the patient's abdomen.

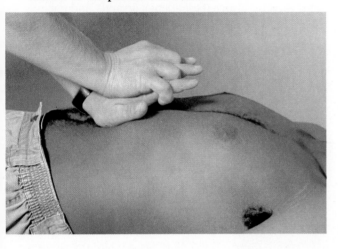

Figure 4-13g. Place one hand on top the other.

8. Apply 6-10 inward and upward thrusts to the patient's abdomen (Figure 4-13h).

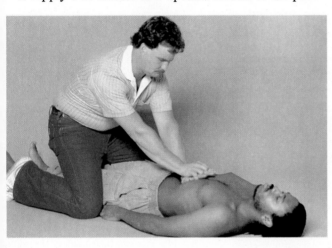

Figure 4-13h. Apply 6-10 inward and upward thrusts.

9. Perform a finger sweep, open the airway, attempt ventilations, and, if ineffective, repeat the thrust sequence from Step 6.

Chest Thrusts

To perform chest thrusts on a conscious patient that is standing or sitting:

1. Stand behind the patient with your arms directly under the patient's armpits and encircle the patient's chest. The patient should be leaning forward (Figure 4-14a).

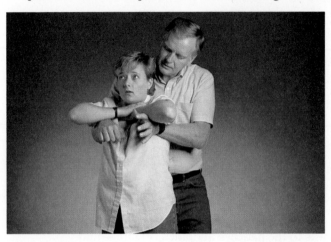

Figure 4-14a. Stand behind the patient and encircle the patient's chest.

2. Place the thumb side of the fist on the middle of the breastbone (the midpoint of the sternum) and grasp the fist with the other hand (Figure 4-14b)

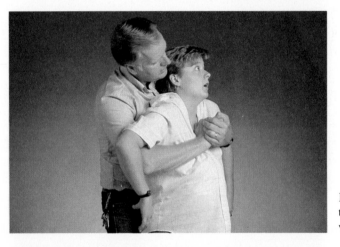

Figure 4-14b. Place the thumb side of the fist on the middle of the breastbone. Grasp the fist with the other hand.

3. Exert backward thrusts (Figure 4-14c).

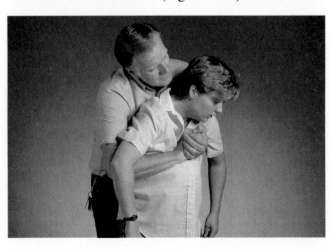

Figure 4-14c. Exert backward thrusts.

To perform chest thrusts on a conscious patient that is lying down:

1. Place the patient on his or her back (Figure 4-15a).

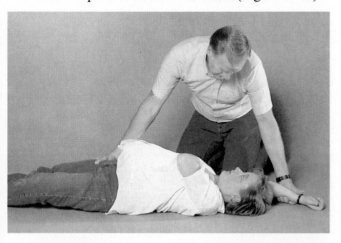

Figure 4-15a. Place the patient on her back.

2. Kneel close to the side of the patient's body (Figure 4-15b).

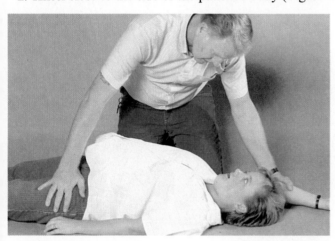

Figure 4-15b. Kneel close to the side of the patient's body.

3. Place the heel of your hand on the lower half of the sternum (two or three fingers above the xiphoid process) (Figure 4-15c).

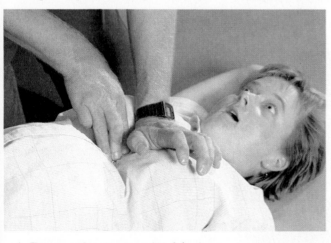

Figure 4-15c. Place the heel of your hand on the lower half of the sternum.

4. Depress the sternum 1½-2 inches.

   NOTE: As hypoxia progresses, previously tense muscles and tissues usually relax, and the techniques to relieve the obstruction may become more effective.

To correct the obstructed airway of the unconscious adult:

1. Establish unresponsiveness by tapping the patient gently or shouting (Figure 4-16a).

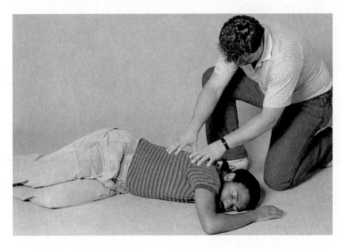

Figure 4-16a. Establish unresponsiveness.

2. Call for help.

3. Place the patient on his or her back (Figure 4-16b).

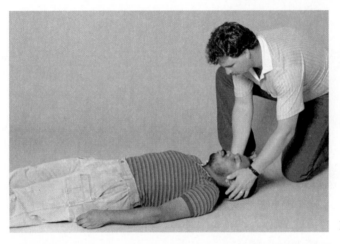

Figure 4-16b. Place the patient on his back.

4. Open the airway (Figure 4-16c).

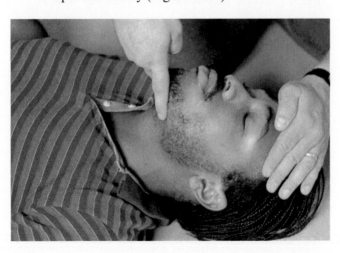

Figure 4-16c. Open the airway.

5. Establish the presence or absence of respiration (Figure 4-16d). If respiration is absent, try to ventilate. If unable to ventilate, quickly perform the following steps:
   a. Reposition the head and try to ventilate again.
   b. If unsuccessful and a second person is available, activate the EMS system.

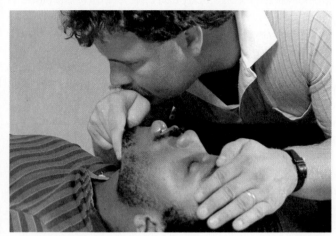

Figure 4-16d. Establish the presence or absence of respiration.

6. Apply 6 to 10 manual thrusts.

7. Apply the finger sweep (if necessary, remove dentures to improve sweep) using the tongue-jaw lift procedure.

MODIFICATIONS FOR INFANTS AND CHILDREN

Airway obstruction is very common among infants and children and is usually caused by foreign bodies or infection.

It is important that you try to differentiate between a foreign body and an infection as the cause of airway obstruction. Treatment of the two conditions differs. Treating an infection as if it were a foreign body obstruction can be dangerous. Recognizing the high-pitched sounds caused by croup or epiglottitis (inflamation of the epiglottis) is important.

Relieving a foreign obstruction in an infant should be done only if the act of obstruction was witnessed or a strongly suspected aspiration has occurred. Observation of increasing respiratory difficulty and ineffective coughing to relieve the problem is reason to consider relief techniques.

If the airway obstruction problem is caused by swelling due to infections like croup or epiglottitis, then you must take immediate steps to get the infant to the nearest hospital.

Variations in size among infants and children require different techniques. The techniques for infants is recommended for any child under 1 year of age. For unconscious children or children that become unconscious during life support procedures, between the ages of 1 and 8, the technique for a child should be used.

The procedures for accessing and opening the airway of an adult applies for infants and children also.

Removing a Foreign Object From an Infant

To remove a foreign object from a conscious infant:

1. Assess the infant for airway obstruction and observe any breathing difficulties.

2. Straddle the infant over your arm. The infant's head should be lower than the trunk. Support the head with your hand around the jaw and chest while resting the infant on your thigh (Figure 4-17a).

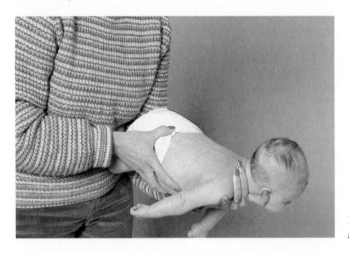

Figure 4-17a. Straddle the infant over your arm.

3. With the heel of one hand between the infant's shoulder blades, deliver four forceful back blows (Figure 4-17b).

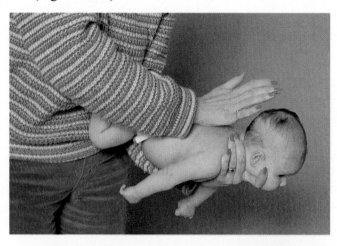

Figure 4-17b. Deliver four forceful back blows.

4. Following the back blows, support the infant by sandwiching the infant between your hands. Turn the infant and place the head lower than the trunk (Figure 4-17c).

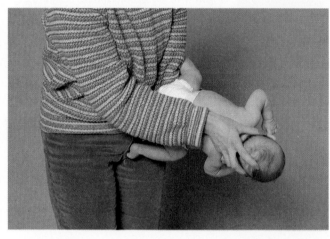

Figure 4-17c. Turn the infant.

5. Deliver four chest thrusts (do not use abdominal thrusts!) to the midsternal region in the same manner as external chest compressions, but at a slower rate (Figure 4-17d).

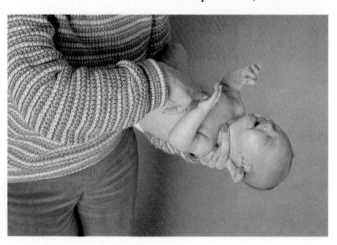

Figure 4-17d. Deliver four chest thrusts.

6. Repeat the procedure from step 3 until the foreign body is expelled or the infant becomes unconscious.

To remove a foreign object from an infant that has become unconscious:

1. Call for help, or if another person is present, have them activate the EMS system.

2. Check for the foreign body by performing the tongue-jaw lift by placing your thumb in the infant's mouth over the tongue. Lift the tongue and jaw forward with your fingers wrapped around the infant's lower jaw (Figure 4-18).

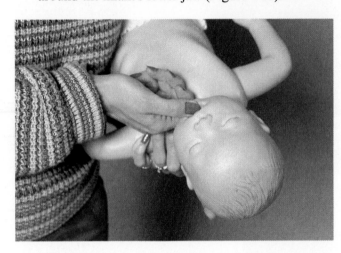

Figure 4-18. Check for a foreign body using the tongue-jaw lift.

3. Remove the foreign body only if you can see it.

   NOTE: Try a finger sweep only if the object is visible. Blind finger sweeps may push the foreign object deeper into the airway.

4. Open the airway using the head-tilt/chin-lift technique discussed earlier in this chapter.

5. Seal the mouth and nose and attempt ventilation (rescue breathing) as described earlier in this chapter.

6. If the airway is still obstructed, deliver four back blows and four chest thrusts.

7. Check for a foreign body as described in Step 2.

8. Open the airway and reattempt ventilation.

9. Repeat Steps 6 through 8 until successful.

To remove a foreign object from an infant that is found unconscious:

1. Perform assessment to determine unresponsiveness.
2. Call for help.
3. Turn the infant on his back, supporting the head and neck.
4. Open the airway using the head-tilt/chin-lift maneuver. Be careful not to hyperextend the head.
5. Look, listen, and feel for breathing.
6. Maintain an open airway and attempt ventilation.
7. If the airway is still blocked, reposition the infant's head and reattempt ventilation.
8. If another person is present, have that person activate the EMS system.
9. Straddle the infant over your arm. The infant's head should be lower than the trunk. Support the head with your hand around the jaw and chest while resting the infant on your thigh (Figure 4-19a).

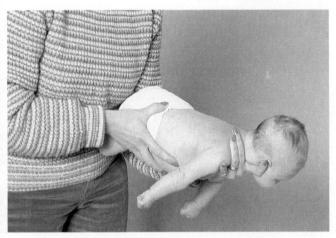

Figure 4-19a. Straddle the infant over your arm.

10. With the heel of one hand between the infant's shoulder blades, deliver four forceful back blows (Figure 4-19b).

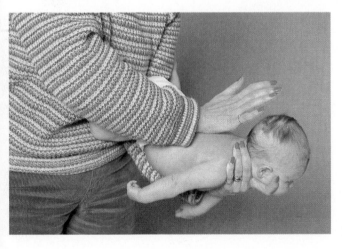

Figure 4-19b. Deliver four forceful back blows.

11. Following the back blows, support the infant by sandwiching him or her between your hands. Turn the infant and place him or her with the head lower than the trunk (Figure 4-19c).

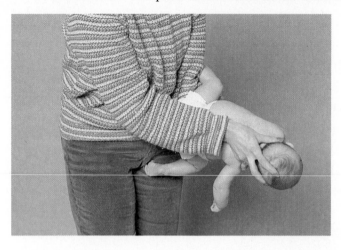

Figure 4-19c. Turn the infant.

12. Deliver four chest thrusts (*do not use* abdominal thrusts) to the midsternal region in the same manner as external chest compressions, but at a slower rate (Figure 4-19d).

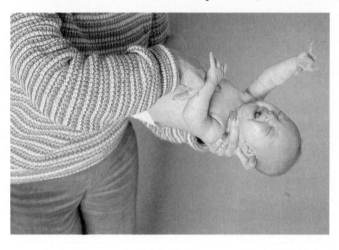

Figure 4-19d. Deliver four chest thrusts.

13. Perform the tongue-jaw lift to check for foreign body by placing your thumb in the infant's mouth over the tongue. Lift the tongue and jaw forward with your fingers wrapped around the infant's lower jaw (Figure 4-19e).

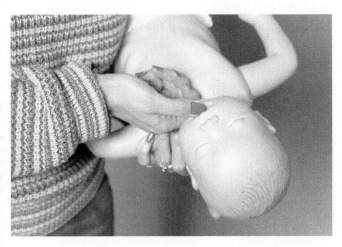

Figure 4-19e. Check for a foreign body using the tongue-jaw lift.

14. Remove the foreign body *only if you can see it*.

   NOTE: A finger sweep should only be attempted if the object is visible. Blind finger sweeps may push the foreign object deeper into the airway.

15. Open the airway using the head-tilt/chin-lift technique discussed earlier in this chapter.

16. Repeat Steps 9-15 until successful.

Removing a Foreign Object From a Child

To remove a foreign object from a conscious child:

1. Determine airway obstruction by asking, "Are you choking?"
2. Perform the Heimlich maneuver if the patient's cough is ineffective and there is increasing respiratory difficulty.
3. Stand behind the patient (Figure 4-20a).

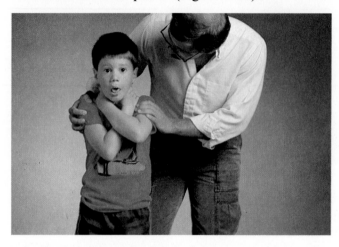

Figure 4-20a. Stand behind the patient.

4. Wrap your arms around the patient's waist.
5. Grasp one of your fists with the other hand. Place the thumb side of your fist against the patient's abdomen in the midline slightly above the navel and well below the tip of the xipyhoid process (Figure 4-20b).

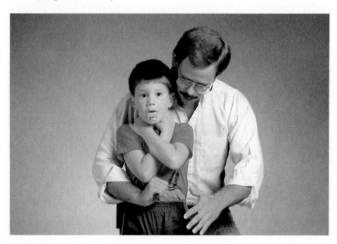

Figure 4-20b. Grasp one of your fists with the other hand. Place the thumb side of your fist against the patient's abdomen in the midline slightly above the navel.

6. Press your fist, using a quick inward and upward thrust, into the patient's abdomen (Figure 4-20c). Each thrust should be distinct and delivered with enough force to relieve the obstruction.

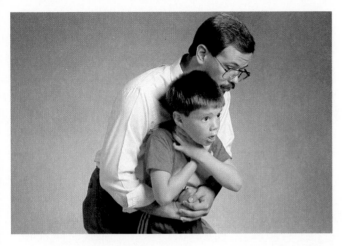

Figure 4-20c. Press your fist into the patient's abdomen using a quick inward and upward thrust.

NOTE: The position of your hands in applying the Heimlich maneuver is important to prevent possible damage to internal organs (Figure 4-20d). Your hands should never be placed on the xiphoid process of the sternum or the lower margins of the rib cage. Be prepared for vomiting to occur as a result of the thrusting effect.

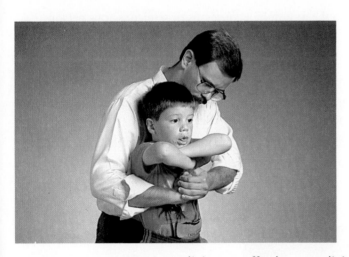

Figure 4-20d. Avoid the xiphoid process or lower margins of the rib cage.

7. Repeat manual thrusts until they are effective or until the victim becomes unconscious. There is no recommended number of initial thrusts.

To remove a foreign object from an unconscious child:

1. Place the patient horizontally on his or her back with the head in the normal anatomical position (Figure 4-21a).

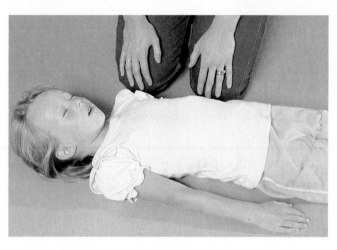

Figure 4-21a. Place the patient on his or her back.

2. Call for help.
3. Perform a finger sweep, using the tonque-jaw lift to check for foreign objects.

Here is the tongue-jaw lift procedure:

NOTE: Never insert your finger into the mouth of a conscious or semiconscious person.

❊ Place the patient's head in its normal anatomical position.

❊ Using your thumb and fingers, open the mouth. Grasp the tongue and lower jaw and lift. This may partially relieve the obstruction.

❊ Insert the index finger of your other hand along the inside of the cheek and deeply into the throat to the base of the tongue and across to the other cheek.

❊ Using a hooking motion, try to dislodge and remove the foreign body in the mouth.

CAUTION: Do not force foreign objects deeper into the airway.

4. Open the airway using the head-tilt/chin-lift technique described earlier in this chapter (Figure 4-21b).

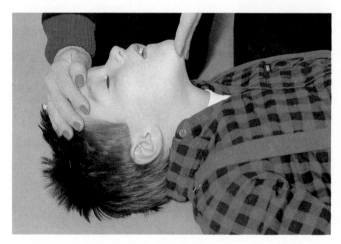

Figure 4-21b. Open the airway using the head-tilt/chin-lift technique.

5. Seal the mouth and nose and attempt ventilation as described in the "Rescue Breathing" section Figure 4-21c).

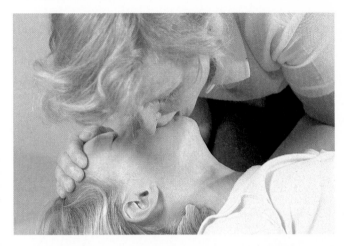

Figure 4-21c. Seal the mouth and nose and attempt ventilation.

6. Apply abdominal thrusts (the Heimlich maneuver) from the feet position of the child, if supine and on the floor (Figure 4-21d) or from the knees if the child is on a table, with the legs dangling over (Figure 4-21e) or astride, if the child's size so indicates.

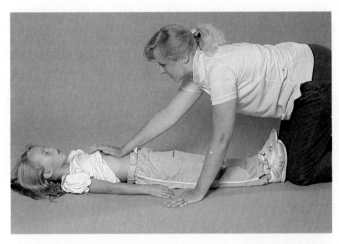

Figure 4-21d. Apply abdominal thrusts from the child's feet.

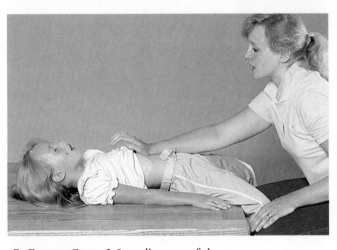

Figure 4-21e. Apply abdominal thrusts from the knees if the child is on a table.

7. Repeat Steps 3-9 until successful.

NEAR DROWNING

When a person has been under water for a long period of time, the cells of the body are deprived of oxygen (hypoxemia). Removing the person from the water is obviously the most important and initial step to take. Rescue attempts should be done safely by some device, e.g., boat, spare tire, personal flotation device (PFD), or other means (Figure 4-22). The rescue attempts should not endanger you.

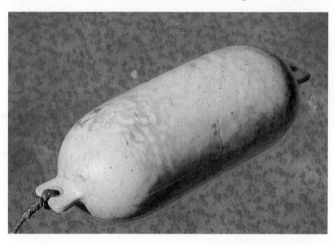

Figure 4-22. Rescue attempts should be done safely.

In the case of a near drowning, try rescue breathing using the mouth-to-mouth or mouth-to-nose techniques described earlier in this chapter. Start rescue breathing as soon as possible, even before the person is removed from the water, provided it is safe for you to do so (Figure 4-23).

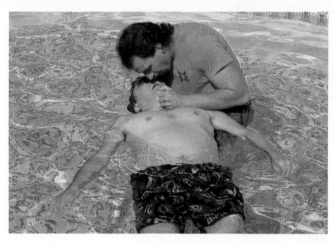

Figure 4-23. Start rescue breathing as soon as possible.

If injury to the neck is suspected, support the neck in a neutral position and float the person on his or her back on a long backboard or other similar device (Figure 4-24). In many near-drowning victims, some water is often aspirated. If you suspect that foreign matter is obstructing the airway, perform abdominal thrusts. Be alert for gastric contents; vomiting and aspiration are a potentially dangerous situation.

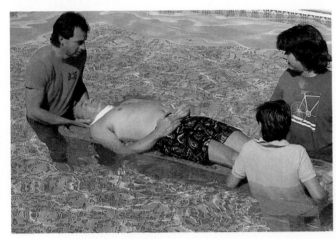

Figure 4-24. If a neck injury is suspected, support the neck in a neutral position and float the patient on a long backboard.

SUMMARY

Brain cells deteriorate when deprived of oxygen. The First Responder must rapidly help a person gain and maintain an airway that allows a sufficient air exchange. Blocking can occur from anatomical changes in the airway or foreign bodies obstructing the airways. Review this chapter to assure you can:

* Open an airway effectively
* Remove foreign obstructions when required
* Position a patient for air exchange
* Breathe for the person using rescue breathing and necessary adjuncts

It has been stated, "If the patient does not have an airway, he or she is going to die." This simple statement sums up the necessity for the First Responder to quickly open an airway and breathe for a sick or injured person whenever required.

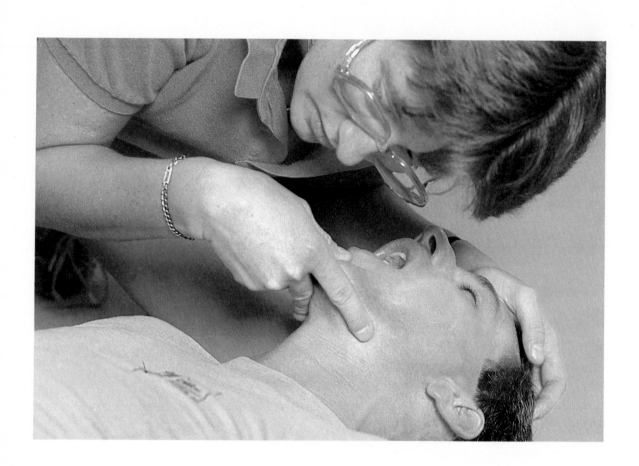

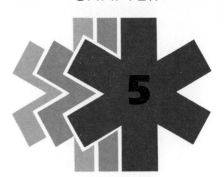

CARDIOPULMONARY RESUSCITATION (CPR)

KEY CONCEPTS AND SKILLS

By the end of this chapter, you will be able to:

✳ Identify the major parts of the circulatory system.

✳ Identify the major parts of the heart.

✳ Describe the flow of blood through the circulatory system.

✳ List the signs of cardiac arrest.

✳ Perform, on a manikin, one-person and two-person adult Basic Life Support (BLS).

✳ List the signs of effective cardiopulmonary resuscitation.

✳ Describe the complications in performing cardiopulmonary resuscitation.

✳ Describe when to stop cardiopulmonary resuscitation.

KEY WORDS

Aorta – The main trunk artery of the body's arterial systems. The aorta is about 1 inch in diameter and carries oxygenated blood from the left ventricle to the arteries and arterioles.

Aortic Valve – A half-moon valve located between the left ventricle and the aorta.

Arteries – The blood vessels that carry oxygenated blood from the heart to all parts of the body.

Arterioles – Small branches of arteries that feed blood into the capillaries.

Atrium – The two upper chambers of the heart that receive blood from the body through the venous system.

Brachial Artery – The main artery of the upper arm.

Brachial Pulse – The pulse of the brachial artery. Feel for this pulse by placing a finger at the inside of the upper arm.

Bradycardia – A heart rate of less than 60 beats/min in an adult.

Capillaries – Small blood vessels that connect the arterioles with the venules. Blood and tissue cells exchange various substances through the capillaries.

Cardiac Arrest – A sudden stoppage of the heart's output and a loss of arterial blood pressure.

Cardiovascular System – The network of structures, including the heart and blood vessels, that pump and send blood throughout the body.

Cardiopulmonary Resuscitation (CPR) – An emergency procedure for life support consisting of rescue breathing and external heart compression.

Carotid Arteries – Arteries that distribute blood to the left and right sides of the head.

Carotid Pulse – The pulse of the carotid artery. Feel for this pulse by placing a finger between the larynx and the neck muscle.

Coronary Arteries – Arteries of the heart that branch from the aorta. These arteries supply the heart with blood.

Diastole – The relaxation stage of heart action.

Mitral Valve – The heart valve located between the left atrium and left ventricle. This valve opens to allow blood flow from the left atrium to the left ventricle.

Plasma – The fluid colorless part of the blood.

Platelets – The smallest cells in the blood. These particles help form clots to stop bleeding.

Pulmonary Valve – A valve located between the right ventricle and the base of the pulmonary artery.

Septum – A wall in the heart that separates the left and right chambers.

Systole – The contraction stage of heart action, which forces blood into the aorta and pulmonary arteries.

Tachycardia – A heart rate of over 100 beats/min in an adult.

Tetani – A muscle spasm or cramp that causes muscles to be in a constant state of contraction.

Tricuspid Valve – A heart valve that separates the right atrium and right ventricle.

Valves – Structures of the heart and vessels that serve as dividers and prevent the backflow of blood.

Veins – The vessels that carry blood back to the heart.

Vena Cava – One of the two large veins that returns blood from the body to the right atrium of the heart.

Ventricle – Either of the two lower chambers of the heart. When these chambers are filled with blood, they contract to push the blood into the vessels.

Venules – The smallest veins. These veins connect blood from the capillaries to the veins.

THE CIRCULATORY SYSTEM

The circulatory system provides the vital transportation of food and oxygen to cells.

✳ Heart

✳ Blood vessels

✳ Blood

The Heart

The heart is the pump of the cardiovascular/circulatory system. In the average adult, the heart beats 60-80 times/min or 100,000 times each day.

The heart pumps blood through some 60,000 miles of tubing consisting of arteries, arterioles, capillaries, venules, and veins. It expels about 3 ounces of blood during each stroke when a person is resting; this amounts to pumping 2,000 gallons every day. During heavy exercise, the heart can increase its output five to six times.

A single phase of systole and diastole takes place in about 1 second. The heart spends at least half of each contraction *(systole)* cycle at rest *(diastole).* The faster a heart beats, the less rest time it has to rest. The term tachycardia refers to a rapid heart rate. In an adult, the rate is over 100 beats/min. *Bradycardia* refers to a slow heart rate. In an adult, this rate is under 60 beats/min. Note that a person in good physical shape, e.g., a jogger, may have a heart rate of 30-50 beats/min (bpm) and still have effective circulation because of conditioning.

The heart is located in the chest (thoracic cavity) beneath the sternum and between the two lungs as shown in Figure 5-1. The adult heart is about the size of a clenched fist and weighs between 11 and 16 ounces.

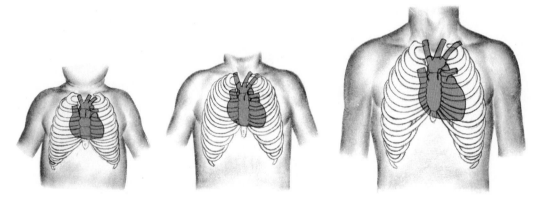

Figure 5-1. The location of the heart. (From Seidel, H.M., et al: Mosby's Guide to Physical Examination, St. Louis, 1987, The C.V. Mosby Co.)

The heart has two sides, divided by a wall called the *septum.* Each side of the heart has two chambers: a small upper cavity *(atrium)* and a larger, lower cavity *(ventricle).* The atrium is the receiving chamber and the ventricle is the pumping chamber. The left ventricle is larger and thicker than the right. It pumps blood to the entire body. The right ventricle pumps blood only through the lungs.

Between each chamber is a one-way valve to keep blood flowing through the heart in the right direction (Figure 5-2).

The right atrium receives blood from the venous system and passes it to the right ventricle. This blood is low in oxygen and high in carbon dioxide. The right ventricle pumps the blood through the pulmonary artery to the lungs to exchange waste gases for oxygen. Oxygenated blood is returned to the heart through the pulmonary vein to the left atrium, then to the left ventricle and then pumped to all parts of the body, including the heart itself. The left ventricle is larger and thicker than the right ventricle. The left ventricle pumps blood to the entire body; the right ventricle pumps blood only through the lungs.

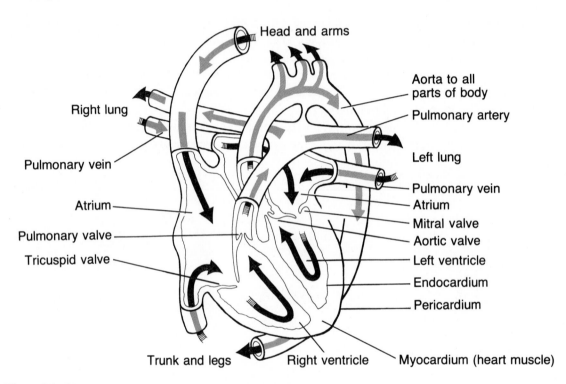

Figure 5-2. The heart. (From Austrin, M.G. and Austrin, H.R.: Young's Learning Medical Terminology, a worktext, 6th edition, St. Louis, 1987, The C.V. Mosby Co.)

Blood Vessels

There are three kinds of blood vessels; arteries, veins, and capillaries. *Arteries* carry blood away from the heart to the capillaries for tissues. *Veins* carry blood toward the heart, away from the body tissues from capillaries. *Capillaries* carry blood from tiny arteries *(arterioles)* into tiny veins *(venules)*.

Arteries, veins, and capillaries differ in structure. Arteries have the property of elastic recoil because of relatively thick muscular walls that exert pressure on the volume of blood. Veins are not as thick as arteries. They are more elastic but not as muscular. You can see veins and arteries but not capillaries. Capillaries are microscopic vessels that pass blood cells through in single file.

Arteries, veins, and capillaries perform different functions. Arteries and arterioles distribute blood from the heart to capillaries in all parts of the body. Venules and veins collect blood from capillaries and return it to the heart. Capillaries control the flow of energy-producing substances flowing in and out of cells. Red blood cells pass through each capillary, one at a time.

Blood

Blood is a liquid tissue that has millions of chemicals suspended in it. The liquid part of blood is called *plasma*. There are three types of blood cells found in blood.

1. Red cells

2. White cells

3. Platelets

Red blood cells transport oxygen and carbon dioxide. White blood cells fight infectious microorganisms that have succeeded in invading the tissues or blood stream. Platelets control the blood loss due to an injury by assisting in clotting.

Cardiac arrest is a sudden and sometimes unexpected cessation of the heartbeat and effective circulation. The two main signs of cardiac arrest are:

1. Lack of pulse in the large arteries (e.g., carotid, femoral, brachial)

2. Lack of respiration

Another important sign of cardiac arrest is profound cyanosis. Most persons in cardiac arrest will not be breathing, but occasionally a patient without a pulse will gasp for air.

Some of the causes of cardiac arrest are (Figure 5-3):

* Acute airway obstruction

* Electric shock

* Reaction to insects, medication, or food

* Trauma to the heart

* Lack of oxygen (anoxia)

* Inhalation of toxic gases

* Drug overdose

* Multiple systems trauma

The signs and symptoms of cardiac arrest include:

* Loss of consciousness

* Absence of palpable carotid pulse in adults and brachial pulse in infants

* Absence of breath sounds or air movement through the nose or mouth

* Dilation of pupils or eyes

* Ashen gray color, cyanosis

Over 650,000 people in the United States die each year from sudden cardiac arrest. When cardiac arrest occurs, basic life support is urgent and must be initiated within 4-6 minutes if the patient is to have a chance for a successful recovery.

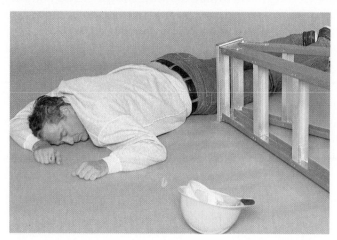

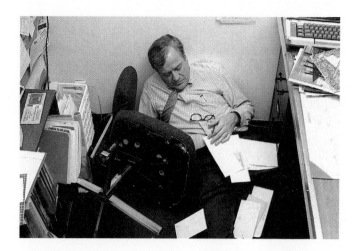

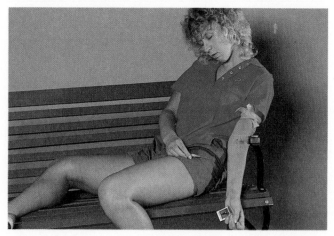

Figure 5-3. Some causes of cardiac arrest. **A,** Electric shock. **B,** Trauma to the heart. **C,** Drug overdose.

CARDIOPULMONARY RESUSCITATION – BASIC LIFE SUPPORT (CPR-BLS)

The purpose of Cardiopulmonary Resuscitation-Basic Life Support (CPR-BLS) is to promptly establish effective circulation and ventilation, and to prevent irreversible cerebral damage.

The principles of CPR-BLS consist of:

✳ Basic ABC (Airway, Breathing,and Circulation).

✳ Maintaining an open airway, providing artificial ventilation by means of rescue breathing, and providing artificial circulation by external cardiac compression.

PROCEDURE FOR CPR-BLS

There are a variety of procedures to perform CPR:

✳ One-person CPR

✳ Two-person CPR

✳ CPR for the child

✳ CPR for the infant

Before performing actual CPR procedures, the First Responder must perform the assessments as outlined in the following 7 steps:

1. Perform assessment for unresponsiveness.

   ✳ Determine unresponsiveness by quickly assessing any possible injury and whether the individual is unconscious. If trauma to the head or neck is suspected, move the person only if absolutely necessary to avoid injury to the spine.

   ✳ Gently tap or shake the person and shout "Are you okay?" This procedure reduces the possibility of attempting BLS on a person who does not require resuscitation (Figure 5-4a).

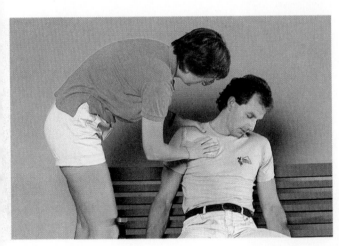

Figure 5-4a. Gently tap or shake the person.

✳ If the person does not respond to these attempts at arousal, *call out for help* (Figure 5-4b). If another person is present, or as soon as someone else arrives, have that person activate the EMS system.

✳ Position the patient so that he or she is supine and on a firm, flat surface (Figure 5-4c).

✳ Kneel close to and at the level of the patient's shoulders (Figure 5-4d).

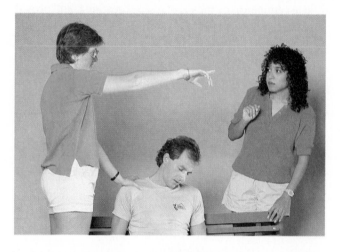

Figure 5-4b. Call out for help.

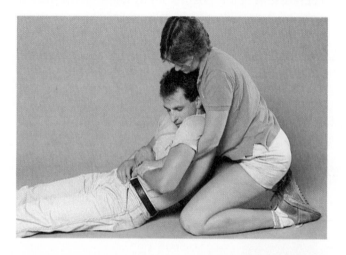

Figure 5-4c. Position the patient on a firm flat surface.

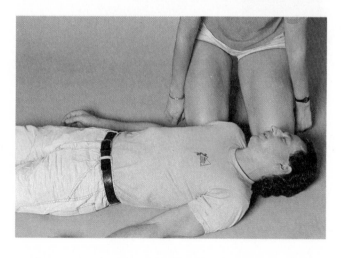

Figure 5-4d. Kneel close to and at the same level as the patient's shoulders.

2. Perform assessment of Airway

✳ Maintain an open airway using the head-tilt/chin-lift technique (Figure 5-a). Refer to Chapter 4 for detailed head-tilt/chin-lift instructions.

NOTE: If neck injury is suspected, the modified jaw-thrust technique (Figure 5-b) is the safest first approach to opening the airway. Refer to Chapter 4 for detailed instructions.

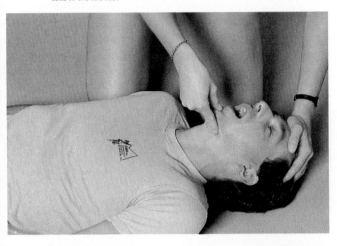

Figure 5-5a. Maintain an open airway using the head-tilt/chin-lift technique.

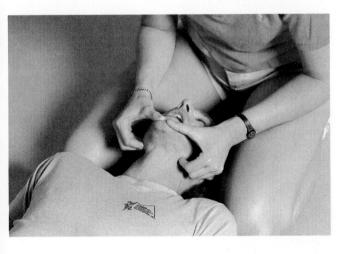

Figure 5-5b. If neck injury is suspected, use the jaw-thrust technique.

3. Perform assessment of *Breathing*

   ✸ Determine if there is an absence of breathing by placing your ear over the patient's mouth and nose and while maintaining an open airway (Figure 5-6a). Look, listen, and feel for the following signs:

   > *Look* for rising and falling of the patient's chest.
   > *Listen* for air escaping during exhalation.
   > *Feel* for a flow of air that can be felt.

   ✸ Perform rescue breathing (Figure 5-6b); delivering two full ventilations of 1-1½ seconds each. Chapter 4 provides detailed instruction for performing rescue breathing.
   If the signs are not apparent, the victim is breathless (This step should not take more than 3-5 seconds.)

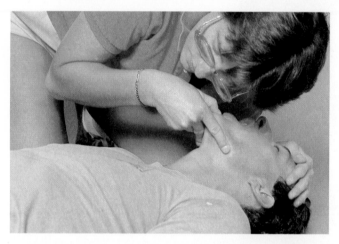

Figure 5-6a. Determine breathlessness.

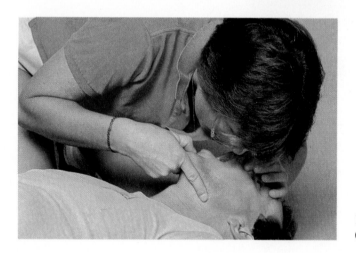

Figure 5-6b. Perform rescue breathing (no mask used).

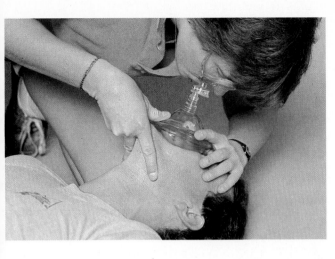

Figure 5-6b. Perform rescue breathing
(mask used).

4. Perform assessment for circulation.

✳ Determine and restore circulation by administering two initial ventilations and maintaining an open airway, then feeling for the carotid pulse (located between the larynx and the neck muscle) for 5-10 seconds (Figure 5-7).

 NOTE: It is very important to determine that the pulse is absent before beginning CPR. Serious medical problems can develop if CPR is performed on a person with a pulse.

✳ If a pulse is present but there is no breathing, perform rescue breathing at a rate of 12 breaths/min (once every 5 seconds after the two initial breaths of 1-1 ½ seconds each).

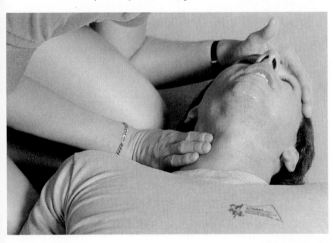

Figure 5-7. Check the carotid pulse.

5. Perform Landmarking

✳ Position the patient in a flat position on the ground and a firm surface as shown in Figure 5-8a.

✳ With the middle and index finger of the hand nearest to the patient's feet, locate the lower margin of the patient's rib cage on the side nearest you as shown in Figure 5-8b.

✳ Run your fingers up along the rib cage to the notch where the ribs meet the sternum in the center of the lower part of the chest as shown in Figure 5-8c.

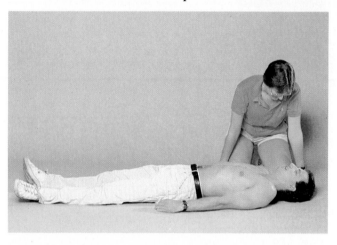

Figure 5-8a. Position the patient on a flat firm surface.

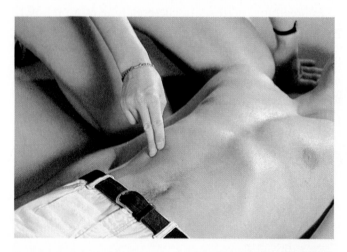

Figure 5-8b. Locate the lower margin of the patient's rib cage on the side nearest you.

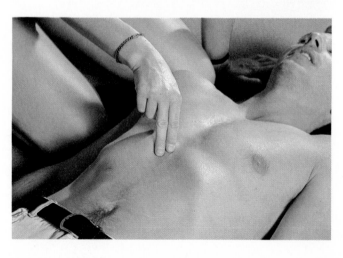

Figure 5-8c. Run your fingers along the rib cage to the notch where the ribs meet the sternum.

✳ With your middle finger on the notch, place the index next to the notch on the lower end of the sternum as shown in Figure 5-8d.

✳ Place the heel of your other hand (which has been used on the patient's forehead to maintain head position) on the lower half of the sternum, next to, but not covering, the index finger that is next to the middle finger in the notch as shown in Figure 5-8e.

✳ Place the long axis of the heel of your hand in the long axis of the patient's sternum as shown in Figure 5-8f. This keeps the main line of the force of compressions on the sternum and decreases the change of rib fracture.

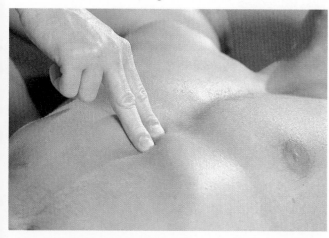

Figure 5-8d. With your middle finger on the notch, place the index next to the notch on the lower end of the sternum.

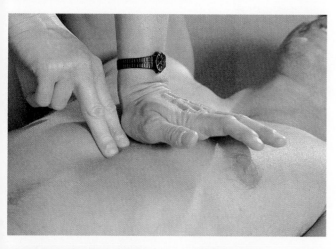

Figure 5-8e. Place the heel of your other hand on the lower half of the sternum next to the index finger.

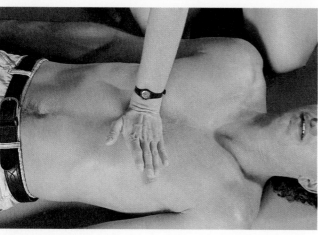

Figure 5-8f. Place the long axis of the heel of your hand in the long axis of the patient's sternum.

NOTE: An alternative method is to grasp the wrist of the hand on the chest with the hand used to locate the lower end of the sternum (Figure 5-8g). This technique may be helpful for those with arthritis of the hand or wrist.

✳ Remove your hand from the notch and place it on top of your other hand on the sternum. The heels of both hands should be parallel with the fingers directed straight away from you as shown in Figure 5-8h. The fingers may be either extended or interlaced but keep them off the chest to avoid damage to the chest and internal organs as shown in Figure 5-8i.

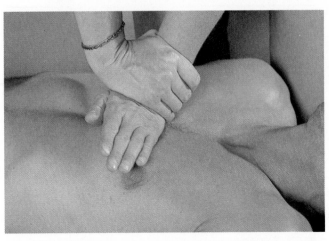

Figure 5-8g. An alternative method is to grasp the wrist with the hand used to locate the sternum.

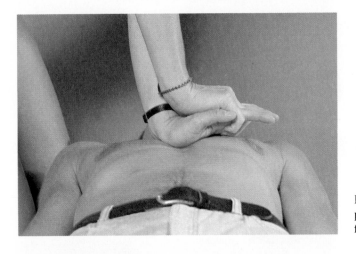

Figure 5-8h. The heels of both hands should be parallel with the fingers directed straight away from you.

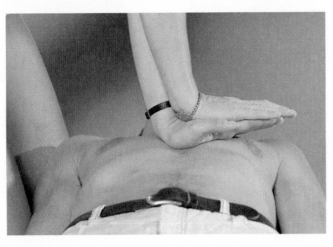

Figure 5-8i. Keep your fingers off the chest to avoid damage to the chest and internal organs.

6. Position your body.

   ✱ Straighten your elbows by locking them and positioning your shoulders directly over your hands so that the thrust for external chest compression is straight down as shown in Figure 5-9a.

   If the thrust is not straight down, the patient's torso can roll, making chest compression less effective and possibly fracturing ribs. Another complication from improper rescuer body position is injury to visceral organs and body structures of the patient (Figure 5-9b).

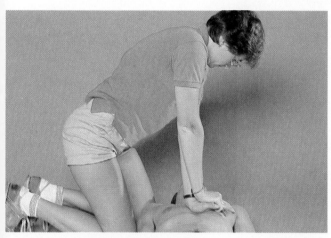

Figure 5-9a. Straighten your elbows so the thrust for external chest compression is straight down.

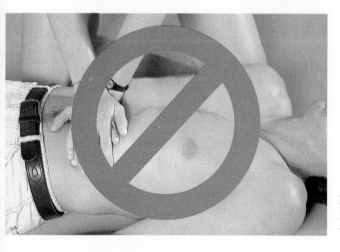

Figure 5-9b. Another complication from improper rescuer body position is injury to visceral organs and body structures of the patient.

7. Perform chest compression.

   ✱ For a normal size adult, apply enough force to depress the sternum 1½-2 inches.

   ✱ After compression, release the pressure completely without removing your hand to allow blood to flow into the heart and the chest to return to its normal position.

   The time permitted for release is equal to the time required for compression.

   NOTE: Do not change hand position during release; doing so may cause you to alter or lose correct hand position.

   If you lose your hand position at any time during compression, relandmarking must be done.

One-Person CPR

If you are the only qualified person to perform CPR, follow the basic assessment ABC's:

✳ Assess for unresponsiveness (Figure 5-10a)

✳ Call for help (Figure 5-10b)

✳ Position the victim (Figure 5-10c)

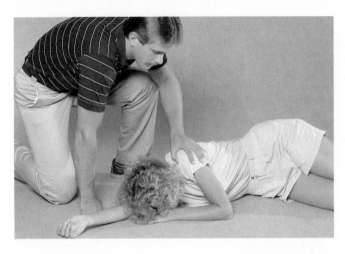

Figure 5-10a. Assess unresponsiveness.

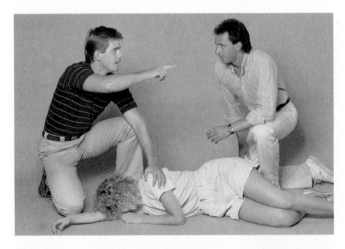

Figure 5-10b. Call for help.

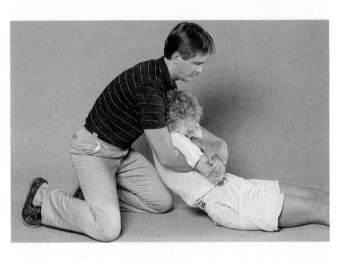

Figure 5-10c. Position the victim.

✳ Open the airway (Figure 5-10d)

✳ Assess breathlessness (minimum of 5 seconds)

✳ If the patient is not breathing, deliver 2 full ventilations of 1-1½ seconds each (Figure 5-10e)

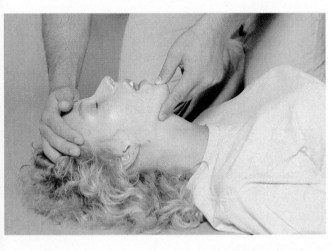

Figure 5-10d. Open the airway.

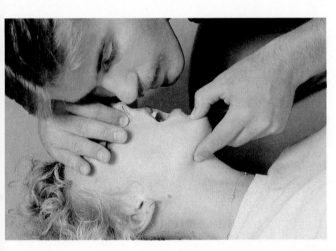

Figure 5-10e. Deliver 2 full ventilations (without mask).

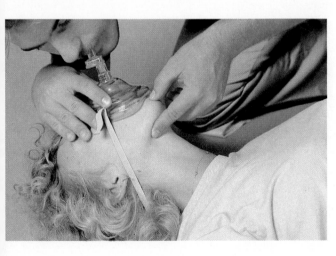

Figure 5-10e. Deliver 2 full ventilations (with mask).

✳ While maintaining an open airway, palpate the carotid pulse for 5-10 seconds to determine the presence or absence of a pulse (Figure 5-10f).

✳ If there is no pulse, begin compression at a rate of 80-100 compressions per minute. The counting rate is one and two and three and four and (up to)...15 (Figure 5-10g).

✳ Breathe. Breathing consists of two full, 1-1½ seconds lung inflations after each series of 15 chest compressions. Allow full exhalation between your breaths (Figure 5-10h).

✳ Continue compression and ventilation at a rate of 15:2.

✳ Check the carotid pulse periodically during CPR to determine effectiveness (Figure 5-10i). It must be checked after the first minute (4 cycles of 15 compressions and 2 ventilations) and every 4 minutes thereafter.

✳ If no pulse is found, ventilate two times and resume compression/ventilation cycles.

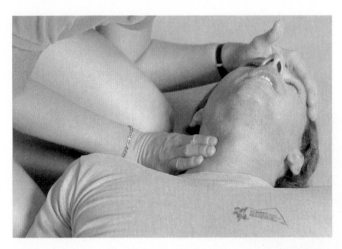

Figure 5-10f. Palpate the carotid pulse.

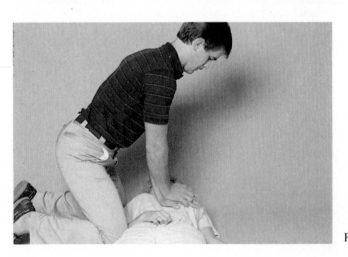

Figure 5-10g. If there is no pulse, begin compre

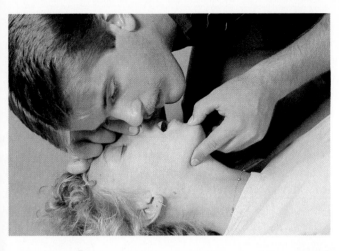

Figure 5-10h. Breathe (without mask).

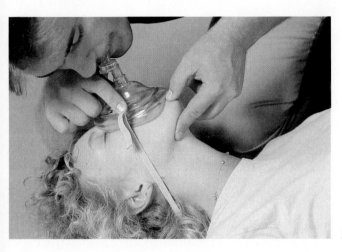

Figure 5-10h. Breathe (with mask).

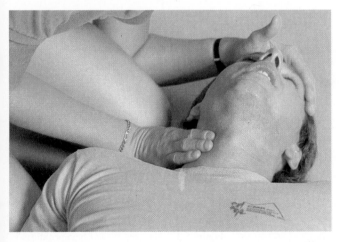

Figure 5-10i. Check the carotid pulse.

Two-Person CPR

The First Responder is an important part of the pre-hospital EMS team. Individuals involved in emergency medical care need to know and be proficient in CPR with two people involved. Two-person CPR is more effective. It allows for the use of mouth-to-mask ventilation, is less fatiguing, and permits rescuers to exchange positions when the person performing chest compression becomes tired. The following 4 steps outline the methods used for two-person CPR.

1. If CPR is in progress by one rescuer, the second rescuer should enter into the process after the first rescuer has completed a full 15:2 cycle.

2. With the first rescuer positioned at the head, open the airway and check for a pulse. The second rescuer locates the proper position for external compression and finds proper hand position (Figure 5-11). This should take 5 seconds.

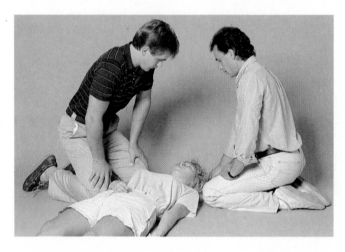

Figure 5-11. Positions for two-person CPR.

3. If there is no pulse, the person at the head (the ventilator states "No pulse," and gives 2 breaths. The compressor begins external chest compression at the rate of 80-100/min as shown in Figure 5-12. The compression-ventilation ratio is 5:1. The count is the same as one-person CPR: one and two and three and four and five.

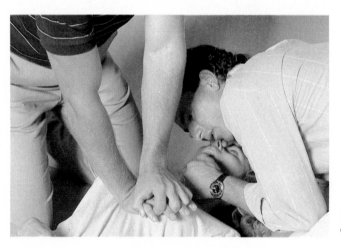

Figure 5-12. The compressor begins external chest compressions (without mask).

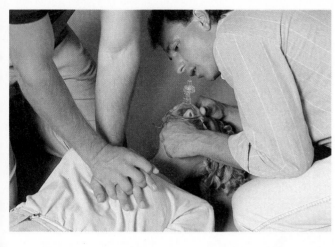

Figure 5-12. The compressor begins external chest compressions (with mask).

4. At the end of the compression cycle, the compressor pauses (keeping his or her hand in a relaxed position) and the ventilator gives 1 full ventilation of 1-1½ seconds.

To change positions during two-person CPR, clearly state that you want to "change." It is recommended that you use the word, "Change and two and three and four and five" and then follow the 7 steps outlined below:

1. The compressor calls for the change and completes the 5th compression (Figure 5-13a).

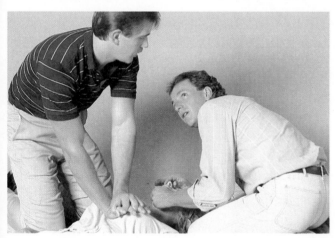

Figure 5-13a. Compressor calls for a change and completes the 5th compression.

2. The ventilator completes ventilation after the 5th compressions (Figure 5-13b).

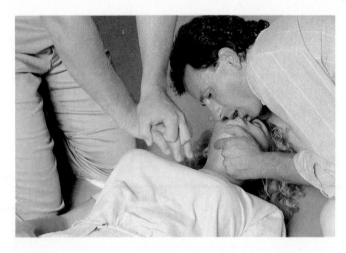

Figure 5-13b. The ventilator completes ventilation (without mask).

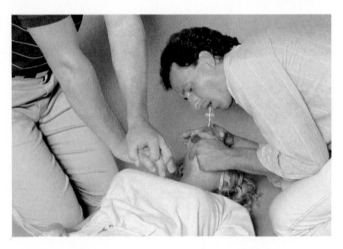

Figure 5-13b. The ventilator completes ventilation (with mask).

3. A simultaneous change is made (Figure 5-13c).

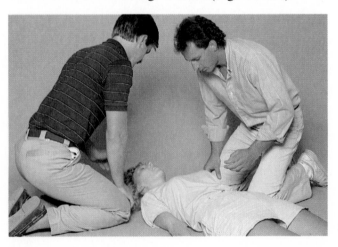

Figure 5-13c. The simultaneous change is made.

4. The ventilator moves to the chest and gets into position for compressions and locates the landmark notch (Figure 5-13d).

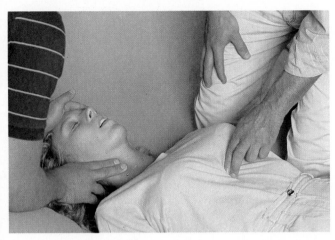

Figure 5-13d. The ventilator moves into position as the compressor and locates the landmark notch.

5. The compressor moves to the head and becomes the ventilator (Figure 5-13e).

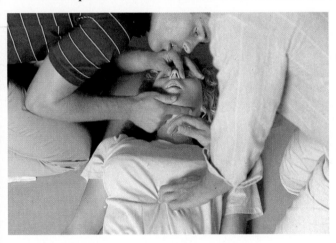

Figure 5-13e. The compressor becomes the new ventilator.

6. The "new" ventilator checks for the carotid pulse (5 seconds) and says "No pulse" if no pulse is found (Figure 5-13f). The other person performs the landmarking procedure.

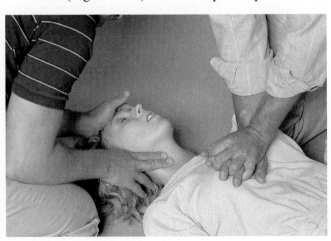

Figure 5-13f. The "new" ventilator checks the carotid pulse.

7. The ventilator gives one ventilation (1-1½ seconds): compressions are started and CPR continued by repeating steps 1-4 of the two person CPR method before change was initiated (Figure 5-13g).

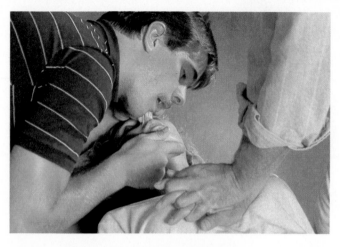

Figure 5-13g. The "new" ventilator gives one ventilation. Compressions are started. CPR continues (without mask).

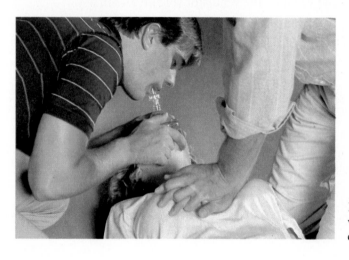

Figure 5-13g. The "new" ventilator gives one ventilation. Compressions are started. CPR continues (with mask).

SPECIAL SITUATIONS AND CONSIDERATIONS

Ordinarily, CPR should not be interrupted for more than 7 seconds. If interrupted for more than 7 seconds, begin the cycle over again.

However, there are special situations or conditions that may cause CPR to become interrupted or may actually inhibit the administration of CPR. Such situations and conditions include:

* The need to change the location of the patient
* Gastric distention
* Chest compressions
* Possible transmission of disease to the First Responder (See Appendix B)
* Traumatic injury
* Electric shock
* Hypothermia

Changing the location of the patient - If a patient is found in a cramped difficult location, do not move them unless absolutely necessary (Figure 5-14) until effective CPR has been started, the patient has a spontaneous pulse, or help arrives so that CPR can be performed without interruption.

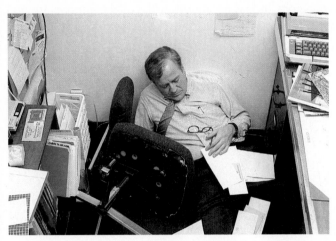

Figure 5-14. Do not move this patient unless absolutely necessary.

When movement of a patient involves going up and down a flight of stairs, perform CPR at the top and at the bottom of the stairs (Figure 5-15). At a predetermined signal, e.g., stop at the next level, CPR is halted, movement to the next level or landing is accomplished and CPR is resumed. Such interruptions should not exceed 30 seconds.

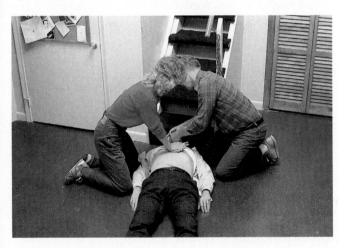

Figure 5-15. Perform CPR at the top and bottom of stairs.

Gastric Distention - Gastric distention may be a problem during CPR. Refer to Chapter 4 for a detailed discussion of gastric distention and related procedures. Do not maintain continuous pressure on the abdomen to prevent distention. This may cause the liver to rupture or regurgitation and aspiration of vomitus.

Chest Compressions - Even properly performed chest compressions can fracture and cause other injuries. Separation of the ribs from the sternum, fractured sternum, laceration of the spleen, and other chest trauma have been reported (Figure 5-16). You can minimize these complications by carefully adhering to performance standards. Compressions should be smooth with equal compressions and relaxation cycles to reduce injury to the patient. Proper hand position is also important to reducing injury during compression.

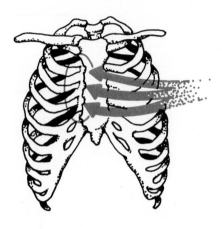

Figure 5-16. Rib fractures caused by improper compressions.

Disease Transmission - Many health care providers are concerned about disease transmission during CPR. For a more complete discussion, refer to Appendix B.

Traumatic Injury - CPR may not be effective if serious injury has resulted in massive blood loss. Rapid transportation to a hospital is necessary. Volume replacement and definitive care must be provided in a hospital. Stabilize the cervical spine for all trauma victims, particularly those with injuries above the clavicles (collar bones). Movement of the head and cervical spine must be minimal. Use the jaw-thrust maneuver without the head-tilt or chin-lift to open the airway.

Electric Shock - Many complications may occur following contact with an energized source. These complications depend upon the amplitude and duration of contact with the source. Other injuries, e.g., burns and fractures, may also occur due to falls or the force of the electric shock. Exposure to electric shock may pose the following complications:

❋ Constant intervention (tetani) of the breathing muscles; this is usually limited to the duration of the current exposure, but if long enough may lead to cardiac arrest secondary to hypoxia.

❋ Prolonged paralysis of the breathing muscles leading to cardiac arrest.

❋ Cardiac arrest; interruption of the electric impulses to the heart may lead to ventricular fibrillation (uncoordinated contraction of cardiac muscle) or other cardiac conditions.

If the area is safe for you to enter, CPR-BLS assessment and care is initiated as with any other patient.

Hypothermia - Caring for a patient with hypothermia is discussed in detail in Chapter 14. Hypothermia, e.g., blood temperature less than 94 °F slows down the heart and causes the blood to be thicker.

ADMINISTERING CPR TO INFANTS AND CHILDREN

The procedures outlined in this section pertain to infants and children under 1 year of age.

In infants and children, cardiac arrest usually is the end result of some other emergency problem often low oxygen level caused by:

* Traumatic injuries
* Foreign body aspiration e.g., toys, candies, or a plastic bag over the head
* Smoke inhalation
* SIDS (Sudden Infant Death Syndrome)
* Infection, particularly of the respiratory tract, e.g., pneumonia, epiglotitis

When performing CPR on an infant or child, first check for a pulse. Because infants often have a short fat neck, the carotid pulse may be difficult to palpate. The recommended pulse for assessing an infant is the brachial artery (Figure 5-17), which is located on the inside of the upper arm, midway between the elbow and the shoulder.

Press the tips of the index and middle fingers lightly toward the upper arm to check for a pulse. If there is no pulse, external chest compressions must be started.

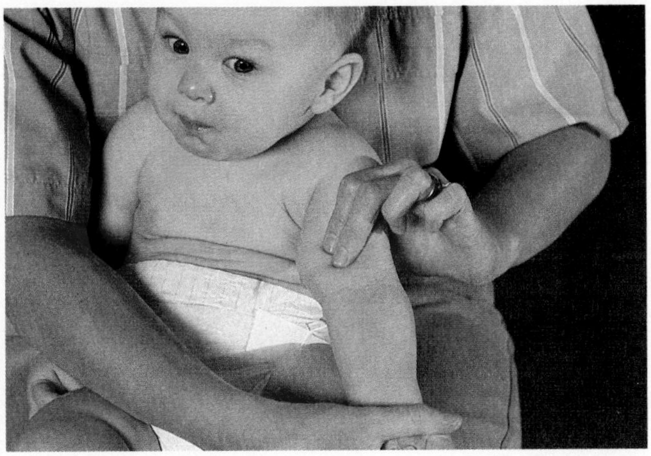

Figure 5-17. The brachial artery is recommended for assessing an infant's pulse.

Location of the Heart

The heart in the infant or very young child is located a little higher in the chest than the adult. The proper area for compressions of the infant is midsternum, with the compressor's fingers being placed 1 finger width below the imaginary intermammary line (Figure 5-18). Compressing the infant's midsternum at the location of the intermammary line will compress the great vessels of the heart and not the ventricles.

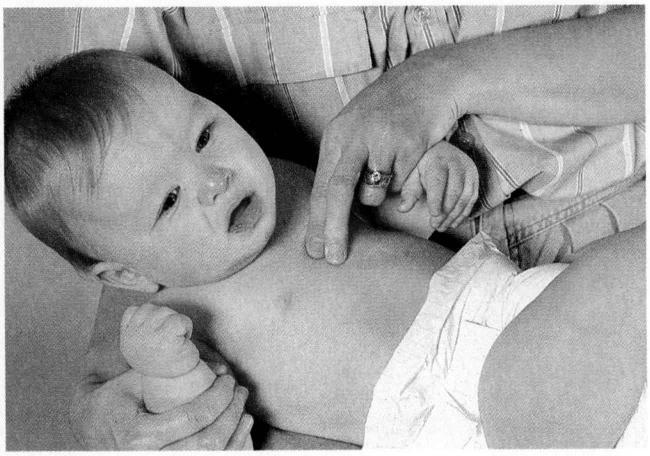

Figure 5-18. Location of the imaginary intermammary line.

The child's heart is located lower than the infant, but not as low as an adult. If you use the adult technique, the notch in the center of the chest is located with the middle finger. The area just above the index finger is the appropriate area for compression in the child (Figure 5-19).

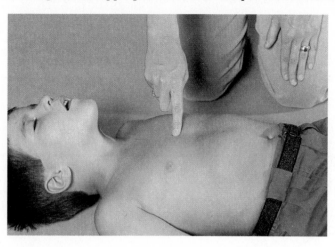

Figure 5-19. The correct area for compression in the child.

Compression

Heart rate is faster in infants and children than adults so the compression rate must be faster. Two hands are *not* necessary for compressions since the chest of an infant or child is smaller and more flexible.

Infants

✱ Using 2 or 3 fingers for compression, place your fingers 1 finger width below the imaginary line on the midsternum (Figure 5-20).

✱ Compress the breastbone ½-1 inch at a rate of at least one hundred compressions/min (5 in 3 seconds or less).

✱ Use 5 compressions to one breath for both one-person and two-person rescue. The counting rate is one, two, three, four, five, breathe.

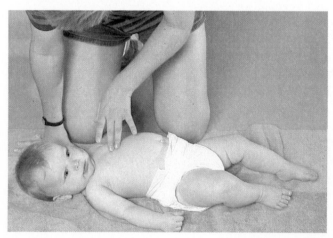

Figure 5-20. Use 2 or 3 fingers for compression placed 1 finger width below the imaginary line on the midsternum.

Children

✳ Using the heel of one hand, compress the breastbone from 1-½ inches as shown in Figure 5-21 at a rate of 80-100 compressions/min (5 per 3 seconds).

✳ Use 5 compressions to one slow breath for both one-person and two-person CPR. The counting rate is one, and two, and three, and four, and five, and breathe.

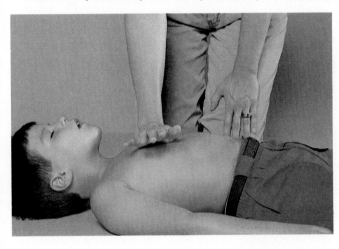

Figure 5-21. Using the heel of one hand, compress the breastbone from 1-½ inches.

The Sequence of CPR for Infants and Children

One-Person CPR - The sequence of steps of CPR for infants and children is similar to that for adults.

✳ Assessment - Determine unresponsiveness and/or respiratory difficulty (Figure 5-22a). Look, listen, and feel.

✳ Call for help.

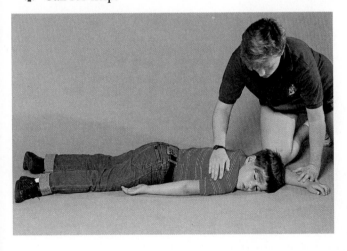

Figure 5-22a. Determine unresponsiveness.

✳ Position the infant or child by turning him or her as a unit, supporting the head and neck (Figure 5-22b).

✳ Open the airway using the head-tilt/chin-lift or jaw thrust (Figure 5-22c). Refer to Chapter 4 for detailed instructions.

✳ Perform breathing assessment by determining if breathing is present or absent (Figure 5-22d). Refer to Chapter 4 for detailed instructions.

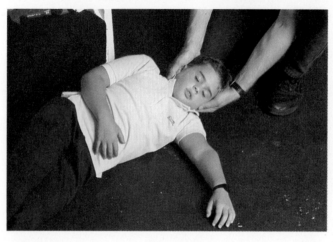

Figure 5-22b. Turn the patient as a unit. Support the patient's head and neck.

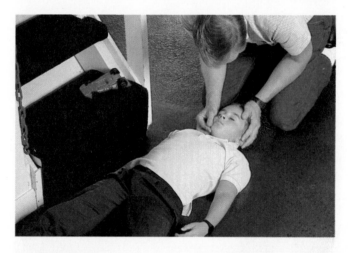

Figure 5-22c. Open the airway.

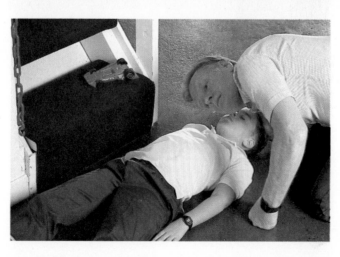

Figure 5-22d. Perform breathing assessment.

✳ Perform a pulse assessment by determining if a pulse is present (Figure 5-22e).

✳ If possible, activate the EMS system.

✳ Landmark for proper chest position (Figure 5-22f & g).

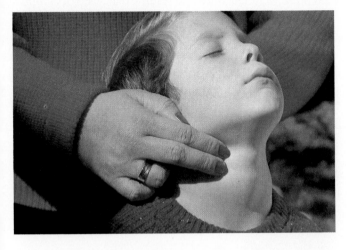

Figure 5-22e. Perform pulse assessment.

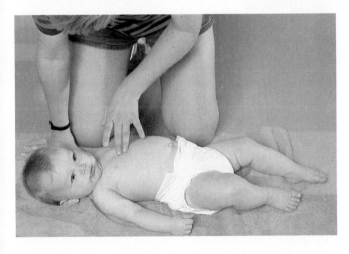

Figure 5-22f. Landmarking chest position for infants.

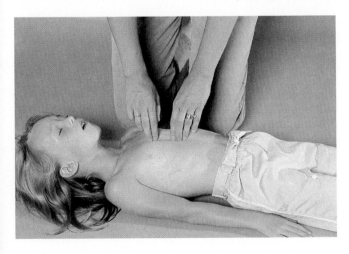

Figure 5-22g. Landmarking chest position for children.

✱ In the infant and child, perform 10 cycles of 5 compressions to 1 ventilation (before stopping to reassess the pulse). Chest compressions must be at least 100/min in the infant (5 in 3 seconds) 80-100/min in the child (5 in 3-4 seconds).

✱ Reassess for pulselessness. If there is no pulse, ventilate once and resume the cycles of compression and ventilation.

✱ The brachial pulse should be palpated every few minutes.

Two-Person CPR - Two-person CPR for the child is the same as for the adult, except for the specific steps outlined e.g., rate, 1 hand for compression. Remember that the compression rate is 80-100/min (5 compressions within 3-4 seconds), and requires less force in compressing the sternum (Figure 5-23).

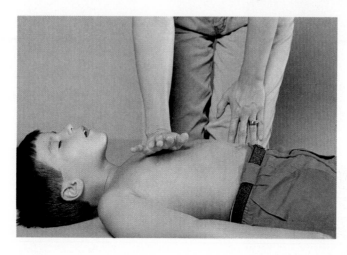

Figure 5-23. Compressions for infants and children require less force.

CESSATION OF CPR-BLS

Once resuscitation is begun, continue until one of the following events occurs:

✱ Effective, spontaneous circulation and ventilation are restored.

✱ Resuscitation efforts have been transferred to another person who continues BLS.

✱ A physician or physician-directed person or team assumes responsibility.

✱ The patient is transferred to a properly trained and designated medical professional or allied health professional charged with responsibilities of EMS.

✱ The rescuer is exhausted and unable to continue resuscitation.

The ultimate responsibility to stop CPR is exclusively that of the physician, when one is available.

SUMMARY

The First Responder is required to perform CPR-BLS whenever a sick or injured person is found unconscious without a pulse.

To best provide this important care, you need to understand the major organs involved with moving blood throughout the body.

Some major signs of cardiac arrest include:

✳ Loss of consciousness

✳ Weak or absent breathing

✳ No pulse

Whenever a patient is found in cardiac arrest, initiate BLS immediately. Practicing the skills outlined in this chapter, you may be able to save a life using BLS on persons of all ages.

CPR should never be discontinued without a physician's order or until the rescuer is too exhausted to continue.

Even when CPR is correctly administered, complications can develop such as rib fractures or lung contusions.

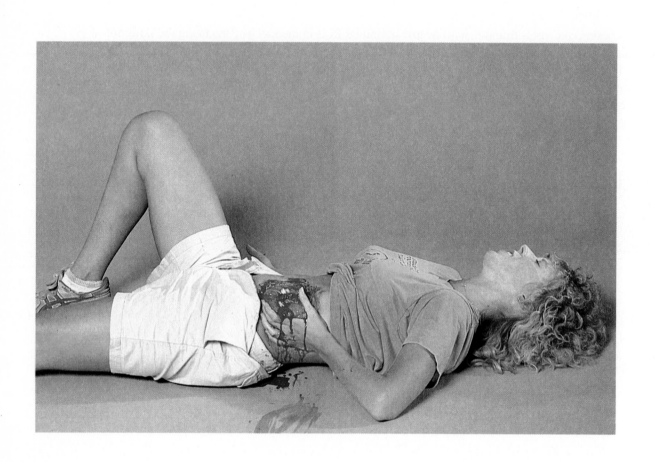

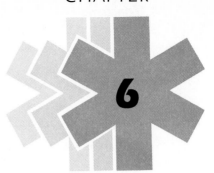

CONTROLLING HEMORRHAGE AND SHOCK

KEY CONCEPTS AND SKILLS

By the end of this chapter, you will be able to:

* List and describe the two basic types of wounds.
* Describe the proper management procedures for treating soft tissue injuries.
* Describe special considerations for treating soft tissue injuries.
* Identify bleeding and visually note the source.
* Describe the control of bleeding (hemorrhage) through use of direct pressure, elevation, pressure points, and the tourniquet.
* Describe the location of the carotid, brachial, radial, and femoral pulses.
* Describe the proper method used to record these pulses.
* Describe and recognize the signs and symptoms of shock.
* Identify the treatment for shock.
* Identify the proper treatment for anaphylactic shock.

KEY WORDS

Abrasion – A scraping, or rubbing away, of a surface by friction, e.g., rope burns.

Anaphylactic shock – An extreme systemic reaction caused by a substance such as venom from a bee sting. This condition requires immediate care.

Anxiety – A state or feeling of apprehension, uneasiness, agitation, and fear resulting from the anticipation of some threat or danger. An imagined threat to one's physical or mental well-being.

Avulsion – The separation, by tearing, of any part of the body from the whole. The avulsion may be partial or complete.

Bandage – A strip or roll of cloth or other material that may be wound around a part of the body to secure a dressing.

Closed Injury – Damage to the internal body structures, tissues, or organs.

Direct Pressure – Application or force, e.g., using a hand to control bleeding.

Dressing – A clean or sterile covering applied directly to wounded or diseased tissue.

Elevation – Lifting an arm or leg to help in the control of bleeding.

Epinephrine – A hormone produced by the adrenal glands. It acts as a cardiac stimulant, a bronchial relaxer, and as a constrictor for the blood vessels. This hormone is often used to treat asthma and acute allergy reactions.

Guarded Abdomen – A condition in which a patient protects his or her abdomen from being examined by stiffening the abdominal muscles.

Hematoma – A mass of usually clotted blood found in a body area. A hematoma may be caused by a break in a blood vessel. Also referred to as a blood blister.

Hives – An eruption of very itchy wheals on the skin caused by an allergic substance.

Hypovolemic Shock – A state of shock caused by low or diminished blood volume.

Immobilization – Making a body part or extremity immovable.

Impaled Object – A foreign body inserted (and not removed) into the body, e.g., a knife.

Incision – A wound characterized by sharp cuts such as one made by a knife, razor blade, or shard of glass.

Laceration – A wound characterized by torn or jagged edges.

Open Injury – A wound that results in the breaking of the skin.

Perfusion – The passage of a fluid through a specific organ or an area of the body.

Pressure Point – A point over an artery where the pulse may be felt. Pressure on this point may help to stop the flow of blood from a wound distal to the point.

Puncture – A wound characterized by a hole caused by a pointed object such as a nail or ice pick.

Shallow Breathing – Light breathing without full expansion of the chest.

Supine – Lying on the back.

Tourniquet – A device used to control hemorrhaging. Using a tourniquet is a drastic measure employed only in life-threatening situations.

WOUNDS

There are two classifications of wounds, closed and open.

Closed Wounds

Closed wounds are not exposed to the outside environment. Minor closed wounds do not require care by a First Responder. Bleeding from minor wounds is absorbed by the body tissue within a short time; usually a few days. A bruise is a closed wound most commonly seen by a First Responder. A bruise begins as a sore blue area on the body. As the tissue absorbs the leaked blood, different skin colors occur. The closed wound changes from blue to red to green and then to yellow before resuming its normal color. If swelling or a mass of blood (hematoma) forms, a pressure bandage may be needed to help control the bleeding and reduce the swelling (Figure 6-1). Ice is sometimes helpful to reduce pain and prevent swelling (Figure 6-2). Ice should never be applied directly to the skin's surface. Wrap the ice in a towel. Elevation may be used to help control bleeding from internal injury caused by minor closed wounds.

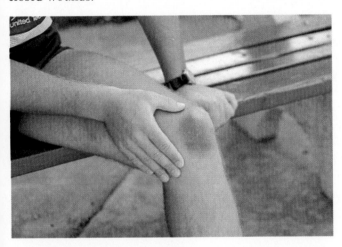

Figure 6-1. The closed wound changes from blue to red to green and then to yellow before resuming its normal color. If swelling or a mass of blood forms, a pressure bandage may be needed to help control the bleeding and reduce the swelling.

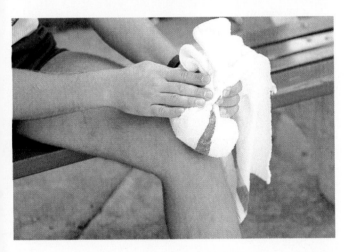

Figure 6-2. Ice is sometimes helpful to reduce pain and prevent swelling.

Be aware of the location of the important body parts beneath each area of the skin. A closed injury to some areas will cause serious injury to underlying tissue. Always suspect injury to underlying organs and treat the patient if any doubt exists by making the patient as comfortable as possible. Maintain an airway, keep the patient warm, and request whatever additional help is needed.

Many closed wounds involve fractures to bones. All fractures should be properly immobilized to prevent further injury to the surrounding tissue and to control bleeding. Immobilizing fractures (splinting) is discussed further in Chapter 7.

Open Wounds

There are several types of open wounds (Figure 6-3):

* Puncture
* Abrasion
* Incision
* Laceration
* Avulsion, including amputation

Puncture wounds are one of the most dangerous wounds inflicted on the body. A puncture wound may look harmless but one must consider the possibility of injury to underlying tissue. As the penetrating object enters the body, foreign material, bacteria, and dirt are often pushed deep into the body. Puncture wounds are made by any object causing an entrance or entrance and exit wound in the skin. Bullets, ice picks, and knives are examples of a few of the objects that most commonly cause puncture wounds.

Abrasion wounds are caused when the skin is forcefully rubbed across a hard surface. These wounds usually involve the most superficial layers of the skin. These wounds are sometimes referred to as "road rash." Their danger lies in the area of the skin involved. Since large areas of the skin are often removed, infection is always a danger when abrasions occur.

Incisions are smooth, clean wounds. They have a tendency to be deep since they are usually caused by a razor blade, knife, piece of glass, or even a sharp piece of metal.

Lacerations are jagged cuts in the skin caused by dull objects coming in forceful contact with the tissue. These types of wounds tend to bleed freely. Many lacerations occur in motor vehicle or industrial accidents.

Avulsions are pieces of tissue that have been cut away from the body. Whenever a piece of tissue is cut off the body or a flap is forcibly removed leaving a small portion still attached, it should always be saved and taken to the hospital with the patient even if completely severed (amputations) from the body. Sharp cutting objects, like lawn mowers, tend to avulse fingers if the hands are placed in the wrong area of the lawn mower.

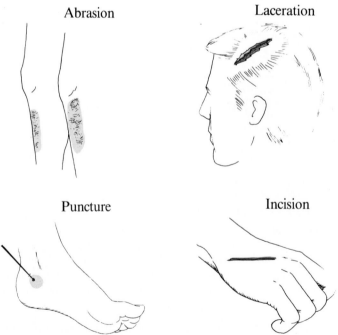

Figure 6-3. There are several types of open wounds. (From Arnheim, D.D.: Modern Principles of Athletic Training, 6e, St. Louis, 1985, The C.V. Mosby Co.)

Treatment of Open Wounds

As a First Responder, you must assure the patient that you are there to help. One important element in treating any patient is to assess the scene. Scene assessment is discussed in Chapter 1 and is also discussed in detail in Chapter 16. Care must always be taken to protect the injured as well as yourself from further harm. There are several steps involved in treating an open wound.

1. Control bleeding using:

   * Direct pressure - place a hand directly on the wound.

   * Pressure points - use one of the pressure points discussed later in this chapter in the arm, leg, or groin.

   * Elevation - raise the wound area higher than the heart if the injury will safely permit.

   * Tourniquets - use only as a last resort.

   * Pressure dressing - use the most sterile material available.

   The techniques to control bleeding are discussed in detail later in this chapter.

2. Have the patient remain still and reassure the patient.

3. Prevent further wound contamination by covering the area with a sterile dressing if available.

4. Immobilize any object penetrating the body.
   Impaled objects must be left in place until internal injuries can be evaluated properly in a medical facility. The impaled objects may have to be shortened, if necessary, to prevent further damage to the tissue from their weight or to allow the patient to be transported.

5. Save any avulsed parts. If any part is avulsed, or any body organ is protruding outside the body, special care must be taken. Wrap any avulsed portion in a moist sterile material and protect it with Saran wrap, or aluminum foil.
   Do not attempt to replace any protruding organs or body parts back into the body. This may add additional contamination inside the patient's body. Simply cover these organs with a very moist dressing like those discussed in the next section, Dressings and Bandages.

6. Splint all broken bones (refer to Chapter 7).

DRESSINGS AND BANDAGES

Any material placed directly on a wound is a dressing and should be sterile if possible. Any clean absorbent material can be used as a dressing. The dressing should cover the wound completely. If the dressing becomes saturated with blood or other fluids, add additional dressings to the original. Do not remove the original dressing. Never touch the area of the material to be laid against the wound.

Some examples of dressings are:

* Gauze pads

* Handkerchieves

* Sanitary napkins

* Large abdominal pads

* Towels

A bandage can be made of many types of material (e.g., strips of cloth, towels, adhesive tape) since it does not come in direct contact with the wound. It should maintain pressure on the wound and hold the compress in place.

If a bandage is to properly stay in place, body surfaces must be considered when anchoring and tying a bandage. Bandages must be tight enough to control bleeding but not impede circulation distal to the injury. Monitor the skin color, temperature, and pulses distal to the bandage site after any bandage has been applied. Body surfaces include:

❋ Round - the head

❋ Flat - the rib cage

❋ Tapered - the forearm

❋ Joint - the elbows

The examples listed are not all inclusive.

To properly anchor a bandage, a flap of the corner of the material must be held in place with the first wrap taken with the bandage (Figure 6-4). Flat areas such as the rib cage can be easily bandaged using circular turns. When bandaging the chest, care must be taken not to restrict breathing. Tapered areas seem to be most difficult to bandage. These areas include the arms, legs, and fingers (Figure 6-5). Joints require the use of figure "8" (Figure 6-6) bandages.

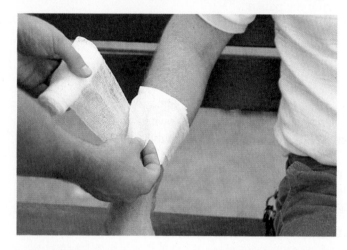

Figure 6-4. To properly anchor a bandage, a flap of the corner of the material must be held in place with the first wrap taken with the bandage.

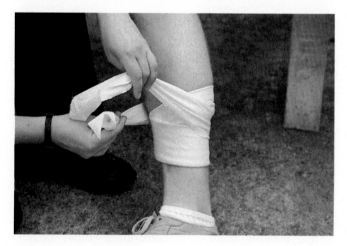

Figure 6-5. Tapered areas seem to be most difficult to bandage.

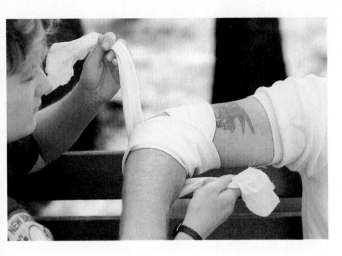

Figure 6-6. Joints require the use of figure "8" bandages.

INTERNAL BLEEDING

The signs and symptoms of internal bleeding are similar to those for shock. A few signs and symptoms of shock include:

* Cold clammy skin
* Rapid weak pulse
* Anxiety
* Thirst
* Weakness
* Nausea

Internal bleeding should be considered with any patient involved in a forceful accident or exhibiting any of the following signs or symptoms.

* Spitting or coughing up bright red or frothy blood (the discharge may be bubbly).
* Vomiting a dark maroon, foul smelling blood mass (coffee ground vomitus).
* Passage of either bright red or dark tarry stool (from bowels).
* Patient expresses pain.
* Tender, guarded abdomen, or other area of the body.
* Any patient with a penetrating wound, especially of the chest or abdomen.

The abdomen and chest areas can hold large amounts of internal blood loss. Bleeding in these areas is of great concern. The signs and symptoms of internal bleeding are the same as those for shock.

Most coughing up of frothy blood is caused by lung damage, while spitting of bright red blood usually involves bleeding in the mouth, nose, or esophagus. Coffee ground vomitus is present when bleeding occurs in the digestive system. This bleeding is usually old bleeding from the stomach or the upper portion of the small intestine. Bright red bleeding from the esophagus and stomach may be present from erosive ulcers of the blood vessels that line the esophagus.

Bright red bleeding from the rectum is usually caused by injury near the opening of the anus. Examples of this bleeding include:

* Cancer
* Inflammation of the colon
* Hemmorhoids
* Tears in the mucosa of the colon-rectum

Tarry stools normally denote old bleeding from further up the digestive system.

Internal bleeding can occur in an extremity. The involved area will swell rapidly. This swelling can usually be controlled with a pressure dressing and a splint. Elevation may help slow the bleeding until the clotting factors can take effect.

Little can be done by the First Responder to control internal bleeding. The prevention of shock must be started as soon as possible. The prevention and treatment for shock is discussed later in this chapter. Some of the steps to be taken include:

* Securing and maintaining the patient's airway

* Placing the patient in a comfortable position

* Giving nothing to eat or drink by mouth

* Keeping the patient comfortable

* Activating the EMS system

Allow the patient to find a comfortable position. However, the trauma patient may have to be stabilized in a less than comfortable position to protect them from further injury. Exercise care with the patient who may have a spinal injury. As a First Responder, you may sometimes become so caught up in the treatment that you may fail to recognize body position as a method of caring for the patient. Many patients with internal abdominal bleeding may control the bleeding by rolling up in a tight ball and applying pressure to their abdominal area.

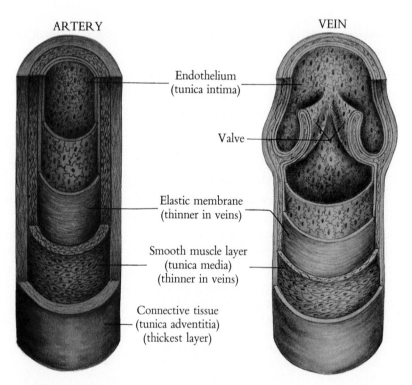

ARTERY VEIN

Endothelium
(tunica intima)

Valve

Elastic membrane
(thinner in veins)

Smooth muscle layer
(tunica media)
(thinner in veins)

Connective tissue
(tunica adventitia)
(thickest layer)

Figure 6-7. Arteries have three major linings and thicker walls than veins. (From Seidel, et al: Mosby's Guide to Physical Examination, St. Louis, 1987, The C.V. Mosby Co.)

EXTERNAL BLEEDING

There are several types of external bleeding:

✳ Arterial - bright red, spurting

✳ Capillary - red to blue in color and oozing

✳ Venous - dark red or bluish, steady flow

Arteries are the more protected vessels in the body. Arteries have three major linings and thicker walls than veins (Figure 6-7). The muscles within the walls of the artery will contract and attempt to control bleeding. If the artery is completely severed, the muscles will contract and seal off the opening. As a First Responder you may still have to control the blood loss.

Capillaries are to cells as alveoli are to lungs (Figure 6-8). These thin-walled vessels allow passage of food products and waste to and from the cell. Capillaries are so thin that they must depend on the clotting mechanism of the body to control their bleeding when injured.

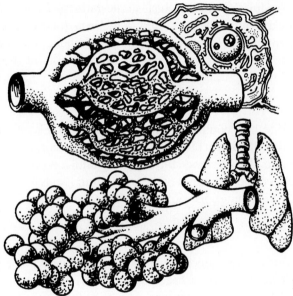

Figure 6-8. Capillaries are to cells as alveoli are to lungs.

Veins are less muscular and do not maintain the pressure of arteries but are thicker than capillaries. The wall thickness, muscles of the body, and a system of valves help them move blood back toward the heart. Veins are usually found closer to the body surface than arteries, and can be more easily compressed to control bleeding.

CONTROLLING BLEEDING (HEMORRHAGE)

Most bleeding can be controlled by applying direct pressure on the wounded area. Blood may take as long as 10 minutes to clot, so it is important to maintain the pressure for a sufficient amount of time. The following techniques will control most bleeding:

* ❋ Direct pressure - hand on wound
* ❋ Elevation - raise the injured part above the level of the heart
* ❋ Pressure points - apply digital pressure
* ❋ Splinting - keep injured parts still
* ❋ Tourniquet - when all else fails

Direct Pressure

A person may bleed to death in a very few seconds. Most bleeding can quickly be controlled with direct pressure. Place a hand on the site of the bleeding. A handkerchief, sterile gauze pads, or any other suitable material may be placed directly on the wound. Speed is important, *Do not* take time to find a sterile material if the bleeding is severe; use your hand (Figure 6-9). However, a bandage may be used to apply direct pressure to the wound and free your hands to execute other important care measures.

Elevation

Elevation of an injured extremity can be used to help control bleeding (Figure 6-10). Elevation quickly deprives distal areas of blood volume. This reduction in blood volume will help to control extremity bleeding. However, if a fracture is suspected, do not elevate the extremity until it is properly splinted. Elevation of the injured extremity should be above the level of the heart. Your hands may be used to splint an extremity if necessary or if a life-threatening condition exists. (Refer to Chapter 7 for detailed instructions on splinting.)

Pressure Points

If bleeding cannot be controlled using direct pressure in conjunction with elevation, especially when an extremity is involved, pressure on a strategic pressure point may be required. The primary pressure points are illustrated in Figure 6-11. There are many pressure points on the body; only two, the brachial and femoral, will be discussed in this chapter. Pressing the arterial walls against bone can diminish blood flow and allow the clotting process to control bleeding at the injury site. Many times direct pressure in conjunction with pressure points is required to control bleeding.

Tissue around a fracture site is usually damaged by the causative trauma. Early splinting of the fracture site and adjacent bone ends is one method to control bleeding (Figure 6-12). Soft tissue damage may be reduced if the splint is applied early.

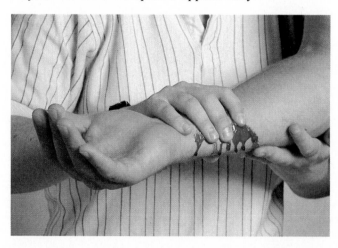

Figure 6-9. Direct pressure will control most bleeding.

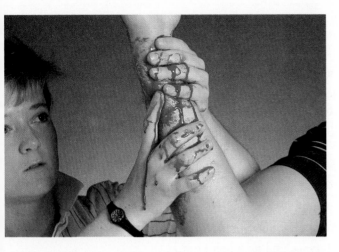

Figure 6-10. Elevation of an injured extremity can be used to help control bleeding.

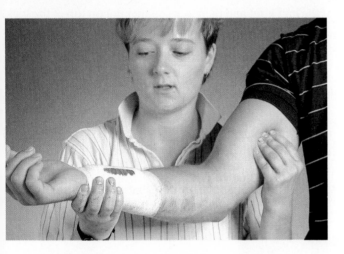

Figure 6-11. A primary pressure point.

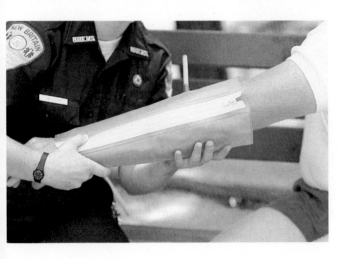

Figure 6-12. Pneumatic splints may be used to control bleeding.

Tourniquet

The tourniquet, which often causes nerve and blood vessel damage should be used to control bleeding only when all other measures fail.

NOTE: Remember the rule, Save a life but lose a limb.

A tourniquet is rarely needed. Most bleeding can be quickly and easily controlled during direct pressure, elevation, and pressure points. If a tourniquet must be used, tighten it until absolute control of bleeding is effective (Figure 6-13). Once in place, do not remove a tourniquet until the patient is in the hospital and under physician's care. When using a tourniquet, always remember the following guidelines:

* Use a thick, 3- to 4-inch wide bandage.
* Place the bandage as close to the wound as practical.
* The bandage should be placed between the injury and the patient's heart.
* Wrap the bandage around the limb twice and tie a half knot.
* Place a 6-inch stick (dowel) on top of the half knot and then tie a square knot on top of the stick.
* Twist the stick in circles until the bleeding stops. Be careful not to pinch any skin beneath the bandage.
* Tie the stick to hold it in place.
* Use lipstick, a felt tip pen, or any other source to write "TK" and the time on the injured patient's forehead.
* Never cover the area where bleeding is being controlled with a blanket or any other material that would prevent constant vision of the tourniquet and the injured area.

NOTE: Do not use the tourniquet unless all other methods to control bleeding fail. A tourniquet prevents circulation distal to the point of application — that distal portion of the limb may die.

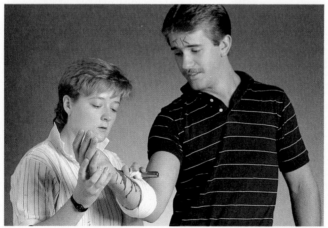

Figure 6-13. If a tourniquet must be used, tighten it until absolute control of bleeding is effective.

HYPOVOLEMIC SHOCK

Perfusion occurs when sufficiently oxygenated blood circulates through an organ of the body. Blood enters all organs through the arteries and is removed through the veins. Hypovolemic shock occurs when circulation and/or perfusion is reduced to the extent that major organs are adversely affected, and the volume of blood is insufficient to support the function of the involved cell. Though many types of shock are discussed, all relate to reduction of perfusion in specific areas of the body. An example of this is psychogenic shock. Psychogenic shock is simple fainting, which occurs when insufficient blood flow to the brain fails to provide enough oxygen to support consciousness.

The body has an elaborate protection system to ensure all major organs of adequate blood supply. The skeletal and digestive systems are the first organs to reduce function when circulation is reduced. There is an insufficient amount of blood to fill all the transport tubes in the body. Blood is then selectively shunted to organs of need. The 4 organs most protected by the body's elaborate blood flow control system are the kidneys, lungs, heart, and brain. We will usually recognize shock when the heart rate is fast or the patient exhibits one of the neurological signs. When the patient appears anxious, the brain may have been significantly deprived of blood flow.

Shock occurs when one or more of the following conditions exists:

* The heart fails to pump enough blood.
* Blood or fluid loss cause an insufficient amount of blood to be circulated.
* Blood vessels become too large for the patient's blood volume.
* A respiratory deficiency causes a reduction of circulating oxygen in the blood.

Anxiety is one of the earliest signs of shock. Restlessness may occur even before pulse or blood pressure changes. Every sick or injured person should be treated to prevent shock before any of the early signs or symptoms are detectable to you.

The following are the signs and symptoms of shock:

* Restlessness or anxiety
* Rapid weak pulse (thready)
* Profuse perspiration (diaphoresis)
* Cold, clammy skin
* Cyanosis or slow capillary filling time
* Pupils dilated; may just appear dull
* Thirst
* Shallow or irregular breathing
* Nausea and vomiting
* Unconsciousness

One method to evaluate the effectiveness of circulating blood is to use a blanch test (Figure 6-14). Here is the procedure for the blanch test:

❋ Gently pinch the patient's fingernail between your thumb and forefinger.

❋ Release this pinch quickly.

❋ Count "one-thousand one, one-thousand two."

If the fingernail of the patient has not returned to the normal pink color in two seconds, circulation is reduced.

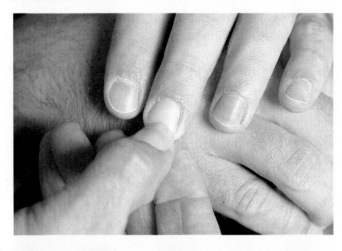

Figure 6-14a. Gently pinch the patient's fingernail between your thumb and forefinger.

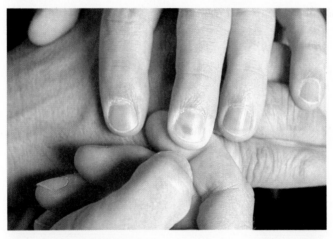

Figure 6-14b. Release this pinch quickly.

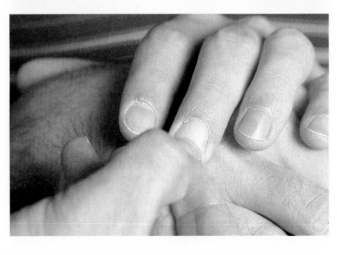

Figure 6-14c. Count, "one-thousand one, one-thousand two." If the patient's fingernail has not returned to its normal pink color in two seconds, circulation has been reduced.

Shock accompanies most traumatic incidents and must be treated as early as practical. Prevention of shock may not be possible, for example, in injuries involving massive internal bleeding. Even so, stabilizing the patient and treating for shock may slow the progression and help the patient to survive. Preventing shock is caring for the whole patient in an efficient, effective, and professional manner.

Follow these steps to care for shock:

✳ Secure and maintain an open airway.

✳ Protect the cervical spine.

✳ Restore breathing and circulation if needed.

✳ Control bleeding

✳ Position the patient properly:
  Place the patient supine if possible, and raise the patient's lower extremities if injuries do not prevent the movement of the extremities.

✳ Avoid rough handling of the patient.

✳ Prevent the loss of body heat.

✳ Splint fractures as needed.

✳ Do not give the patient anything to eat or drink.

✳ Administer oxygen if available (see Appendix A).

✳ Arrange for transportation by EMSS to a medical facility.

Prevention of shock cannot be over emphasized, since shock may quickly cause death. Organs are rapidly destroyed when harmful waste products increase in the cells and this waste cannot be removed by the circulatory system. Early detection is the key since shock, if untreated, may reach a point where it cannot be reversed. When this point is reached, the patient cannot be saved.

Pulses

One of the more effective methods to evaluate the circulatory system without adjunctive equipment is to use various pulses to estimate blood pressure.

As described in Chapter 3, the heart is a two-stage pump, with one side supplying blood to the lungs, and the other supplying blood to the rest of the body. With each contraction (systole) of the ventricles, a pulse can be felt throughout the body. Pulse palpitation is an effective tool to measure adequacy of circulation.

The carotid pulse may be one of the more reliable pulses since it is the last to be felt as systolic pressure falls. A patient must have a systolic pressure of approximately 60 mmHg for a carotid pulse to be felt. It is usually not covered with clothing and is one of the easiest pulses to locate. The pulse is found by sliding the fingers laterally into the groove between the trachea (windpipe) and the muscle at the side of the neck (Figure 6-15). Do not feel for both carotid pulses at the same, since you may close off a major portion of the blood supply to the brain.

Another very reliable pulse is the femoral. The femoral pulse is found on the anterior side of the leg, in the groin (Figure 6-16). This pulse may be a little harder to locate because of clothing. The patient requires a systolic pressure of approximately 70 mmHg for this pulse to be palpable. It can often be found quickly and effectively on children.

In infants and small children, the brachial pulse is the pulse of choice. This pulse is often preferred since the carotid may be hard to palpate due to the child's short, fat, flexible neck. The brachial artery is located on the inside of the upper arm (humerus), midway between the elbow and the shoulder (Figure 6-17).

A generally accessible, and most frequently used pulse is the radial. The radial pulse is located in the wrist proximal to the thumb. It is felt when the radial artery is pressed against the radius. The radius is the bone of the forearm ending at the thumb side of the wrist (Figure 6-18). However, unless the patient has a systolic pressure of approximately 80 mmHg, the radial pulse may not be palpable.

Approximate minimum systolic pressures for an adult are:

* Carotid — 60 mmHg
* Femoral — 70 mmHg
* Radial — 80 mmHg

When taking a patient's pulse, remember you have a pulse in your thumb. Be sure to locate all pulses using the tips of your fingers. Take a pulse every few minutes until the patient arrives at the medical facility, since the pulse is one of the better measures of the circulatory system.

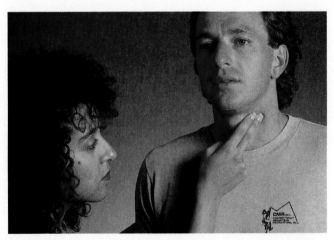

Figure 6-15. The carotid pulse is found by sliding the fingers laterally into the groove between the trachea (windpipe) and the muscle at the side of the neck.

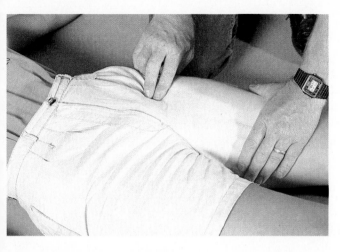

Figure 6-16. The femoral pulse is found on the anterior side of the leg, in the groin.

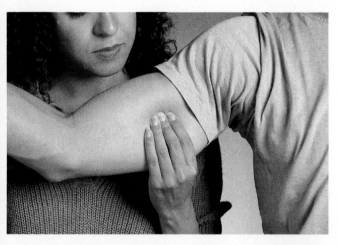

Figure 6-17. The brachial pulse is located on the medial side of the upper arm (humerus), midway between the elbow and shoulder.

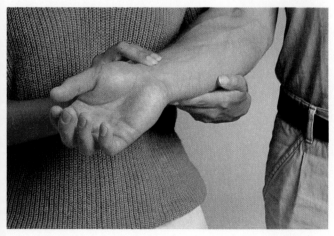

Figure 6-18. The radial pulse is located in the wrist proximal to the thumb.

ANAPHYLACTIC SHOCK

One specialty area of shock may need further explanation since additional treatment is required. Anaphylactic shock is an acute allergic reaction that can progress rapidly into death for the patient. One of the more common causes is the bee sting, although ant bites, ingestion of shellfish, and medications, like penicillin, can cause anaphylactic shock. Any allergic response causing the body to release large amounts of histamine may trigger anaphylactic shock.

The following are signs and symptoms of anaphylaxis:

* Hives, rashes, or redness around the mouth
* Swelling about the face
* Swelling of the tongue or mouth, which may close the airway
* Tightness in the throat
* Difficulty breathing - shortness of breath
* Sneezing, wheezing, or coughing
* Tightness in the chest
* Itching
* Abdominal cramps
* Rapid pulse
* Low blood pressure
* Apprehension
* Unconsciousness

One, all, or any of these signs and symptoms may occur after (Figure 6-19) contact with the allergic substance causing anaphylaxis. A good patient history surrounding the incident and a medical history will help you recognize anaphylactic reactions.

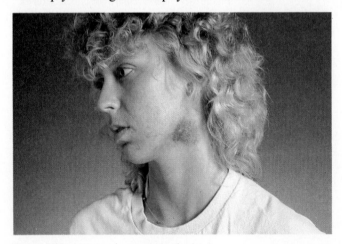

Figure 6-19. A person in anaphylactic shock.

The patient must be rapidly treated. Some highly allergic persons carry epinephrine or a chewable antihistamine with them at all times. Anaphylactic death can occur rapidly without antihistamic treatment. In general these patients have had serious reactions in the past. Local medical protocols must be followed when providing care for this patient. You can assist the patient take an epinephrine injection if the patient is conscious. Do not give the unconscious patient anything to chew or swallow. Immediate transportation to a medical facility is required. Activate the EMS system as early as possible for transportation and treatment.

Care for anaphylactic reactions include:

✳ Establishing an airway; oxygen should be administered, if available, in as high a concentration as the patient can tolerate. (Refer to Appendix A.)

✳ Checking diagnostic signs; take a blood pressure if the equipment is available. Follow other local protocols.

✳ Removing the stinger if possible but do not cause further injury to the wound site. If the sting site is on an extremity apply a proximal constricting band. Do not seal off the pulses distal to the bite site. Ice may be applied but not directly to the skin. The ice may be wrapped in a towel or other suitable material to protect the patient's skin from further injury.

✳ Arranging for immediate transportation to a medical facility, or when the EMS system provides advanced life support, assure they are contacted early for definitive treatment and transportation.

SUMMARY

External hemorrhage must be rapidly controlled since it is an important factor care in shock. Most bleeding can be controlled using direct pressure. If direct pressure does not effectively control bleeding, use elevation, pressure points, or a tourniquet. Bandaging is a simple process to help apply direct pressure, control bleeding, assist in the clotting process, and prevent contamination of an open wound.

Shock treatment is one of the major responsibilities of the First Responder. Whatever the cause, shock will result in an inadequate blood flow to important areas of the body. Assuring sufficient flows to the brain, heart, lungs, and kidneys is a primary responsibility of the First Responder.

Anaphylactic shock occurs as a generalized reaction in persons sensitive to certain allergens. When anaphylaxis occurs rapid intervention is needed to preserve life.

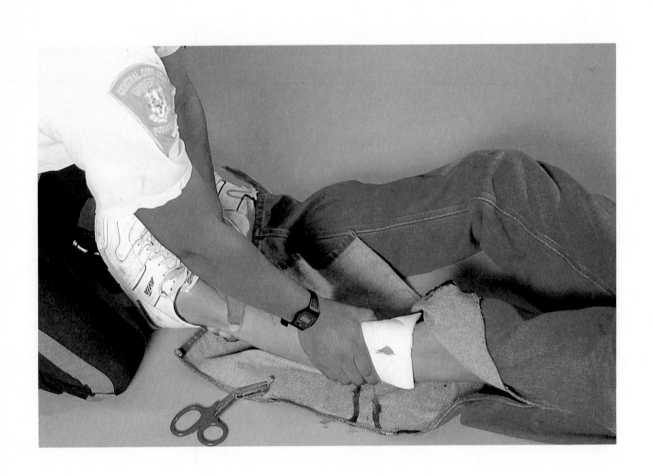

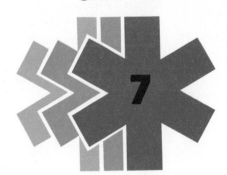

INJURIES TO BONES, JOINTS AND MUSCLES

KEY CONCEPTS AND SKILLS

By the end of this chapter, you will be able to:

❋ Define the function of the musculoskeletal system.

❋ Identify the three kinds of injuries to muscles, joints, and bones, and the mechanisms of each.

❋ Define and identify the two types of fractures — open and closed.

❋ List the signs and symptoms of strains, sprains, dislocations, and fractures.

❋ State the primary reasons and general rules for splinting.

❋ State the reasons for splinting.

❋ State what is done and why assessment procedures are performed on extremity injuries.

❋ Perform an assessment to discover injuries to bones, joints, and muscles.

❋ Identify and describe appropriate care for injuries to bones, joints, and muscles.

KEY WORDS

Adduction – The movement of a limb toward the center of the body.

Air Splint – A plastic inflatable splint used to immobilize a fractured limb.

Amputation – The complete cutting or tearing off of the extremities or limbs.

Angulated – Cornered or angled.

Bone – The dense, hard connective tissue that makes up a human skeleton. There are 206 bones in the human skeleton.

Crepitation – A sound that resembles the crackling noise heard when bone fragments rub together.

Dislocation – Displacement or disarrangement of bone ends from their junction.

Ecchymosis – Discoloration of an area of the skin or mucus membrane due to bleeding into the tissues. The color is blue-black and changes to brown or yellow in several days (bruising).

Fixation Splint – A device that immobilizes a fracture. An example is a board splint used to immobilize a fracture of the lower arm.

Fracture – A break in a bone structure either open or closed.

Joints – Any one of the junctions of the bones. Each type of joint is classified according to structure and how it moves. Joints may include more than two bone ends.

Muscle – A kind of tissue made up of fibers that contract, and shorten, causing and allowing the movement of the structures and organs of the body.

Paralysis – An abnormal condition characterized by the loss of muscle function or the loss of sensation or both, often caused by injury or disease to the nervous system.

Sprain – An injury to the tendons, muscles, or ligaments around a joint, characterized by pain or swelling or discoloration of the skin over the joint.

Strain – An injury caused by overexertion or stretching of a muscle.

Traction Splint – A device used to exert and maintain pull and stabilization.

FUNCTIONS OF THE BONES, JOINTS AND, MUSCLES

Bones, joints and muscles provide the body with a system of support, protection, and allow movement.

Bones serve as a mineral reservoir for calcium and phosphorous. Blood cell formation takes place in the red marrow of the body's major bony structures, e.g., the thigh bone (femur).

The skeleton is a supportive and protective structure composed of 206 bones (Figure 7-1). Some bones encase and protect organs, e.g., the thoracic cage shields the heart and lungs.

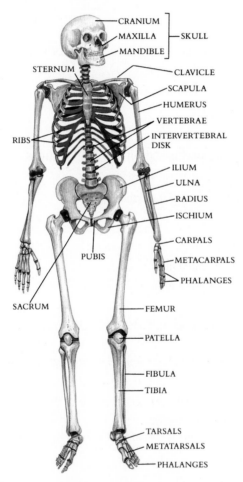

Figure 7-1. The skeleton. (From Raven, P.H. and Johnson, G.B.: Biology, St. Louis, 1986, The C.V. Mosby Co.)

Joints are generally divided into three groups. One group is made up of "hinge-like structures" that allow bones to move in relation to one another. An example of this type of joint is the knee (Figure 7-2). Another group is the "ball-in-socket" found in the shoulder allowing a wide range of motion in more than one place. Other joints, known as immovable joints, like the ones in the skull do not permit any movement, but join parts of the cranium together.

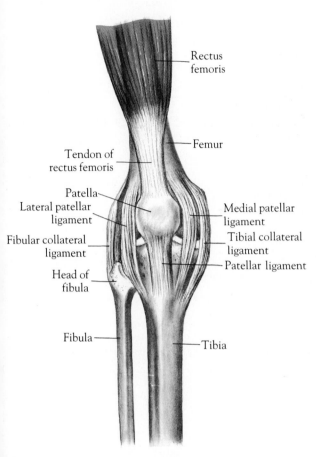

Figure 7-2: The knee joint. (From Seidel, H.M., et al: Mosby's Guide to Physical Examination, St. Louis, 1987, The C.V. Mosby Co.)

Muscles which are classified as voluntary and involuntary, provide for movement of the organs or parts of the body. In fact, all movement of any part of the body is accomplished by muscles. Although some minor control may be exercised over involuntary muscles, these muscles are not subject to conscious control. Examples are muscles that make up the heart and intestines (Figure 7-3). Voluntary muscles are subject to conscious control. Examples are the muscles found in the legs and arms (Figure 7-4).

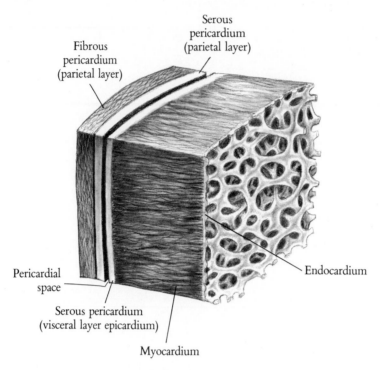

Figure 7-3: An example of involuntary muscles. (From Seidel, H.M., et al: Mosby's Guide to Physical Examination, St. Louis, 1987, The C.V. Mosby Co.)

ANTERIOR

POSTERIOR

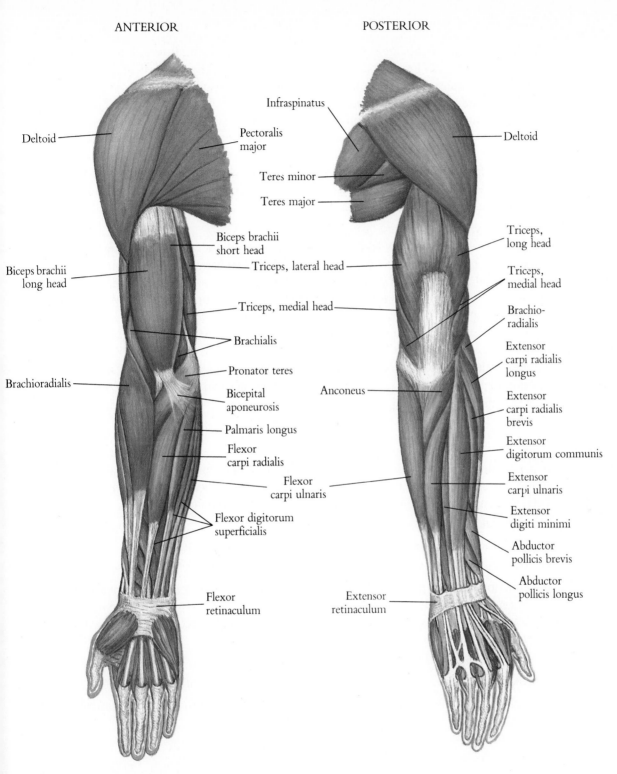

Deltoid

Infraspinatus

Pectoralis
major

Deltoid

Teres minor

Teres major

Biceps brachii
short head

Triceps,
long head

Biceps brachii
long head

Triceps, lateral head

Triceps,
medial head

Brachio-
radialis

Triceps, medial head

Extensor
carpi radialis
longus

Brachialis

Pronator teres

Brachioradialis

Anconeus

Bicepital
aponeurosis

Extensor
carpi radialis
brevis

Palmaris longus

Flexor
carpi radialis

Extensor
digitorum communis

Flexor
carpi ulnaris

Extensor
carpi ulnaris

Flexor digitorum
superficialis

Extensor
digiti minimi

Abductor
pollicis brevis

Flexor
retinaculum

Extensor
retinaculum

Abductor
pollicis longus

Figure 7-4. An example of voluntary muscles. (From Seidel, H.M., et
al: Mosby's Guide to Physical Examination, St. Louis, 1987, The C.V.
Mosby Co.)

MECHANISMS OF INJURY

Muscles, joints, and bones are subject to injury due to their form, function, and structure.

Muscles can only exert limited pull, stretch, or lifting force. When the task attempted exceeds the muscle's ability, strains, sprains, or more serious injury may result.

Joints have similar limits. Only a particular range of motion is allowed. When a joint is forced to move in a direction that is physically impossible, the surrounding involved tissues will suffer injury. This injury may be a sprain, dislocation, or even a combination of the two, in addition to bone damage.

Bones have limited ability to withstand excessive stresses of bending, twisting, or pressure. When these stresses exceed the capability of the bone, the bone fractures in a number of ways.

TYPES OF BONE INJURIES

Injuries to the extremities involving muscles, joints, and bones rarely present the First Responder with life-threatening conditions. These injuries may look bad because of distortion of the body parts or bleeding, and often are given more attention than deserved — at least at the immediate moment. Only a few fractures represent a threat to life, such as pelvic fracture where massive bleeding may occur as a result of injury to the major blood vessels.

Injuries to the extremities must take second place to life-threatening or potentially life-threatening conditions assessed by the First Responder during the primary survey. If severe bleeding from a fracture is present, it should be observed by the First Responder during the first several seconds of primary survey and treated right away, assuming the ABC's have been attended to first. Look at the mechanism of the injuries to muscles, joints, and bones. Remember the "C" in ABC stands for both circulation and bleeding control in managing the trauma patient.

Strains

A strain, sometimes called a pulled muscle, is the result of overstretching a particular muscle (or a group of muscles). Bending improperly and attempting to lift heavy objects may cause a strained muscle. Swelling, rupturing, and tearing of the muscle may also occur.

The signs and symptoms of strain are:

✳ Tenderness - Ask the patient if the affected area feels tender to touch.

✳ Swelling - Look at the area; feel it gently. The swelling occurs because of internal bleeding.

✳ Function - Ask the patient if there is a loss of function to the area, but do not ask the patient to try any physical activity to bring on this symptom. If rupture to the muscle has occurred, no function will be possible. Stiffness and black-and-blue marks (ecchymosis or ecchymoses) usually occur several hours later.

The emergency care for strain is as follows:

✳ Keep the patient still, avoiding movement that involves the affected area.

✳ Apply ice wrapped in a cloth or cold compress to the area to help reduce swelling and pain (Figure 7-5).

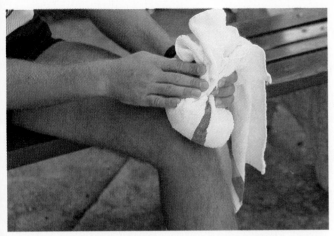

Figure 7-5. Apply ice wrapped in a cloth or cold compress.

Sprains

Most sprains are produced by overextension of a joint, causing a partial tearing of the ligaments (Figure 7-6). Sprains usually swell early following the trauma.

The signs and symptoms of a sprain are:

✳ Pain in the affected area - Ask the patient where it hurts.

✳ Possible inability to use the affected joint. Most sprained joints can still function, but use is painful. Ask the patient if movement is possible.

NOTE: An injury severe enough to cause a sprain may also involve damage to surrounding bones. Be careful about manipulating the joint. In severe sprains that involve tearing and rupturing of the joint parts, functional use may be impossible. In these instances, the joint usually appears very swollen and distorted.

✳ Swelling - Look for puffiness and a swollen area.

✳ Discoloration resulting from bleeding and other tissue damage is a sign that usually appears after several hours or the following day.

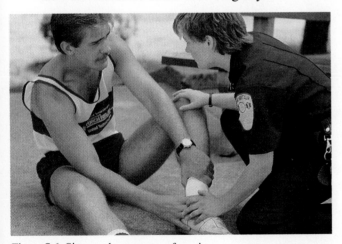

Figure 7-6. Signs and symptoms of sprains.

The emergency care for a sprain is as follows:

✳ Treat the sprain as if it were a fracture and immobilize the sprained area. The wrist may be stabilized in an air splint, a board splint, or with a pillow (Figure 7-7a).

✳ For an ankle sprain, a pillow or blanket may be placed around the foot and ankle (Figure 7-7b).

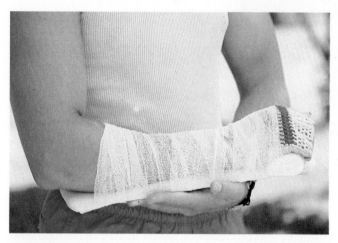

Figure 7-7a. Stabilization of the wrist.

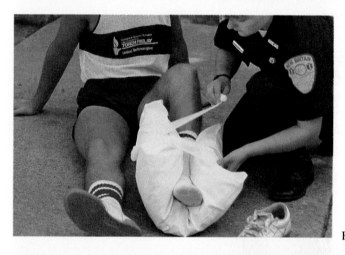

Figure 7-7b. Stabilization of the ankle.

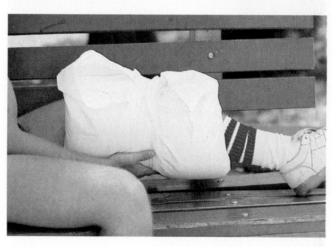

Figure 7-7c. Immobilizing the knee using a pillow.

✳ The knee may be immobilized by a pillow (Figure 7-7c), an inflatable full leg splint (Figure 7-7d), or a long padded board (Figure 7-7e).

✳ To immobilize the shoulder, a sling and swathe may be used (Figure 7-7f).

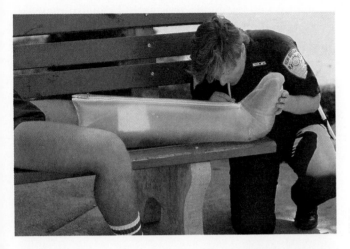

Figure 7-7d. Immobilizing the knee using an inflatable full leg splint.

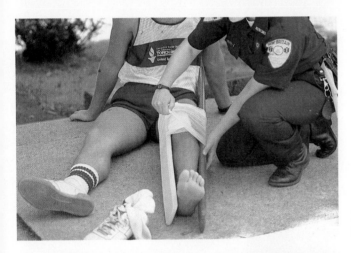

Figure 7-7e. Immobilizing the knee using a long padded board.

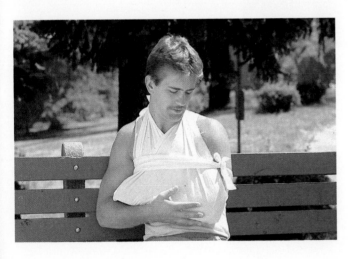

Figure 7-7f. Immobilizing the shoulder using a sling and swathe.

✳ Elevate the sprained part, if possible, to reduce any swelling (Figure 7-8).

✳ Apply ice wrapped in a cloth or a cold compress to help reduce any swelling and reduce pain (Figure 7-9).

   CAUTION: *DO NOT* straighten the joint if you encounter resistance. Doing so may cause severe injury to nerves, blood vessels, and other structures in the joint area.

✳ Keep the patient still by avoiding movement or use of the injured joint.

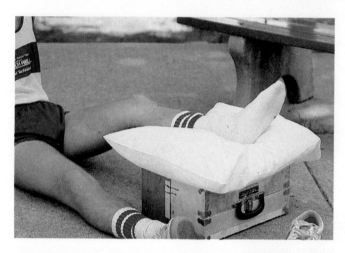

Figure 7-8. Elevate the sprained part to reduce any swelling.

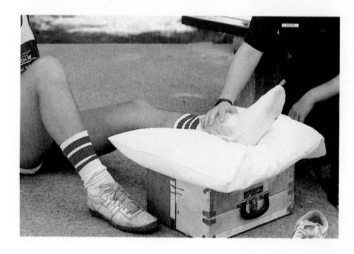

Figure 7-9. Apply ice wrapped in a cloth or cold compress to help reduce swelling.

Dislocations

Dislocations are similar to fractures. Occasionally, fractures occur because the bones around the joint were broken by the stress applied when the joint was dislocated (Figure 7-10). A dislocation injury is usually a result of a severe force that has torn the ligaments around the joint (Figure 7-11). Other dislocations may occur as a result of birth defects or arthritic conditions.

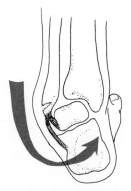

Figure 7-10. Fracture caused by stress on dislocated joint. (From Arnheim, D.D.: Modern Principles of Athletic Training, St. Louis, 1985, The C.V. Mosby Co.)

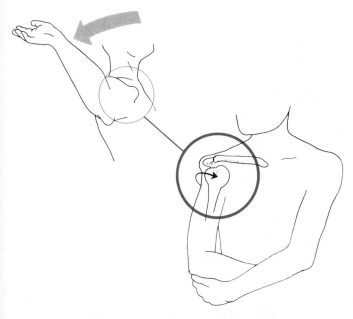

Figure 7-11. Severe force causes torn ligaments around joint. (From Arnheim, D.D.: Modern Principles of Athletic Training, St. Louis, 1985, The C.V. Mosby Co.)

The signs and symptoms of a dislocation are:

❋ The joint looks longer - Examine the area, see if the bony structures are in their normal anatomical position (Figure 7-12).

❋ Pain - Pain is usually severe. Ask if the patient is in pain.

❋ Swelling - Swelling occurs quite rapidly (within 15-20 minutes). Look at the injured area.

❋ Discoloration - The area involved quickly turns a bluish color due to blood leaking into the surrounding tissue.

❋ Function - Usually the joint is immovable and the patient cannot attempt motion. Ask the patient how the injured area felt when motion was attempted. The joint may also be "locked," i.e., the patient is unable to move at all. If this is the case, *do not* attempt to straighten the injured extremity.

❋ Neurovascular damage - There may be damage to both nerves and blood vessels. Check for sensation and pulse *at a point distal* from the injury (Figure 7-13a). Ask the patient if the touch of your hand below the involved area can be felt (Figure 7-13b). If there is no pulse or sensation, the condition is serious and requires prompt attention at a medical facility.

The emergency care for a dislocation is as follows:

❋ Treat a dislocation as if it were a fracture.

❋ Protect and stabilize the dislocated area with as little manipulation as possible. Use a sling and swathe, pillows, blankets, or similar materials (Figure 7-14).

❋ After stabilizing the dislocation, recheck the sensation and pulse of the affected area. Note any changes and advise the EMS unit.

❋ Do not attempt to relocate the joint. You may cause serious damage.

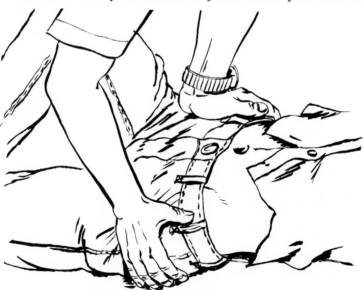

Figure 7-12. Check to see if bony structures are in their normal anatomical position.

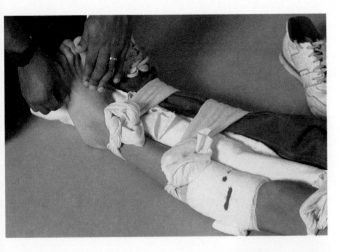

Figure 7-13a. Check for pulse and sensation a point distal from the injury.

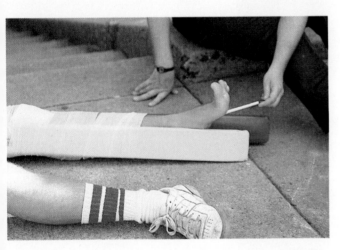

Figure 7-13b. Ask the patient if the touch of your hand can be felt below the involved area.

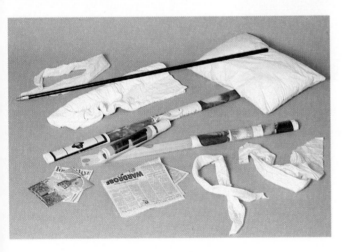

Figure 7-14. Some examples of materials which may be used as splints.

Fractures

A fracture is a break in a bone. This injury results from the stresses of physical forces that are too great for the bone to withstand. When the knee hits the dashboard of a motor vehicle during an accident, excessive force is applied to the thigh and may cause the bone to fracture (Figure 7-15). Similarly, a heavy object dropped on the forearm may cause the bone to fracture (Figure 7-16).

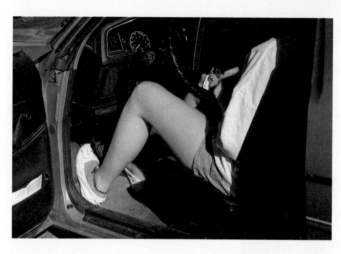

Figure 7-15. Deceleration injury to the thigh.

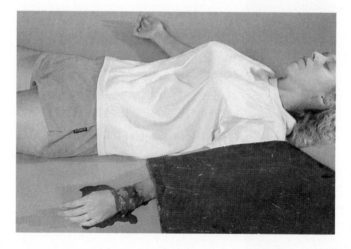

Figure 7-16. A crush injury to the forearm.

As noted earlier, most fractures rarely present a life-threatening situation. Some fractures involving the spinal column can be life-threatening. See Chapter 8 for a complete discussion of spinal injuries. Some fractures, though, together with other injuries, can cause permanent disability. Early recognition and care, after attending to primary life support needs, may well reduce the possibility of long-term disability and hasten healing.

Fractures for classification purposes are either closed or open. A closed fracture is often easier to treat, because the skin over the fracture is unbroken (Figure 7-17a). In this case, there is no direct contact with the outside environment. An open fracture has an open wound at or near the fracture site (Figure 7-17b). The opening may be caused by any number of mechanisms of injury, e.g., sharp bone ends, a bullet, or a piece of pipe penetrating the skin.

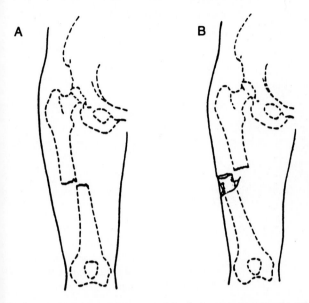

Figure 7-17. A closed fracture (A) is easier to treat because the skin over the fracture is unbroken. An open fracture (B) has an open wound at or near the fracture site. (From Sorrentino, S.A.: Mosby's Textbook for Nursing Assistants, 2nd edition, St. Louis, 1987, The C.V. Mosby Co.)

Certain injuries to the arms and legs and their adjoining structures are considered life-threatening because of the following associated factors:

❋ Massive, open fractures with many lacerations and foreign materials that have entered the wound (Figure 7-18).

❋ Fracture of both femurs because of blood loss, either open or closed (Figure 7-19).

❋ Crushing injuries to the abdomen and pelvis; pelvic fractures (Figure 7-20).

❋ Injuries to the blood vessels in the knee or elbow areas (Figure 7-21).

❋ Amputations to the arm or leg (Figure 7-22).

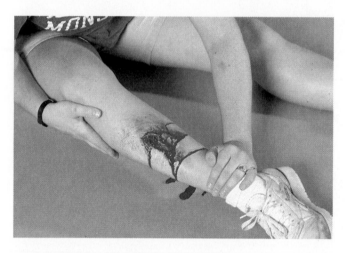

Figure 7-18. Massive, open fractures with many lacerations and foreign materials which have entered the wound are considered life-threatening.

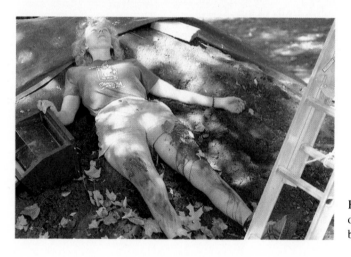

Figure 7-19. Fractures of both femurs, either open or closed, are considered life-threatening because of blood loss.

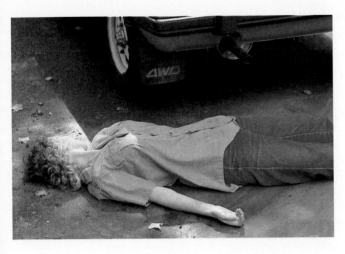

Figure 7-20. Injuries which crush the abdomen or pelvis are considered life-threatening.

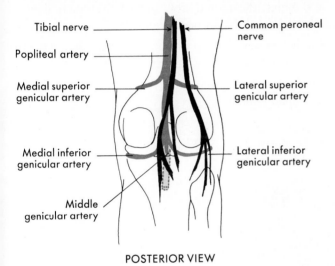

POSTERIOR VIEW

Figure 7-21. Injuries to the blood vessels in the knee or elbow areas are life-threatening. (From Arnehim, D.D.: Modern Principles of Athletic Training, St. Louis, 1985, The C.V. Mosby Co.)

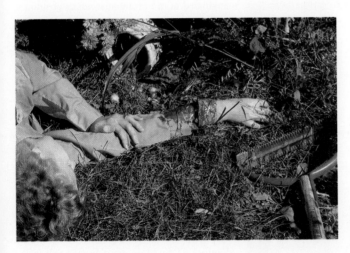

Figure 7-22. Amputations of the arm or leg are considered life-threatening.

The signs and symptoms of a fracture are:

❋ Deformity - The extremity is shortened and angulated in its normal anatomical position (Figure 7-23).

❋ Swelling, discoloration, bruising - Observe the limb (Figure 7-24).

❋ Spasms - Check to see whether any muscles are twitching.

❋ Wounds - Check to see whether the fracture is open. Also, look for surrounding tissue injuries (Figure 7-25).

❋ Circulation - Feel for a pulse in the extremity; perform a capillary blanch test by squeezing the nail bed of the fingers or toes. If the nail bed does not turn pink quickly, circulation is somehow impaired (Figure 7-26). A true emergency exists if pulses distal to the fracture site are absent. Record the time the absence was first noticed, immobilize the fracture, and arrange for immediate transfer of the patient to a medical facility.

❋ Crepitation - Feel for a grating sound upon movement, but feel *very gently*.

❋ Sensation - Gently pinch or otherwise stimulate the injured area, and ask the patient if it was felt. Lack of sensation indicates some neurological impairment (Figure 7-27).

❋ Function - See whether the patient can move the injured limb without difficulty. Do not ask the patient to move an obvious fracture. This action may cause further damage.

❋ Temperature - Feel the limb area to see whether it is warm or cold. A cold limb, in the absence of hypothermia, is a sign of circulatory impairment.

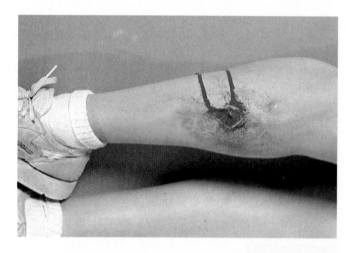

Figure 7-23. The extremity is shortened and angulated in its normal anatomical position.

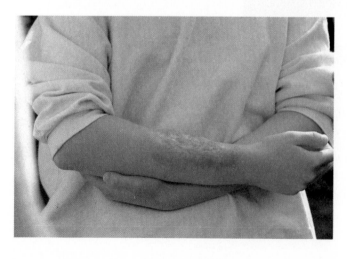

Figure 7-24. Swelling, discoloration or bruising are signs of a fracture.

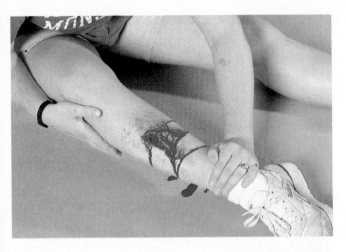

Figure 7-25. Check to see whether the fracture is open. Also check for surrounding tissue injuries.

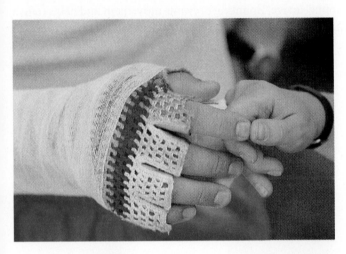

Figure 7-26. Squeeze the nail bed of the fingers or toes. If the nail bed does not turn pink quickly, circulation is somehow impaired.

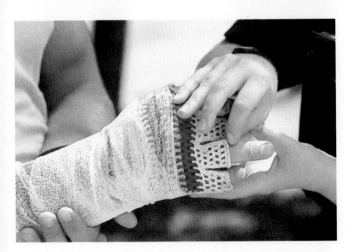

Figure 7-27. Lack of sensation indicates some neurological impairment.

One quick method of assessment for fracture is the 5 Ps. If any or all of the 5 Ps exist, a fracture is likely. The 5 Ps are:

1. *P*ain. Is there severe pain in the affected structure?

2. *P*uffiness. Is the affected area swollen?

3. *P*aralysis (full or partial). Is there a loss of sensation.

4. *P*allor. What is the color of the limb: normal, pale, cyanotic?

5. *P*ulslessness. Is there a distal pulse?

The emergency care for fractures is as follows:

Fractures should be immobilized and then splinted. Splinting prevents movement of the fractured bone or dislocated joint and prevents or reduces the possibility of further injury to the involved extremity. In addition, splinting reduces pain and usually assists in the control of bleeding.

Splinting by the First Responder should be considered *only* if the injured patient has to be moved or if there is a long delay before EMS personnel arrive. Splinting prevents movement and helps reduce the possibility of the broken bone ends damaging one another, or the blood vessels, nerves, or muscle.

The general rules for splinting are:

✳ Do not move the patient before splinting, unless absolutely necessary. The rule is, "Splint where they lie." In life-threatening conditions, the patient may have to be moved before splinting (Figure 7-28).

✳ Take a pulse and check for sensation below the fracture site before and after splinting (Figure 7-29).

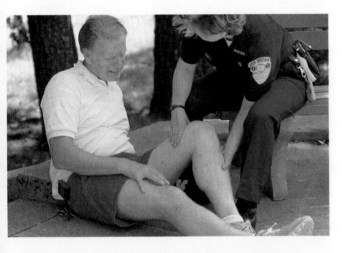

Figure 7-28. Do not move the patient before splinting, unless absolutely necessary.

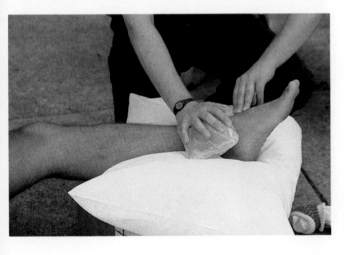

Figure 7-29. Take a pulse and check for sensation below the fracture site before and after splinting.

✳ Cut or remove clothing from the site. Always remove or cut away as much clothing as necessary to allow a viewing area around the suspected fracture site. Areas covered by clothing cannot be properly splinted (Figure 7-30).

✳ Treat for shock.

✳ Do not reposition protruding bones.

✳ If a dislocation is involved, splint it in the positon in which it is found.

✳ Gently align angulated fractures before splinting, if necessary. *Do not force the bones if any resistance is felt.*

✳ The neck may be gently straightened only if the airway is compromised (see Chapter 8 for a full discussion about the care of the spine).

✳ Pad each splint carefully. Padding material may be newspapers, trauma pads, towels, etc. 7-31).

✳ The splint must immobilize the bone ends as well as the joints above and below the fracture site (Figure 7-32).

Apply the splint as soon as practical, taking as much care as possible. Do not move the injured area any more than necessary.

REMEMBER: Always check the pulse and sensation distal to the fracture site before after splinting. Notify responding emergency personnel of the pulse and sensation.

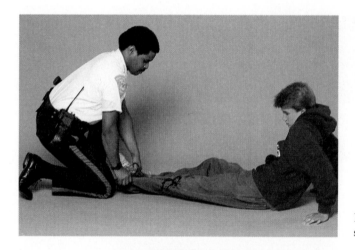

Figure 7-30. Cut or remove clothing from the site.

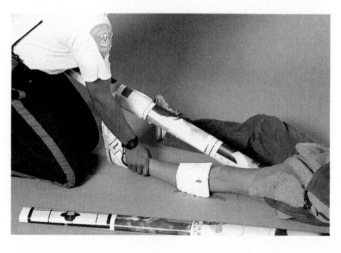

Figure 7-31. Pad each splint carefully.

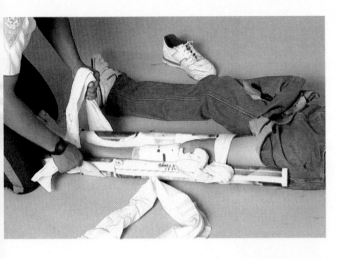

Figure 7-32. The splint must immobilize the bone ends as well as the joints above and below the fracture site.

Splinting material does not have to be fancy. The patient's clothing can be used for a sling and swathe (Figure 7-33). Makeshift items like a rolled newspaper, magazine, broom handle, shovel, or almost any lightweight, firm object can be used to immobilize a fractured bone (Figure 7-34).

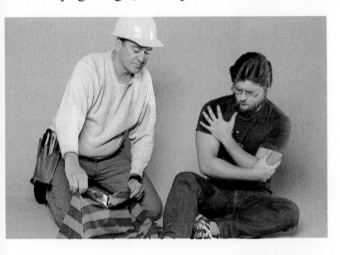

Figure 7-33. The patient's clothing may be used for a sling and swathe.

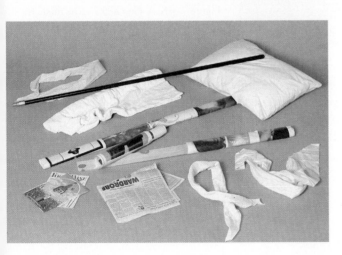

Figure 7-34. Makeshift items may be used to immobilize a fractured bone.

EMERGENCY CARE FOR UPPER EXTREMITY FRACTURES

The Collarbone

One of the most frequently fractured bones is the collarbone (clavicle) (Figure 7-35a). This injury occurs more often in children than in adults.

A sling and swathe made from a strong cloth or patient's shirt can usually be used to immobilize the injury until the patient reaches a medical facility (Figure 7-35b).

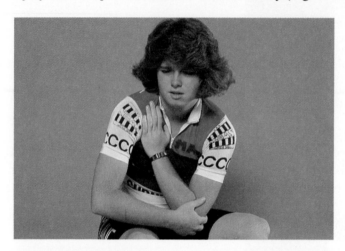

Figure 7-35a. One of the most frequently fractured bones is the clavicle (collarbone).

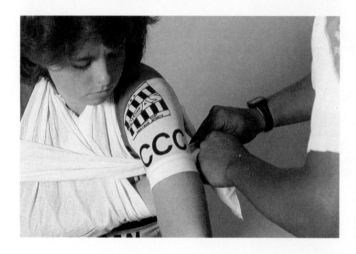

Figure 7-35b. A sling and swathe made from strong cloth or the patient's shirt can usually be used to immobilize the injury.

Do not underestimate this injury, since severe force may have also caused the fracture of the first rib. First rib fractures are extremely dangerous, because this rib protects the major arteries and veins in the upper chest. Additionally, any injury to the clavicle or above may have been forceful enough to have injured the cervical spine. The clavicle can move in towards the trachea and cause airway problems.

The Shoulder Blade

A fractured shoulder blade (scapula) is rare. It is treated exactly as the fracture of the collarbone. Most shoulder injuries involve either dislocation of the upper arm (humerus) from the socket or fracture-dislocation of the same area (Figure 7-36a). This joint allows a good range of motion. Most shoulder displacements, whether or not a fracture exists, allow gentle placement of the arm across the chest.

A sling and a swathe, or the patient's clothing, will adequately secure this injury. If the arm cannot be moved painlessly, it should be splinted in the position in which it was found (Figure 7-36b).

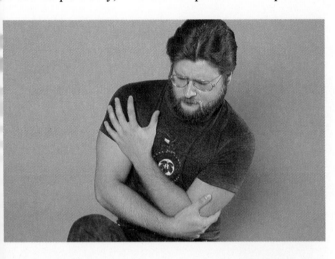

Figure 7-36a. Most shoulder injuries involve either dislocation of the upper arm from the socket or fracture-dislocation of the same area.

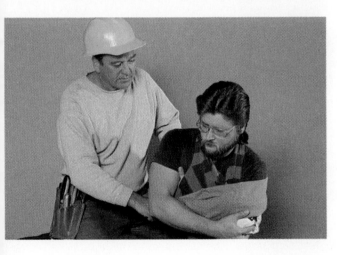

Figure 7-36b. If the arm cannot be moved painlessly, it should be splinted in the position in which it was found.

The Upper Arm (Humerus)

Immobilize the arm by splinting it to the body with a sling and swathe (Figure 7-37a). If the arm is unstable, other splints can be applied (Figure 7-37b).

If dislocation of the upper arm causes the arm to be locked above the body, place a pillow between the patient's arm and head and tie the arm to the head (Figure 7-38).

Occasionally, the affected arm is locked out and away from the body. In this case, secure the arm in

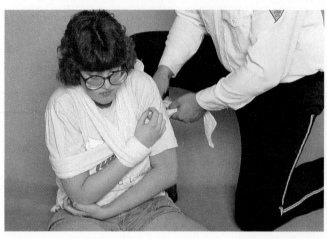

Figure 7-37a. Immobilize the arm by splinting it to the body with a sling and swathe.

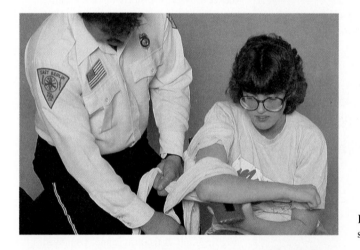

Figure 7-37b. If the arm is unstable, other splints can be applied.

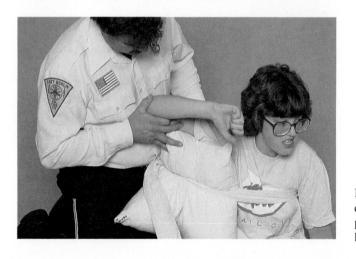

Figure 7-38. If dislocation of the upper arm causes the arm to be locked above the body, place a pillow between the patient's arm and head and tie the arm to the head.

place with a lightweight splint attached to the patient's body. This splint is to hold the arm in the position in which it was found (Figure 7-39).

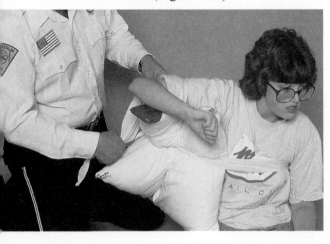

Figure 7-39. If the arm is locked out and away from the body, secure the arm in place with a lightweight splint attached to the patient's body.

The Elbow

Fractures that appear to involve the joint at the elbow should be splinted at the position in which it was found (Figures 7-40a and 7-40b).

Do not attempt to realign or adjust the elbow position if *any* resistance is present. The nerves and blood vessels to the hand are protected in this joint, and serious damage can be done by moving the fracture or dislocation.

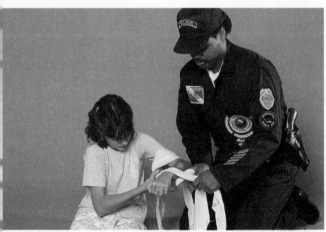

Figure 7-40. Fractures that appear to involve the joint at the elbow should be splinted at the position in which it was found (a) and immobilized (b).

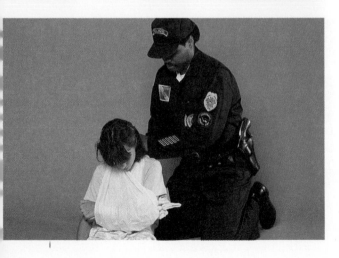

The Forearm

Fractures of the forearm (ulna and radius) may involve one or both bones. If the fracture is not near the wrist or elbow, gently realign the arm and splint it with a firm object, e.g., a board, magazine, newspaper, or a pillow (Figure 7-41a and 7-41b). To use an inflatable splint, perform the following steps:

✳ Select the proper size inflatable splint. The fingertips should be inside the splint (Figure 7-42a).

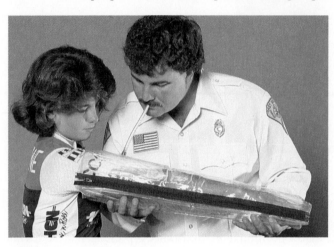

Figure 7-41. If the fracture is not near the wrist or elbow, gently realign the arm and splint it with either an air splint (a) or another firm object (b).

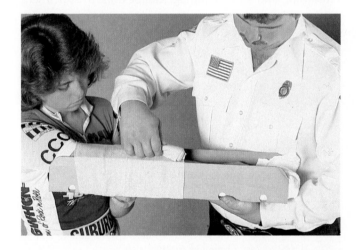

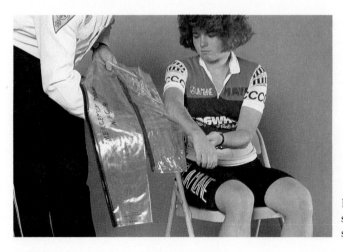

Figure 7-42a. Select the proper size inflatable splint. The fingertips should be inside the splint.

- Dress any open wounds with sterile dressings (Figure 7-42b).
- Remove or cut clothing away from the injured extremity. Remove rings, watches, bracelets, etc. (Figure 7-42c).
- Check the affected site before and after splinting for sensation and observe the color of the skin; if the splint is inflated to much circulation may be reduced.
- Apply the splint, unzipped and uninflated. Grasp the patient's hand while your partner or a bystander holds the limb gently in alignment (Figure 7-42d).

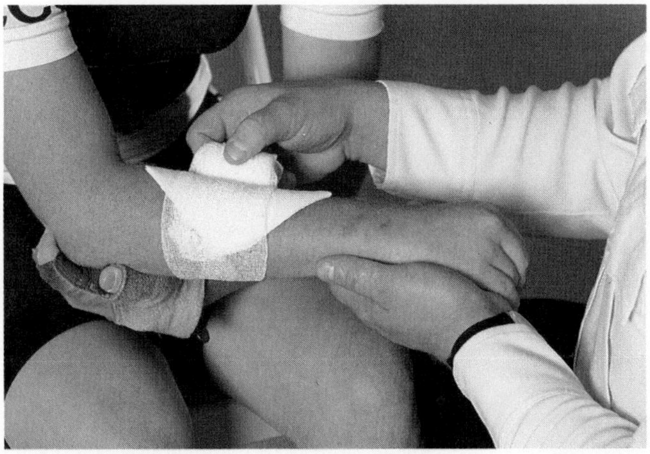

Figure 7-42b. Dress any open wounds with sterile dressings.

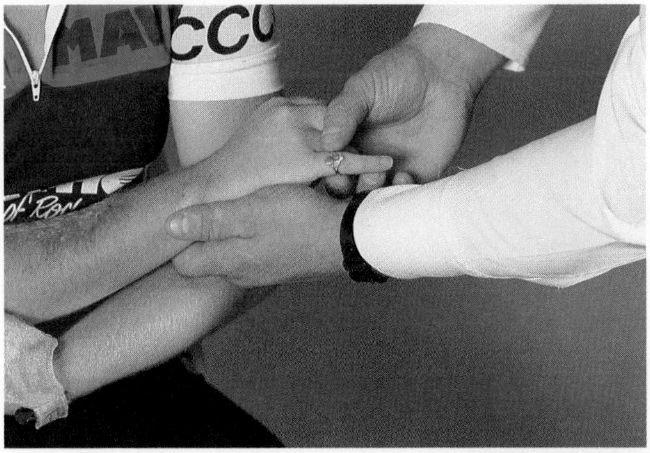

Figure 7-43c. Remove or cut clothing away from the injured extremity. Remove any jewelry.

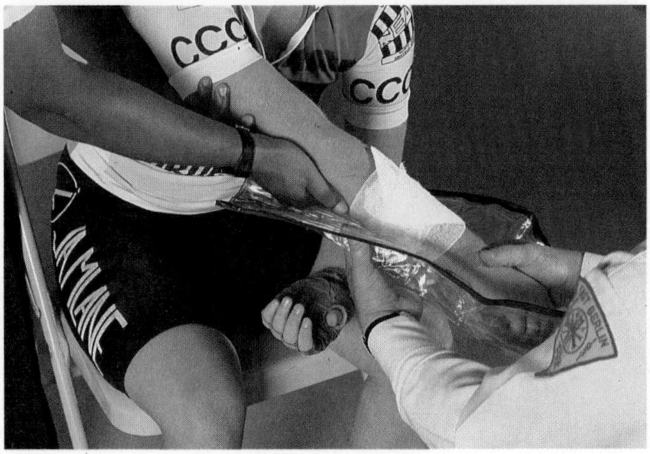

Figure 7-42d. Apply the splint, unzipped and uninflated. Grasp the patient's hand while your partner or a bystander holds the limb gently in alignment.

✳ Slide the splint over your hand onto the patient's hand and arm (Figure 7-42e).

✳ The splint should extend one joint above and below the suspected fracture (Figure 7-42f).

✳ The splint should extend beyond the patient's fingers to prevent a constricting band effect, which reduces circulation (Figure 7-42g).

✳ Continue to maintain gentle alignment while your partner or a bystander inflates the splint (Figure 7-42h).

✳ Inflate the splint to the point where your finger can still make a slight dent in the splint (Figure 7-42i).

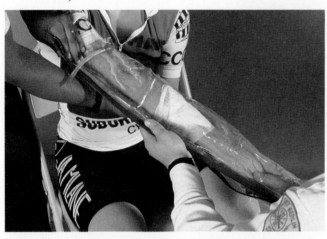

Figure 7-42e. Slide the splint over your hand onto the patient's hand and arm.

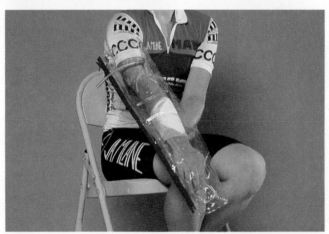

Figure 7-42f. The splint should extend one joint above and below the patient's hand and arm.

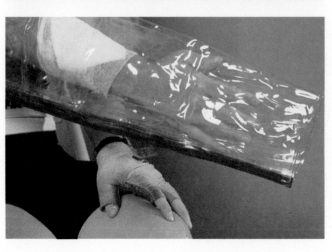

Figure 7-42g. The splint should extend beyond the patient's fingers to prevent a constricting band effect.

✳ Monitor pulses and sensation (Figure 7-42j).

✳ Check the splint occasionally to see that it remains properly inflated, especially when hot environments are a factor.

To use a fixation splint:

✳ Select a splint that is longer than the distance from the elbow to the fingertips.

✳ Pad the splint.

✳ Secure the splint to the arm so that both adjacent joints are stabilized.

REMEMBER: Immobilize the adjacent joints and always monitor distal pulses.

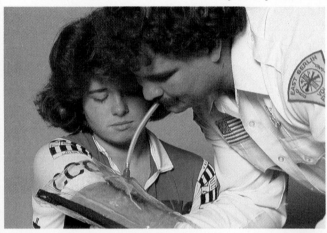

Figure 7-42h. Continue to maintain gentle alignment while your partner or a bystander inflates the splint.

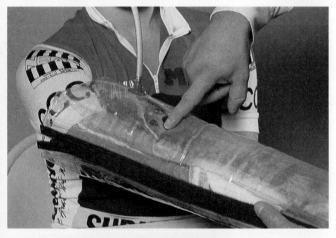

Figure 7-42i. Inflate the splint to the point where your finger can still make a slight dent in the splint.

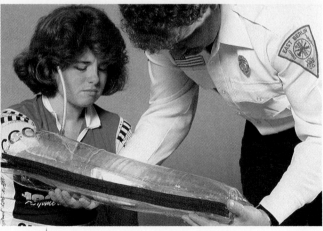

Figure 7-42j. Monitor pulses and sensations.

The Wrist And Hand

Splint fractures of the wrist and hand in the position in which you find them. To splint a wrist or hand, use the following guidelines:

✳ Place a roll of gauze in the hand, and splint the hand in the position of the function, with the fingers slightly flexed as if holding a round object in the palm of the hand (Figure 7-43a).

✳ The hand should always be splinted in a comfortable position (Figure 7-43b).

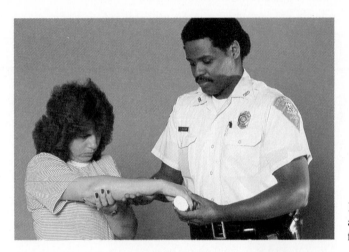

Figure 7-43a. Place a roll of gauze in the hand and splint the hand with the fingers lightly flexed.

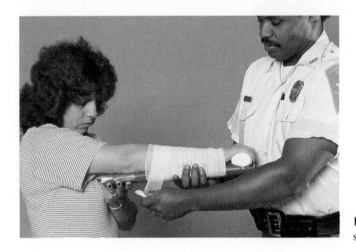

Figure 7-43b. The hand should always be splinted in a comfortable position.

✽ Do not attempt to realign fractures of this area.

✽ Both adjacent joints (wrist and elbow) must be splinted past the elbow to prevent motion of the fractured bone ends (Figure 7-43c).

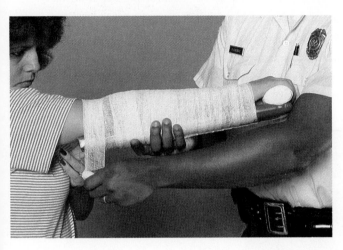

Figure 7-43c. Both adjacent joints must be splinted past the elbow to prevent the motion of the fractured bone ends.

EMERGENCY CARE FOR LOWER EXTREMITY FRACTURES

The Pelvis

Pain on compressions is the principal sign of a fractured pelvis. Feel for pain as follows:

✳ Place one hand on each hip bone (ilium) and press medially (Figure 7-44a).

✳ Press on the pubic bones (Figure 7-44b).

✳ Make a fist and place it between the patient's knees; ask the patient to squeeze your fist. If the femur and hip are stable, the patient will be able to accomplish this task. Pain will be experienced by the patient at the fracture site (Figure 7-44c).

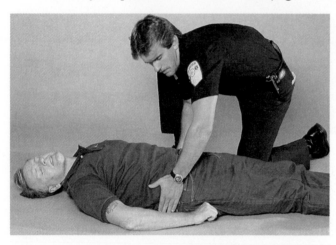

Figure 7-44a. Place one hand on each hip bone and press medially.

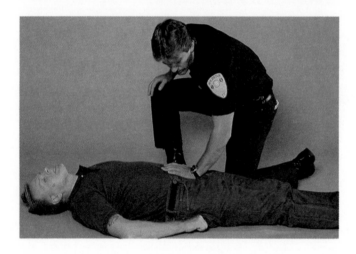

Figure 7-44b. Press on the pubic bones.

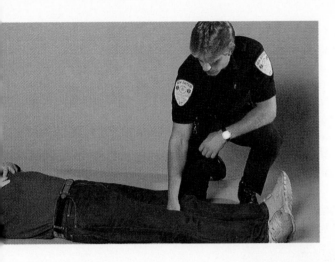

Figure 7-44c. Make a fist and place it between the patient's knees; ask the patient to squeeze your fist.

If any or all of these methods cause pain around the pelvic girdle, assume that this area is fractured. The First Responder can make the patient comfortable, by padding the area with blankets or pillows, restricting the patient's movement, and treating for shock, since a large volume of blood may be lost in the pelvic cavity. These patients should be transported gently to a medical facility.

The Hip

Most hip fractures must be splinted in the position in which they are found. If the socket of the hip is involved, the patient may be unable to straighten the leg. If too much pain is caused by the patient's attempt to straighten the leg, allow the patient to sit up and be transported in a position of comfort.

If the patient must be moved, 2 rescuers are needed. A small, flat board, such as a piece of plywood or a small back board is also needed (Figure 7-45a). The rescuers stand on either side of the patient (Figure 7-45b). As the patient puts an arm around the neck of each rescuer, the patient is lifted (Figure 7-45c) and the board is slipped underneath (Figure 7-45d). The patient can then be lifted from the bed or the floor onto the board. Use pillows or blankets to pad around the hip and buttocks (Figure 7-45e).

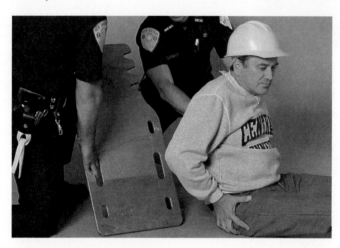

Figure 7-45a. A small, flat board, such as a piece of plywood or a small backboard is needed.

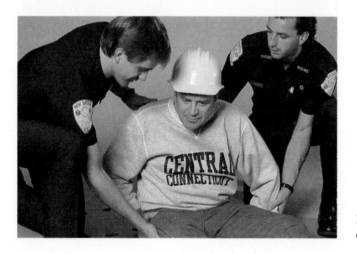

Figure 7-45b. The rescuers stand on either side of the patient.

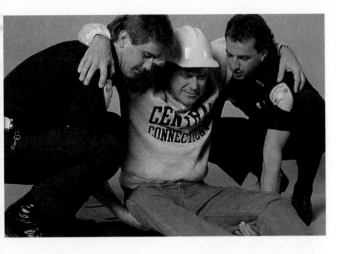

Figure 7-45c. As the patient puts an arm around the neck of each rescuer, the patient is lifted.

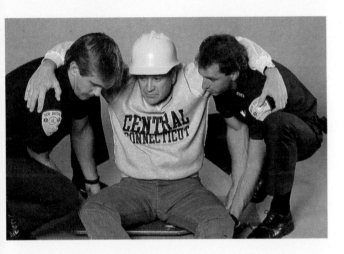

Figure 7-45d. The board is slipped underneath the patient.

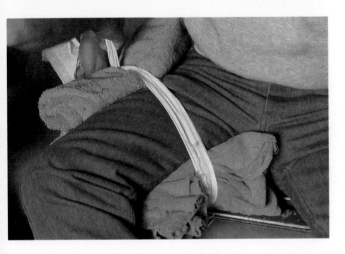

Figure 7-45e. Use pillows or blankets to pad the area.

A patient with posterior dislocation of the hip joint, the most common type, will have a flexed knee and leg adducted toward the midline of the body (Figure 7-46a). This dislocation can be splinted by placing a pillow or blanket in the flexed portion of the leg and securing the leg to prevent movement (Figure 7-46b). Use pillows or blankets to pad around the hip and buttocks.

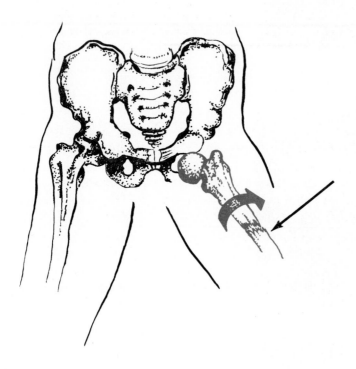

Figure 7-46a. A patient with posterior dislocation of the hip joint, the most common type, will have a flexed knee and leg adducted toward the midline of the body.

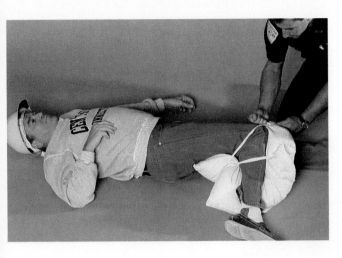

Figure 7-46b. This dislocation can be splinted by placing a pillow or blanket in the flexed portion of the leg and securing the leg to prevent movement.

The Femur

Fractures to the shaft of the femur, the longest and largest bone of the body, are severe because of the mass of extremely long muscles in the upper leg. These muscles can exert tremendous force against the fracture or dislocation site.

Most femur fractures show the usual signs in addition to being adducted away from the midline of the body. Marked shortening of the leg may occur (Figure 7-47). Blood loss in this part of the leg may be extensive whether the fracture is open or closed. Shock is always a possibility with this type of fracture.

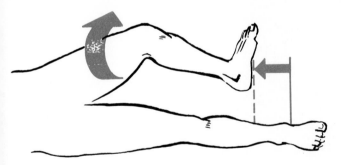

Figure 7-47. Marked shortening of the leg may occur with femur fractures.

A traction splint is the splint of choice. Commercial traction splints such as, Hare ®, Sager®, and Thomas, are available. Since many First Responders may not have this type of splint, or be trained in their use, traction instruction is not provided here. Rely on medical instructions for use of these devices.

If boards are available:

❋ Pad the boards (Figure 7-48a).

❋ Place one board on the inner aspect of the injured leg (Figure 7-48b).

❋ Place one board on the outer aspect of the injured leg (Figure 7-48c).

❋ Tie the boards together using cravats snugly around the leg (Figure 7-48d).

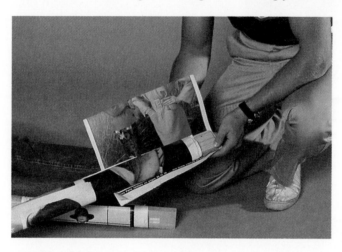

Figure 7-48a. Pad the boards.

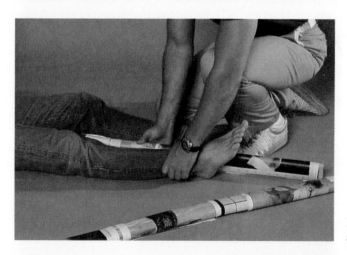

Figure 7-48b. Place one board on the inner aspect of the injured leg.

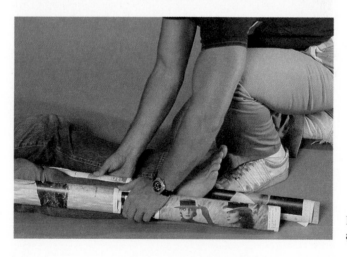

Figure 7-48c. Place one board on the outer aspect of the injured leg.

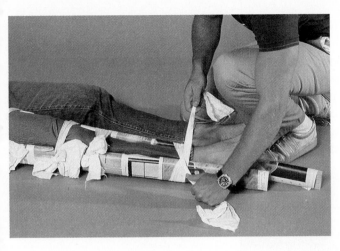

Figure 7-48d. Tie the boards together using cravats snugly around the leg.

NOTE: Check sensation and the pulses in the foot before and after splinting the leg. Perform a capillary blanch test by squeezing the nail beds of the toes. The pulses in the foot can be found on the medial side of the ankle posterior to the knob of the ankle (posterior tibial pulse) and on top (dorsalis pedis) of the foot (Figure 7-49a). The foot is sometimes a difficult place to locate a pulse. Once found, place an X on the spot with a pen (Figure 7-49b). This will allow quick reassessment later.

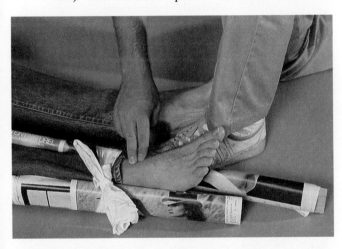

Figure 7-49a. The pulses in the foot can be found on the medial side of the ankle posterior to the knot of the ankle on top of the foot.

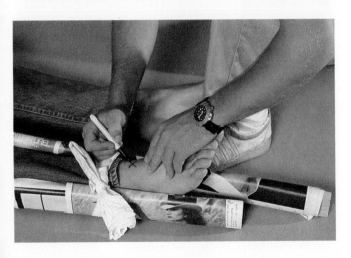

Figure 7-49b. Once found, place an X on the spot with a pen to allow quick reassessment later.

The Knee

Splint fractures or dislocations in the area of the knee as they are found unless distal pulses are absent (Figure 7-50a). A pillow or blanket makes an adequate splint (Figure 7-50b). Occasionally the knee is dislocated. When this happens the kneecap (patella) will be displaced laterally and medially. If this occurs the leg should be gently straightened to reduce pain and prevent further injury. A fracture or dislocation of the kneecap can be rendered less painful by extending the leg. This condition reduces the distance between the femur and tibia, which causes less stress on the muscles, tendons, and ligaments surrounding the knee. If the knee appears locked, splint it in the position in which it was found.

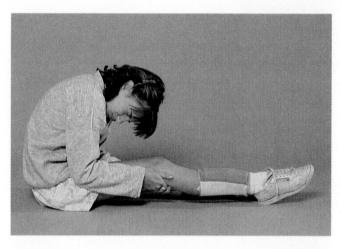

Figure 7-50a. Splint fractures or dislocations in the area of the knee as they are found unless distal pulses are absent.

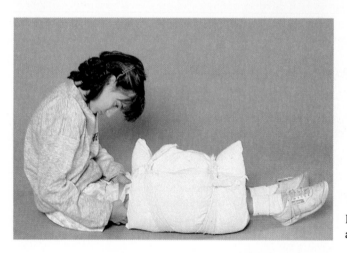

Figure 7-50b. A pillow or blanket makes an adequate splint.

The Lower Leg And Foot

Fractures of the 2 bones of the lower leg (tibia and fibula) can be splinted by simple fixation as with the femur described in the "Fractures" section. The use of an inflatable splint is as follows:

✻ Select the proper size inflatable splint (Figure 7-51a).

✻ Dress any open wounds with sterile dressings (Figure 7-51b).

✻ Remove or cut clothing away from the injured extremity (Figure 7-51c).

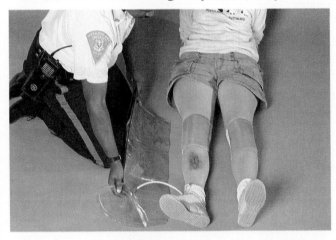

Figure 7-51a. Select the proper size splint.

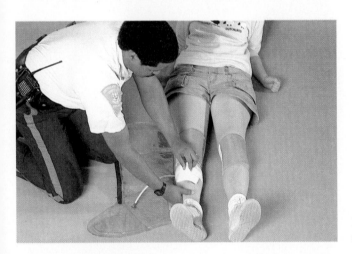

Figure 7-51b. Dress any open wounds with sterile dressings.

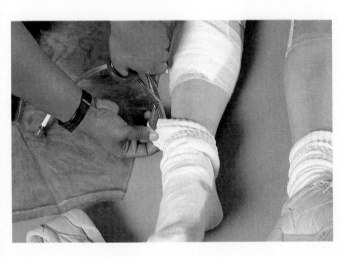

Figure 7-51c. Remove or cut clothing away from the injured area.

❋ Check the affected site for sensation and pulse before and after splinting.

❋ Apply the splint, unzipped and uninflated. Grasp the patient's foot while your partner or a bystander holds the limb in alignment (Figure 7-51d).

❋ Slide the splint over your hand onto the patient's foot and leg (figure 7-51e).

❋ Extend the splint one joint above and below the suspected fracture (Figure 7-51f).

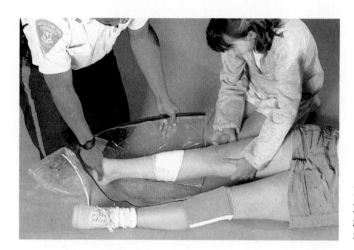

Figure 7-51d. Grasp the patient's foot while your partner or a bystander holds the limb in gentle alignment and apply the splint unzipped and uninflated.

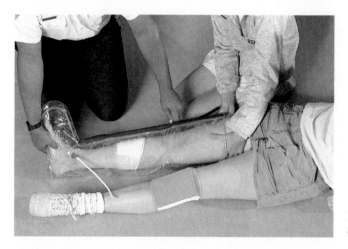

Figure 7-51e. Slide the splint over your hand onto the patient's foot and leg.

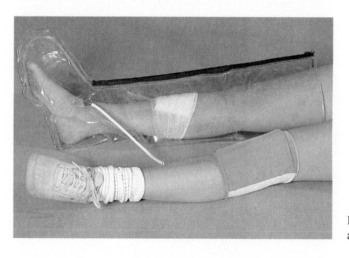

Figure 7-51f. Extend the splint one joint above and below the suspected fracture.

✱ The splint should extend beyond the end of the patient's toes to prevent a constricting band effect., thereby reducing circulation (Figure 7-51g).

✱ Continue to maintain gentle alignment while your partner or a bystander inflates the splint (Figure 7-51h).

✱ Inflate the splint to the point where your finger can still make a slight dent in the splint (Figure 7-51i).

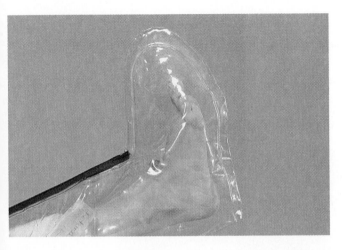

Figure 7-51g. The splint should extend beyond the end of the patient's toes to prevent a constricting band effect.

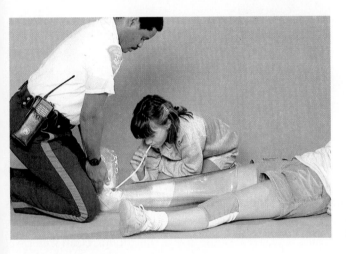

Figure 7-51h. Continue to maintain gentle alignment while your partner or a bystander inflates the splint.

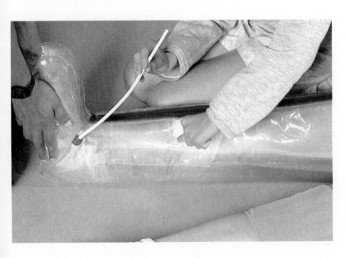

Figure 7-51i. Inflate the splint to the point where your finger can still make a slight dent in the splint.

✳ Observe the color of the extremity for an indication of circulatory status.

✳ Check the splint occasionally to see whether it is properly inflated, especially when hot and cold environments are a factor.

To use a fixation splint:

✳ Select a splint that is longer than the distance from the elbow to the fingertips.

✳ Pad the splint.

✳ Secure the splint to the arm so that both adjacent joints are stabilized.

REMEMBER: Check pulses in the foot before and after splinting. Always immobilize the adjacent joints.

The Ankle And Foot

Fractures involving the ankle or foot can be easily splinted with a pillow or blanket (Figure 7-52). Fractured toes can be splinted to adjacent toes by using adhesive tape.

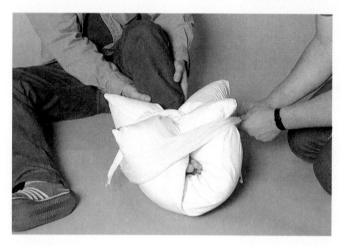

Figure 7-52. Fractures involving the ankle or foot can easily be splinted with a pillow or blanket.

Amputations

Amputation is a serious extremity injury that involves the loss of a limb or extremity. Bleeding control and shock management must be initiated immediately. After life-threatening conditions have been attended to and the open wound has been bandaged, the amputated part must be cared for as follows:

✳ Clean the amputated part of gross debris. Use sterile saline, if available; if not, clean water will do (Figure 7-53a).

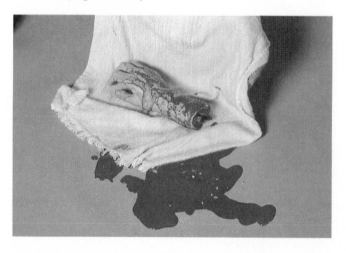

Figure 7-53a. Clean the amputated part of gross debris.

✳ Wrap the part in clean, moistened sterile material, if available; if not, a clean, moist towel will do (Figure 7-53b).

✳ Place the amputated part in a plastic bag in a cooler with ice water, being careful not to freeze the part (Figure 7-53c).

✳ The amputated part must be transported with the patient to a medical facility.

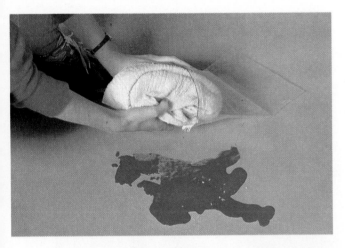

Figure 7-53b. Wrap the part in a clean, moistened sterile material.

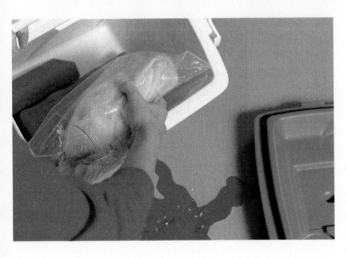

Figure 7-53c. Place the amputated part in a plastic bag in a cooler with ice water.

SUMMARY

An understanding of the musculoskeletal system is required to treat the traumatized patient. Fracture, both open and closed, strains, sprains, and dislocations are all caused by force applied to specific body areas. The severity of the injury determines the required care needed.

Treat any injury to an extremity as if the bone in the affected area were fractured. Be gentle if the patient must be moved or the extremity aligned to prepare for comfortable stabilization of the injury site. Remember to take a pulse below the fracture site before and after splinting. Gentleness cannot be overstressed.

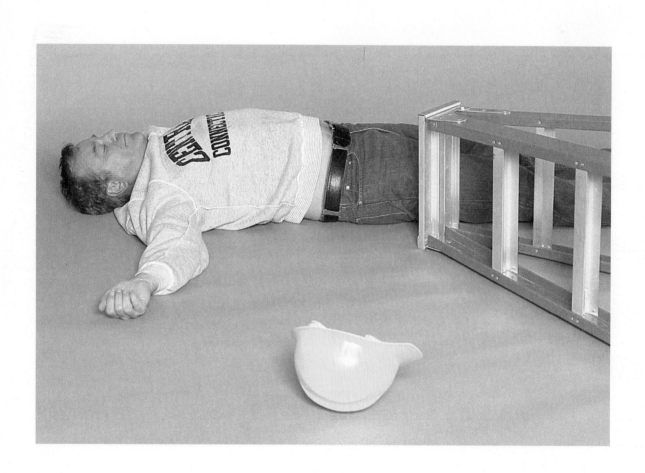

INJURIES TO THE SKULL, FACE AND SPINE

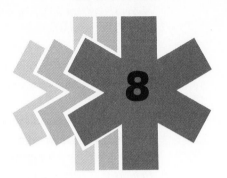

CHAPTER

8

KEY CONCEPTS AND SKILLS

By the end of this chapter, you will be able to:

✳ Identify and describe the function of the two major portions of the skull.

✳ Identify and describe the function of the nervous system.

✳ Describe the care for an eye injury.

✳ Describe the signs and symptoms of a head injury.

✳ Describe the signs and symptoms of a spinal injury.

✳ Describe a patient examination for a head or facial injury.

✳ Describe a patient examination for a spinal injury.

✳ Describe the proper care for a patient with a head or facial injury.

✳ Describe the required assistance for a patient with a spinal injury.

KEY WORDS

Battle's sign – Black and blue markings behind the ear that may indicate a fracture at the base of the skull.

Cerebrospinal fluid – A fluid cushion that protects the brain and spinal cord from shock, and provides nourishment.

Cervical spine – The first 7 vertebrae of the spinal column found in the neck.

Clavicles – The collar bones.

Concussion – An injury to the soft structure of the brain; usually due to violent jarring or shaking caused by a blow to the head; may involve loss of consciousness.

Cornea – The clear, transparent membrane on the outer portion of the eye.

Diaphragmatic breathing – Breathing that is characterized by slight movement of the abdomen. This type of breathing may indicate possible injury at cervical vertebrae C3-C7. Cyanosis is often present.

Extension – The movement that brings the parts of a body part, e.g., a limb, into or toward a straight condition.

Flexion – The act of bending or a condition of being bent in contrast to extension.

Hyperextend – To extend beyond the usual limit of movement.

Lucid interval – A period of mental clarity between periods of irrational behavior. This condition sometimes occurs during seizures.

Lumbar spine – The 5 vertebrae of the spinal column found in the lower back between the sacrum and the thoracic vertebrae. The lumbar spine helps support the lower body trunk.

199

Nervous system – The complex network of structures that activate, coordinate, and control all functions of the body. The nervous system has two major portions, the central nervous system and the peripheral nervous system.

Neurogenic shock – A form of shock that is caused by injury to the nervous system.

Paralysis – Temporary suspension or permanent loss of function, especially loss of sensation or voluntary motion.

Paraplegic – A person with paralysis of the lower limbs.

Positive pressure breathing – Ventilation of a patient using a device to provide pressure that is greater than that found in the atmosphere.

Priapism – A continued, and often painful, erection of the penis; seldom associated with sexual arousal, sometimes present in cervical spine injury.

Quadriplegic – A person with paralysis of the body from the neck to the toes.

Raccoon eyes – Black and blue coloration around the orbit of the eyes caused by injury; also referred to as Panda eyes.

Rotation – The turning on an axis.

Spasm – An involuntary muscle contraction.

Thoracic spine – The 12 vertebrae of the spinal column found in the back; because these vertebrae are attached to the ribs, they have limited movement.

Vertebrae – Any of the 33 bones that make up the spinal column.

Vitreous fluid – The clear, colorless substance that fills the cavity of the eyeball.

THE NERVOUS SYSTEM

The nervous system is the major control appartatus of the body and is responsible for:

* Conscious and unconscious acts.
* The ability to sense things through sight, hearing, smell, touch, and taste.
* The regulation of vital functions.

The parts of the nervous system are the brain, the spinal cord, and the numerous nerves of the body. The brain and spinal cord are called the central nervous system. Similarly, the usual designation for the nerves of the body is the peripheral nervous system because nerves extend to outlying or peripheral parts of the body.

The nervous system transmits information by means of impulses conducted from one nerve cell to another. Therefore, trauma or disease in any part of the nervous system can significantly affect a patient.

STRUCTURES OF THE CENTRAL NERVOUS SYSTEM

Skull

The skull provides protection for the brain. The bones of the skull are fused together to help prevent injury to the central nervous tissue. The bones of the head are divided into two sections. (Figure 8-1). The face can be divided from the cranium by drawing an imaginary line across the face at the level of the eyes. The facial bones protect the eyes, airway, and mouth. These bones also assist in breathing, speaking, chewing, and swallowing.

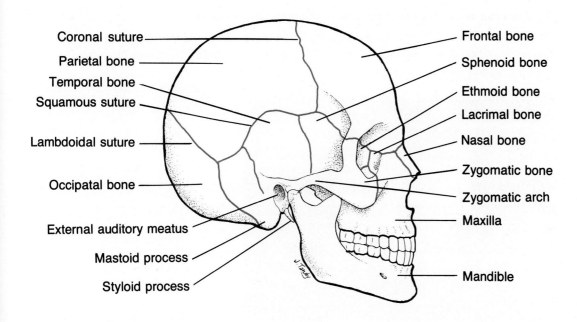

Figure 8-1. The skull. (From Austrin, M.G. and Austrin, H.R.: Young's Learning Medical Terminology, a worktext, 6th edition, St. Louis, 1987, The C.V. Mosby Co.)

Spinal Column and Cord

The spinal cord is protected by tough membranes, the meninges, that contain cerebrospinal fluid. The spinal meninges form a tube-like covering around the spinal cord and line the vertebrae. The spinal cord is encased by 33 irregularly shaped bones called vertebrae. These vertebrae form the spinal column. The spinal cord acts as a communication link between the brain and the periperhal nervous system.

The spinal cord is the conduit through which messages are transmitted to all parts of the body via sensory and motor neurons.

INJURIES TO THE SKULL

The skull, like all other bones of the body, can be fractured. The fractures may occur when objects strike the head. Open fractures are often caused when the head is struck by a penetrating object such as a bullet or glass (Figure 8-2). Signs of skull fracture include:

❋ Deformity such as skull depressions.

❋ Bleeding from the eyes, ears, or nose.

❋ Drainage of cerebrospinal fluid from the eyes, ears, or nose.

❋ Bruising around the eyes (Raccoon or Panda eyes), or behind the ears (Battle's sign), are the result of blood pooling in these areas (Figures 8-3a and 8-3b). Note that bruising seen around and behind the ears is usually a late sign of skull injury.

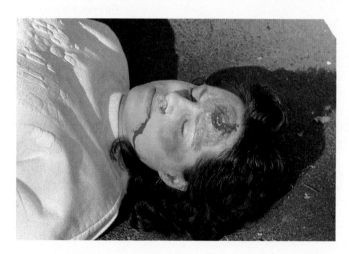

Figure 8-2. Depressed skull fracture.

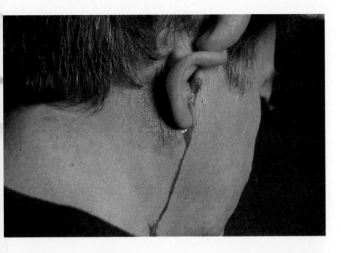

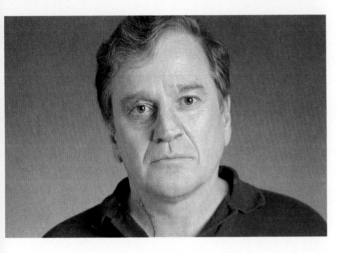

Figure 8-3. **A,** Battle's sign. **B,** Panda or raccoon eyes.

The skull may be difficult to palpate because of the patient's hair. Be careful when feeling the head of an injured person since small bone fragments may be pushed into the brain tissue.

Bleeding from the eyes, ears or nose should be closely evaluated. Look carefully for the source of bleeding. Many times the blood is coming from visible wounds outside or near the eyes, ears, or nose. This bleeding can be easily controlled by applying direct, but gentle, pressure to the wound.

Cerebrospinal fluid can only drain from orifices if the protective coverings of the brain are torn. This fluid is a clear liquid that protects the brain from injury and helps transport nutrients through the central nervous system.

Cerebrospinal fluid will cause the blood draining from the openings of the head to appear thin and watery. If felt between the index finger and thumb, it will feel slick to the touch.

The bruising seen around and behind the ears (Battle's sign) is caused by bleeding occurring within the lower portion of the brain case. When fractures occur in the cranium, the areas behind the ears and below the eyes will most commonly display the signs of bruising (Raccoon or Panda eyes).

INJURIES TO THE BRAIN

Brain injuries can occur without the skull being fractured. A fall or any force striking the head can damage the brain or its protective covering. *Alteration of consciousness* is the hallmark of injury to the brain.

Level of Consciousness

The patient who has a head injury must be evaluated to determine their level of consciousness and orientation. These patients must be monitored closely to ensure that they are not becoming increasingly confused. As a First Responder, you must always relate findings concerning the patient's mental status to the medical team. Any changes should also be reported.

Use the following examples as guidelines to determine the level of consiousness:

✳ *Conscious:* Is the person oriented to name, time, place, and events; awake, alert, and respond appropriately to verbal commands. Ask questions similar to the following to help you determine a patient's orientation:

> What is your name?
> Where are you?
> What is the date? Time?
> What were you doing?
> Where are you?

✳ *Unconscious:* The person is asleep, not alert, and command response may vary. The person may only respond to:

> Verbal command
> Light touch
> Pain
> Loud noise

✳ *Coma:* The person is asleep, not alert, does not respond to any commands, but has a pulse and is breathing.

Any easy scale using the acronym AVPU can be used to assess the level of consciousness. The scale consists of:

A = *A*lert to name, time, place, and orientations.

V = Responds to *V*erbal commands.

P = Responds to *P*ainful stimuli.

U = Is *U*nresponsive.

Note the AVPU level when the patient is first seen, as well as any changes that may occur during your care; report these findings to the medical response team.

A patient may report having been unconscious but may appear alert when you arrive. Watch these patients closely since they may again lose consciousness. The level of consciousness should be clearly assessed and documented at regular intervals.

CONCUSSION

The mildest form of brain injury is a concussion. This short-term condition is caused when the brain is forcibly moved around in the skull. A fall or an object striking the patient's head can cause a concussion. The side opposite, as well as the side of the head struck may sustain some damage. This is caused by the brain being forced against the other side of the skull and then forcefully bouncing back against the side from which the head was hit.

The signs and symptoms of concussion are:

* Confusion
* Anger or inappropriate behavior
* Dizziness
* Loss of consciousness
* Loss of memory
* Visual distortion, often with one pupil dilated
* Headache
* Nausea
* Vomiting

The patient may display some or all of these signs and symptoms. The more severe injuries have a greater effect on consciousness. Anyone sustaining a concussion should be evaluated and tested in a medical facility even though the injuries are short-term and usually cause no permanent damage.

Bleeding in the skull can be due to many causes. Strokes resulting from hypertension can cause blood vessels in the brain to rupture. A blow to the head can tear blood vessels, or a penetrating object can strike a blood vessel and cause bleeding in the skull. Bleeding within the enclosed skull is always serious, since bleeding can cause pressure in the skull and cause further damage to the brain.

Illnesses, such as fever or cancer, can cause swelling to occur within the skull and damage brain tissue. Epilepsy is almost always the result of damage to brain tissue, or an irritable area of cells that become uncontrollable without the help of medication.

The signs and symptoms of brain injury may include:

* Confusion
* Restlessness
* Anger or inappropriate behavior
* Alteration or loss of consciousness
* Paralysis or weakness of one side of the body
* Unequal pupils (be alert because both pupils may dilate)
* Irregular breathing patterns

Always gather the necessary information to assure a competent patient care decision based on the mechanism of injury, the signs, and, the symptoms.

INJURIES TO THE NECK AND SPINE

The spinal cord is approximately 3/8 inch (10mm) in diameter; the diameter inside the vertebrae column is only 5/8 inch (15mm), leaving about 1/8 inch (5mm). A very slight shift of the patient's body during an accident or emergency can cause permanent damage if the cord or nerve roots are trapped between the vertebrae. A severed spinal cord is permanent.

Most spinal cord injuries occur in persons under 30 years of age involved in motor vehicle accidents. The second most frequent cause are accidents, e.g. falls, involving the elderly. Diving and penetrating (bullets, knife wounds) injuries rank third and fourth, respectively.

Signs and symptoms of spinal injury include:

✳ Deformity

✳ Pain in the affected area

✳ Trauma in the affected area, e.g. cuts and bruises

✳ Paralysis

✳ Loss of sensation below the injury site; numbness or tingling

✳ Muscle spasms near the affected vertebrae

✳ Loss or reduction in reflexes

✳ Loss of muscle tone

✳ Abdominal bleeding

✳ Lack of bladder or bowel control

✳ Priapism (uncontrollable erection of the penis)

Assessing an Injury to the Head, Neck, or Spine

When assessing a patient, always think of the mechanism of injury. A "starburst" pattern in the windshield of a car, an injury produced by high speeds, low water in the pool, or a football player who was blocked from the side should cause you, as a First Responder, to consider spinal injury. In fact, any injury above the shoulders may produce spinal injury.

Assessment of the head injury includes:

✳ Gently palpate the entire head feeling for lumps, depressions, cuts, and bleeding. Because of the patient's hair it may be difficult to do this, or blood may have "matted" the hair making it hard to feel areas.

✳ Look at the patient's eyes for leaking fluid, bleeding or dilation.

✳ Check the patient for bruises. In a suspected head injury, look behind the ears for Battle's sign and around the eyes for Panda signs (Figure 8-3).

✳ Ask the patient if there is pain and, if so, ask the location of the pain.

CERVICAL SPINE

The head sits on the spinal column like a basketball on a broom handle making the cervical region susceptible to injury. Any blow to the skull causing flexion or extension may damage the cervical spine. One can almost touch their shoulder with their ear, their chin to their chest, and the back of the head to their seventh cervical area. These lateral, extension, and flexion movements are exaggerated during injuries involving deceleration and acceleration forces. A whiplash is an example of the action of these forces on the injured person's neck (Figure 8-4). The spinal column can sustain violent movements without injury, but all patients involved in a forceful accident should be treated as if they had sustained a neck injury until evaluated in a medical facility.

Assessment of neck and spinal injuries includes:

✱ Tell the patient not to move unless told to do so. Do not ask "yes" or "no" questions unless manual traction has been applied.

✱ Determine the state of the patient's airway; gently obtain good air exchange.

✱ Secure the head in a neutral position.

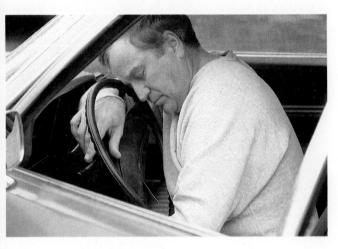

Figure 8-4. A whiplash is an example of the action of these forces on the injured person's neck

❋ Gently feel the back of the neck for deformity, swelling, and bleeding. If any of these signs are found, immediately stablilize the head and neck, by hand if necessary (Figure 8-5).

❋ Re-evaluate breathing to determine sufficient air exchange by looking, listening, and feeling for air flow at the mouth and nose. Damage to the cervical spine may cause stoppage or difficulty with breathing. Some patients will require full ventilatory support. Spinal nerves exiting the spinal column between cervical vertebrae 3 and 5 innervate the diaphragm.

❋ Have the patient press each foot against your hand if you suspect spinal injury to check for movement capability.

❋ Pinch each foot if you suspect spinal injury. Make sure that sensation is equal for each foot.

❋ Check both hands by asking the patient to move their fingers, squeeze your hand, and to lift each hand (Figure 8-6).

❋ Compare the responses on each side of the body. They should be equal from side to side.

❋ If the patient is unconscious, gently pinch the soles of the feet. Observe for movement or other responses. Evaluate each limb separately. Then repeat the pinching in the palm of each hand. If the patient can spread his fingers, the damage is probably below the level of the cervical spine.

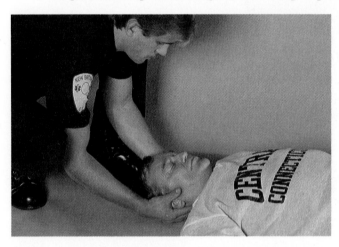

Figure 8-5. Stabilize the neck.

Assessing the Thoracic Spine

The vertebrae found along the posterier portion of the thoracic cavity are somewhat protected by the ribs and are not as movable as the cervical vertebrae. They are occasionally injured, but not as often as the cervical and lumbar spine.

Signs and symptoms of thoracic spinal injuries include:

❋ Pain

❋ Deformity

❋ Paralysis or numbness below the injury site

Care includes evaluation of the patient's entire body. Look around you to determine the mechanism of injury. Other parts of the spine could be involved. Stabilize the back and arrange transportation to a medical facility.

Assessing the Lumbar Spine

The junction of the thoracic and lumbar spine is a point of frequent injury. This area is poorly protected. Most injuries below this point do not cause total loss of sensation in the legs and feet.

As with the thoracic spine, evaluate the patient carefully to make sure that no other areas of the spine are involved. Stabilize the entire spine and arrange transportation to a medical facility.

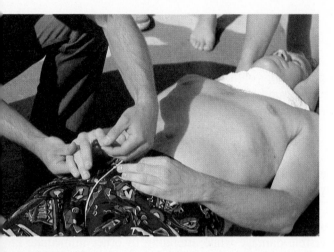

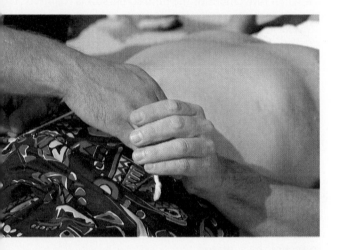

Figure 8-6. A sensory check of the upper extremity.

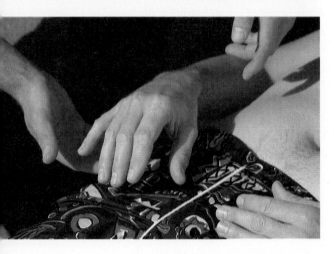

NEUROGENIC SHOCK

Be alert for spinal shock (neurogenic shock) whenever the spinal cord is injured. When the walls of the blood vessels lose nervous control they do not maintain a constant state of constriction. Blood will pool in the extremities causing insufficient circulating volume. The body always attempts to maintain sufficient blood flow to major life-supporting organs. When blood pools, insufficient amounts are available to provide nourishment or remove wastes from the heart, brain, lungs, or kidneys.

EMERGENCY CARE FOR HEAD, NECK, AND SPINAL INJURIES

Emergency care for head, neck, and spinal injuries includes careful, efficient handling of the patient to prevent further damage while constantly supporting effective breathing. Many head injury patients will not effectively exchange air. One very important sign of head injury may be a reduced breathing rate, volume, or grossly irregular breathing pattern. Patients with head or neck injuries must be carefully supported to prevent further irreversible damage while attending to other immediate life-threatening injuries. Always protect the neck when movement of the injured person is required. Do not allow free movement of the head and neck. Support both carefully with your hands or a piece of equipment.

This may include:

* Sandbags
* Towels or sheets
* A car sunvisor
* A board
* Tape

Any of these objects may be used to secure the injured person's head and neck. Sandbags, towels, or sheets may help maintain alignment of the head and neck. A car sunvisor may be placed between the injured person's shoulders and the back of the head to prevent flexion, rotation, or extension of the neck. It may be secured by the shirt collar at the shoulders and tied to the forehead with a circular turn. A sock may also be placed over the head to secure the sunvisor.

The person can be placed on a long or short board. This technique is discussed in Chapter 6. The board does not need to be a professional appliance. Always tape the head to prevent an inadvertent movement that may injure the neck. Paralysis may occure if proper care is not given to securing and moving of an injured person's head or neck.

A patient with a suspected head or neck injury should not be moved prior to evaluation unless a life-threatening situation exists.

If the patient with a head or neck injury is having difficulty breathing, start the following procedures:

* Place the neck in a neutral position while stabilizing the cervical spine (Figure 8-7).
* Use the modified jaw thrust without tilting the patient's head. *Never* hyperextend unless breathing cannot be effectively accomplished in any other manner. Be extremely careful if the neck must be moved.
* Give rescue breathing if required using the proper method described in this text. Use an approved oxygen administration appliance as described in Appendix A.
* Use extreme care to maintain neck and head alignment. It may be necessary to carefully adjust the airway of the injured person to allow sufficient air exchange.

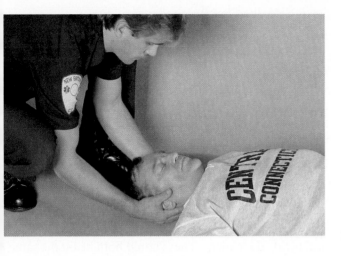

Figure 8-7. Keep the neck in a neutral position.

Cut clothing away to view any injured areas. *Never* remove garments over the person's head; cut them away.

The head, neck, or spinal injured person should always be transported on a firm surface. A spine board or other suitable material, like a door may be used for this purpose. The patient may be placed on the board using a long axis slide as described in Figure 8-8, or if sufficient manpower is present, a lateral log roll and slide may be used (Figure 8-9). Always assure the patient is never moved sideways.

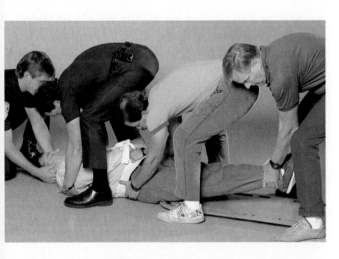

Figure 8-8. Patient being moved using long axis slide

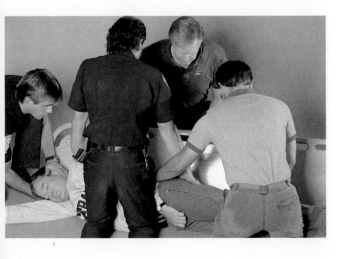

Figure 8-9. Lateral log roll.

To place a person on a board using a long axis slide, the First Responder should:

❊ Use one person to protect the injured person's head and neck from rotating, flexing, or extending by carefully grasping the injured neck with his hands. The person supporting the patient's head should be in command.

❊ Use one person to straddle the person and grasp under their body.

❊ Place the board on long axis at the patient's feet.

❊ Gently lift the patient and slide the board under.

A log roll may be used to place an injured person on a board if the following steps are followed:

❊ One person grasps the injured head and neck to prevent head or neck flexion, extension, or rotation. The person supporting the patient's head should be in charge.

❊ Make sure the patient is flat on his back.

❊ Have two other First Responders kneel beside the patient. They should both be on the same side, one at the torso and the other at the patient's legs (Figure 8-10a).

❊ One reaches across the patient and grasps the hip and shoulder of the injured person.

❊ Another grasps the injured patient's waist and knee on the side across from which they are kneeling (Figure 8-10b).

❊ Roll the patient up gently on the count of three.

❊ Move the body as unit (log).

❊ Have one First Responder slide the board behind the patient up against the injured person's back. The board should extend about 8 inches above the patient's head (Figure 8-10c).

❊ On the count of three, gently roll the patient onto the board while lowering both the board and the patient.

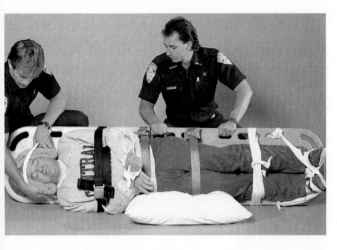

Figure 8-10a. The first responders should be on the same side of the patient.

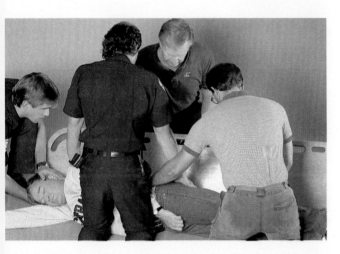

Figure 8-10b. Grasp the waist and knee on the side across from you.

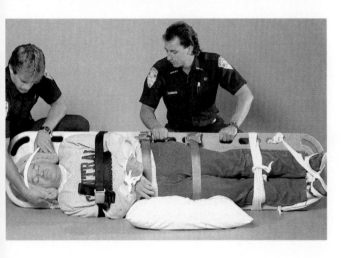

Figure 8-10c. Slide the board behind the patient. The board should rest 8 inches above the patient's head.

A major problem with the log roll is the requirement for a sufficient number of trained First Responders to work together as a team.

A team must practice to become sufficient when log rolling a patient. Three to four experienced First Responders are required to properly move an injured person using this method. Other methods requiring less people power will more commonly be required and may be as effective.

Once the injured person is on the board, tape (Figure 8-11) or straps may be applied to hold the patient in place. The First Responder may want to wait for the medical team for final securing of the patient to the board. The temporary securing is only for protection and should always be completed before the person is moved. The head of the board may need to be elevated 6-8 inches to assist the patient's breathing and help reduce cerebral swelling or bleeding.

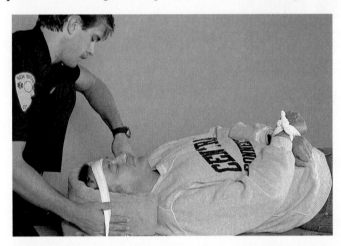

Figure 8-11. Tape may be used to keep the patient in place.

Reassess the patient. This is a good time to check for further injury.

Place all unconscious persons without head and neck injury or with proper neck stabilization on their sides to help protect their airway. This position will help keep the airway clear of liquids. The left coma position, i.e., with the patient on the left side (Figure 8-12), will help protect the airway of the unconscious but otherwise uninjured patient. A patient properly secured to the board will allow board and patient to be placed on his or her side (Figure 8-13).

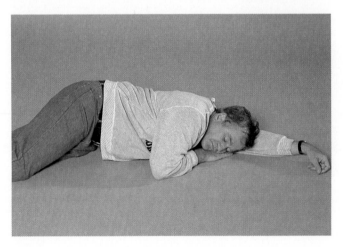

Figure 8-12. Place the unconscious patient in the left coma position.

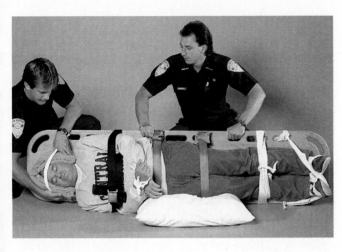

Figure 8-13. The board and patient may be placed on his side.

Head injured patients often vomit or have seizures. Care must be taken to properly secure them to prevent further head or neck injury and if they vomit or have a seizure. The head injury patient may develop an extremely high fever (105 °F, 40.6 °C). Treatment for elevated temperatures is discussed in Chapter 14.

Immobilize all patients with head injuries and expected neck injuries. Protect the patient's airway, place them in a safe comfortable position, and be prepared to relate all findings to the medical response team.

Most head lacerations tend to bleed, but this blood can usually be controlled by using direct pressure to the site of the injury. Blood loss can be extensive especially in children. Care should be taken to make sure that pressure is firm enough to control bleeding but not firm enough to push bone tissue into the cranial vault. Dress and bandage the wounds of the head that do not show the presence of cerebrospinal fluid. This clear fluid will cause the blood to appear weak in color and will be extremely slick to the touch.

Although bleeding should be controlled, *do not* control drainage of cerebrospinal fluid from the nose, eyes, or ears. If cerebrospinal fluid is not allowed to flow from the skull, pressure within the skull may increase and cause damage and even death.

Few head or neck injury patients have low blood pressure. Very little blood can be lost in the cranial cavity. If brain damage is the major injury, the patient's pulse pressure should widen and the pulse rate should reduce. If a patient is cold and clammy, has low pressure and/or a fast pulse, suspect major hemorrhage elsewhere in the body. Maintain spinal stabilization until the emergency care team treats the patient.

Neck

Most neck bleeding can be controlled by positioning the patient with his or her head and neck elevated. Apply direct pressure to the bleeding site. Use great care when moving or caring for a patient with bleeding neck injury since the cervical spine may also be injured. If bleeding from one of the major vessels occurs, apply pressure on the involved vessel above and below the wound. Control bleeding with hand pressure. *Do not* apply a pressure dressing to the neck since this may occlude the patient's airway.

Cheek and Mouth

A wound involving the cheek or mouth is difficult to treat. These wounds tend to bleed freely and tax the resources of the First Responder to control bleeding effectively. The patient's airway must always be maintained.

Use a gauze square or any other suitable piece of material and apply direct pressure to the wound. Remove any foreign objects that completely penetrate the cheek only when bleeding or the airway cannot be controlled. After carefully removing the object, place as dressing both inside and outside the cheek. Hold firm pressure until the clotting controls the flow of blood. Pack the cheek and use a cloth (cravat) or absorbent gauze cloth roll like Klinger® bandage to apply pressure (Figure 8-14). This same bandage can be used to secure a fractured jaw.

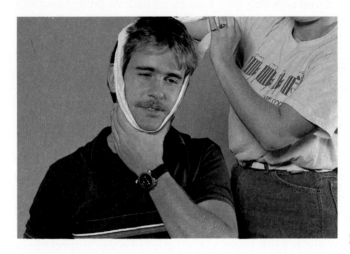

Figure 8-14. Klinger bandage used to apply pressure.

Nose bleeds

Nose bleeds are a common emergency. These are usually harmless and can be controlled by elevating the nose and pinching the nostrils. A nosebleed, especially in adults, can be a life-threatening situation due to the First Responder's inability to effectively measure the amount of blood that has been lost. The difficulty in measuring the blood loss is due to much of the blood being swallowed.

If the patient has been involved in trauma, suspect cerebrospinal fluid is leaking with the blood until proof can be obtained that only blood is presenting. *Do not* control drainage containing cerebrospinal spinal fluid. Always remember that neck injuries commonly occur with trauma involving the face.

Additional causes of nosebleed in adults, other than trauma, are hypertension and sinus infection. Bleeding not caused by trauma can be controlled by elevating the patient's nose and applying direct pressure by pinching the nostrils (Figure 8-15). An ice pack applied to the nose may decrease the time required for blood to clot. Most nosebleeds are minor and can be easily controlled.

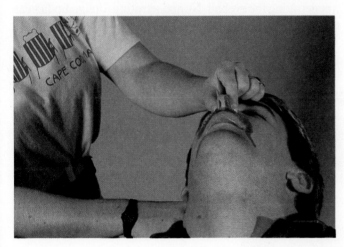

Figure 8-15. Care for nose bleeds.

Eye Injuries

The primary types of eye injury are those that:

✳ Penetrate the layers of the eye covering

✳ Involve the eye lid

Extensive bleeding may occur when the eyelid is lacerated. This bleeding usually can be controlled by using gentle, direct pressure if the First Responder is sure the eyeball is not involved. After bleeding is controlled, apply a soft gauze pressure dressing to maintain the gentle pressure to the eyelid. If the eyeball is involved or clear fluid is leaking from the eye, do not apply pressure since this will increase the leaking of vitreous fluid and cause permanent blindness in the involved eye.

Treatment of eye injuries is as follows:

✳ For foreign bodies:

Do not attempt to remove a body penetrating the eyeball. Nonpenetrating foreign bodies can be removed by using the corner of a gauze pad. If necessary fold the upper lid over as shown in Figure 8-16 to allow a larger working area.

Loose foreign bodies may be flushed from the eye with water.

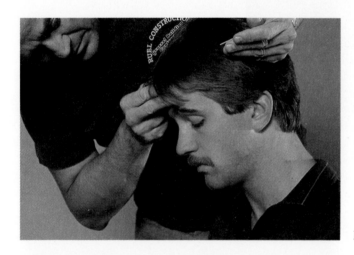

Figure 8-16. Steps to evert the eyelid.

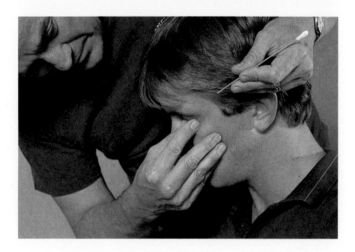

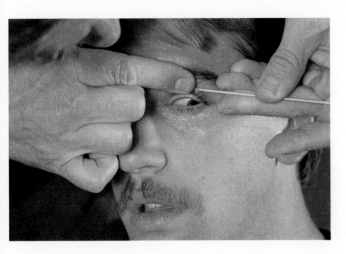

* For chemical burns:

    Flush with water (Figure 8-17).

    Do not use a neutralizing or antagonizing substance; either may cause greater harm to the eye.

* For any eye injury:

    Instruct the patient to close both eyes; since both eyes move together, bandage both of them.

    If there is a penetrating object still in the eye, place a paper cup, or other object that will not apply pressure, over the affected area.

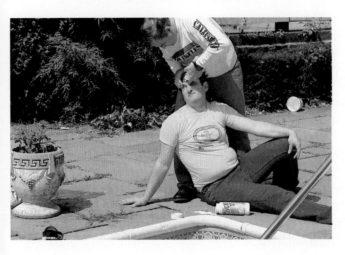

Figure 8-17. Flushing chemicals from the eyes.

Always remember that eye bandages render the patient temporarily blind since both eyes must be bandaged (Figure 8-18).

Explain to the patients that both eyes are bandaged rendering them temporarily blind. Tell them you will stay with them. Continue talking to the patient. After the eyes are bandaged stay with the patient and maintain body contact. A hand on the patient's arm will be reassuring.

If the patient is unconscious, close their eyelids. Drying of these tissues may damage the cornea and cause blindness. Tears constantly bathe the eyes to provide moisture and lubrication. Damage often occurs when this necessary fluid is not present on the eye.

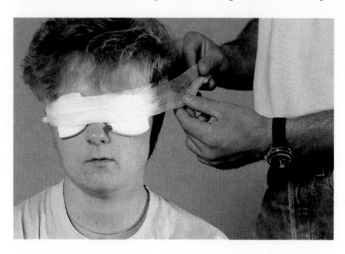

Figure 8-18. Dressing for an injured eye.

SUMMARY

All injuries to the head require airway maintenance, control of bleeding, and protection of the nervous system. Airway maintenance may be difficult, especially with injuries to the face or cheek. Those injuries involving the eyes require careful bleeding control and gentle bandaging to protect the vitreous fluid in the eye. Most bleeding is from the eyelid. Always bandage both eyes since they work together and close the eyelids of the unconscious to prevent drying of the cornea. Control bleeding and remove only those penetrating objects in the cheek if bleeding cannot be controlled and an airway maintained.

Injuries to the spine involve stabilization of the spinal column. Do the muscles have tone? Is the chest rising and falling with each breath? Are there involuntary muscle contractions or is there deformity, muscle spasm, or prominence to any spinal segment? If any of the preceding conditions exist, suspect spinal damage and protect the patient accordingly. Lifesaving actions, if required, must come first, but always protect the spine as much as possible. Airway management and sufficient breathing are always priorities for the First Responder. *Do not* move a patient with a spinal injury unless both your life and the patient's are endangered by uncontrollable circumstances at the scene. Patients suspected of spinal injury must always be secured to a firm device such as a backboard. These patients must be splinted from head to foot on a firm surface with their neck secured with a firm device.

INJURIES TO THE CHEST, ABDOMEN, AND GENITOURINARY ORGANS

CHAPTER

9

KEY CONCEPT AND SKILLS

By the end of this chapter, you will be able to:

❋ Describe an external or internal injury to the organs in any of the following areas:

Chest

Abdomen

Genitourinary organs

❋ Describe the proper care of injuries to the genitourinary regions.

KEY WORDS

Absorbent Material – Substances that take up fluids or gases.

Flail Chest – A condition in which two or more ribs are fractured in two or more places.

Great Vessels – The major conduits of the circulatory system, e.g., the aorta.

Hemothorax – Blood in the thoracic cavity.

Multitrauma Dressing – A large, absorbent material used to cover an injury of extensive size, e.g., chest.

Paradoxical Respiration – A section of the chest wall that moves in the opposite direction of respiration.

Peritonitis – Inflammation of the lining of the abdominal cavity produced by bacteria or irritating substances introduced into the abdominal cavity by penetrating wounds or perforation of an organ.

Pneumothorax – Collection of air or gas in the pleural space.

INJURIES TO THE CHEST

The chest is formed by the rib cage and the diaphragm, with one outlet, the trachea (Figure 9-1). Any trauma that affects the continuity of the chestwall, airway tubes, or alveoli (air sacs) will restrict the patient's ability to exchange air.

You should always consider the possibility of damage to the heart and great vessels when the chest is injured. Trauma to the internal organs of the chest can occur with or without external marks on the chest.

When the airway passages or air sacs are ruptured during injury, the lungs collapse, causing air to be trapped in the chest. This pressure can increase with breathing and compress a lung. The trapping of air in the chest cavity outside the lung is known as *pneumothorax*. Since the lung area is extremely vascular, massive bleeding may occur with lung damage. The presence of blood in the chest cavity is called a *hemothorax*.

As a First Responder, you should be able to identify signs of chest injury. The most common signs of chest injury include:

* Difficult breathing
* Pain in the chest at the site of the injury
* Pinpoint pain in the chest at the site of the injury, particularly during inhalation
* Uneven chest expansion (flailed chest)
* The patient is spitting or coughing up blood, usually bubbly, pink, or bright red in color.
* Rapid, weak pulse
* Lowered blood pressure
* Cyanosis
* Open chest wound
* Trauma

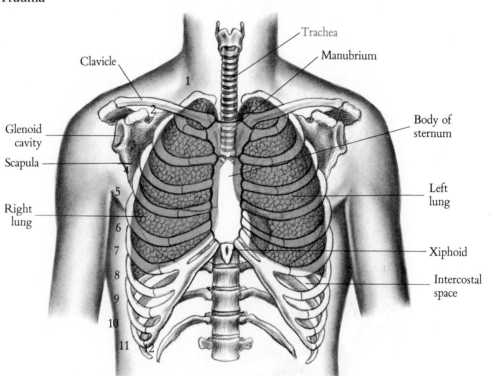

Figure 9-1. The respiratory system. (From Seidel, et al.: Mosby's Guide to Physical Examination, St. Louis, 1987, The C. V. Mosby Co.)

Rib Fractures

Ribs are commonly fractured when the chest is injured. The most common symptom of rib fracture is pain at the fracture site during inhalation. If a fracture of the rib is suspected you should:

✳ Question the patient about how the accident happened.

✳ Question the patient concerning pinpoint chest pain.

✳ Survey the mechanism of the injury as discussed in Chapter 2.

✳ Ask the patient if the pain increases with breathing.

✳ Ask the patient to cough gently.

Most closed fractures involving one rib do not need special attention. The injured person automatically splints the injury by using the chest muscles around the fracture site and reducing the intake of air. However, underlying injury may also exist.

If a patient has multiple rib fractures, make them more comfortable by firmly attaching the arm of the affected side to the body with a sling and swathe as shown in Figure 9-2. Before tightening the swathe, ask the patient to exhale. If breathing difficulty occurs when the chest is bound, loosen the bindings slightly to allow better air exchange.

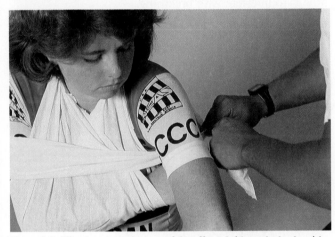

Figure 9-2. Firmly attach the arm of the affected side to the body with a sling and swathe.

When two or more ribs are fractured in two or more places, the chest is said to be *flailed*. This injury results in a condition known as *paradoxical respiration*. The section of the rib that is flailed moves in during inspiration and out during exhalation (Figure 9-3). The term paradoxical describes the chest wall motion. Paradoxical respiration is a serious condition where major quantities of air move but the flow is not sufficient to provide good air exchange. The pain associated with these injuries makes it difficult for the patient to breathe.

The signs and symptoms of flailed chest include:

* Sharp pain in the chest cavity
* Uneven chest expansion
* Shallow, rapid respirations
* Decreased breath sounds

Patients with these signs and symptoms need emergency help quickly and should be one of the first transported from the scene.

Make the patient comfortable until the patient can be transported by following these steps:

1. Secure a pillow or a *multidrama dressing* to the injured side of the chest to prevent paradoxical motion. Do not bind the chest so tightly as to interfere with breathing.

2. Place the patient on the injured side to help stabilize the flailed section.

3. Assist the patient in breathing. (Procedures for breathing assistance are described in detail in Chapter 4.)

4. If oxygen is available, administer it to the patient (refer to Appendix A).

This patient needs emergency care quickly and should be one of the first patients transported.

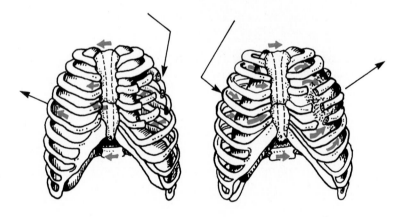

Figure 9-3. When two or more ribs are fractured in two or more places, the chest is said to be flailed. This results in a condition known as paradoxical respiration. The section of the rib that is flailed moves in during inspiration and out during exhalation.

Open Chest Wounds

Penetrating or sucking chest wounds occur when a foreign object is driven forcefully through the chest wall (Figure 9-4).

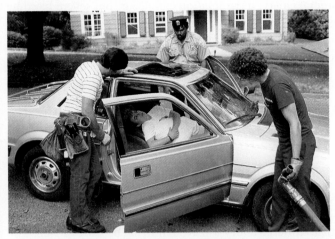

Figure 9-4. Penetration or sucking chest wounds occur when a foreign object is driven forcefully through the chest wall. A pillow may be used to splint the chest wall.

Examine the patient for entrance and exit wounds. An opening in the chest wall will severely impair breathing. The wound will suck air in when the patient inhales but will not expel air on exhalation. A sucking sound may be heard during inspiration.

Control of an open chest wound can be accomplished by sealing off the wound. Plastic wrap, your hand, petroleum gauze, or any other suitable many-layed, air-occlusive dressing can be secured to the wound. This allows air to pass in and out of the chest cage only through the trachea. The dressing should be sealed on three sides of the injury. Taping on three sides of the dressing makes an improvised flap-valve device and may prevent tension pneumothorax from developing (Figure 9-5).

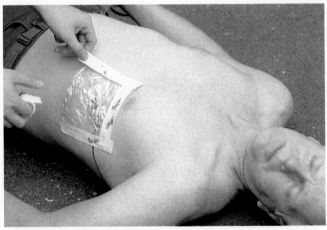

Figure 9-5. Taping on three sides of the dressing makes an improvised flap-valve device and may prevent tension pneumothorax from developing.

Severe complications can occur when a patient has a chest injury. For example, volumes of blood filling the chest cavity or collapsing one lung and rapidly occluding the other lung.

Provide emergency care to a chest injured patient as described below:

✳ Check the airway to be sure it is open

✳ If supplemental oxygen is available, use it (Refer to Appendix A).

✳ If necessary, perform rescue breathing as discussed in Chapter 4.

✳ Control bleeding and treat for shock as discussed in Chapter 5.

✳ Arrange for prompt transportation to the hospital.

INJURIES TO THE ABDOMEN

Two classes of organs are found in the abdomen, solid organs and hollow organs. The pancreas and liver are examples of solid organs, the intestine and gall bladder are hollow organs. If the contents of hollow organs are emptied into the abdominal cavity, inflammation can occur, but severe bleeding usually occurs with the rupture of solid organs.

Evaluating injuries to the abdomen is not easy. It is sometimes easier to recognize and treat open wounds. Closed wounds may prove more difficult since the outward signs may be minimal. The mechanism is the most important factor when evaluating the extent of injury. Signs and symptoms of abdominal injury include:

* Pain - Most common symptom. Ask the patient where the pain is located.

* Nausea - Ask the patient if they feel sick to their stomach. Patients with abdominal injury will often vomit or experience nausea.

* Localized abdominal tenderness - Palpate the abdomen gently for tenderness.

* Abdominal pain and distension may indicate internal bleeding. Look for distention and gently feel for rigidity.

* Difficulty in moving; the patient with abdominal injury will avoid moving because of pain. You may find the patient with knees drawn toward the chest (Figure 9-6). This maneuver helps reduce pressure on the abdominal area and makes breathing easier.

* Altered vital signs: low blood pressure, rapid pulse, and rapid, shallow respirations.

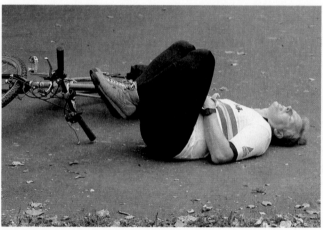

Figure 9-6 The patient with an abdominal injury may be found with their knees drawn toward the chest.

Emergency Care for Abdominal Injury

A closed injury should be treated by making the patient comfortable, if possible, and by monitoring vital signs. Maintain an open airway and treat the patient for shock.

In an abdominal injury, the only additional care is to prevent contamination. You can prevent contamination by bandaging the wound.

Do not attempt to reinsert any body parts that are protruding outside the abdominal cavity. Cover these parts with a moist sterile dressing if available. Do not apply a tight bandage because this will prevent blood from entering these organs and cause them to die. Any portion of the patient's body that is avulsed should be covered with a moist dressing and transported to the emergency care facility with the patient.

In either closed or open injuries there is a great possibility of vomiting. Keep the throat clear of vomited material and if there is no spinal injury, keep the head to one side, lower than the chest.

In suspected spinal injury, the body must be turned on its side as a unit.

GENITOURINARY INJURIES

Genitourinary injuries include injuries to the major urinary organs which include the kidneys, ureters, bladder and urethra. Also discussed are male and female genitalia.

Injuries to the Urinary Organs

The kidneys are well protected and injuries to them are rare. An injury usually results when a blunt or penetrating trauma has occurred. However, the most likely cause of injury to the kidney is a direct blow to the side of the body just below the rib. Patients with fractures of the lower rib cage, lower thoracic, or upper lumbar vertebrae may also sustain an injury to the kidneys. Signs and symptoms of kidney injuries include:

* Pain - Ask the patient how severe the pain is and where the pain is located. In addition to pain in the flank area, pain may sometimes be referred to in the groin.

* Bruising or lacerations in the flank area - Examine the back of the patient since evidence of kidney injury is hard to determine. Look for swelling and discoloration.

* Shock - Significant blood loss may occur from a kidney injury.

Signs and symptoms of injury to the urinary bladder, ureters, or uretha include:

* Severe pain in the abdomen - Ask the patient where the pain is located.

* Rigidity and tenderness of the abdomen - Gently palpate the abdominal area for rebound tenderness as urine may be present in the abdominal cavity.

* Inability to urinate - Ask when the last time was that the patient was able to void urine.

* Significant blood loss may occur from a kidney injury - Ask the patient if there has been any discharge of blood during urination.

* Shock - Signs and symptoms of shock may be present.

Emergency Care for Urinary Organ Injuries

The signs and symptoms of injury to the urinary bladder, ureters, or urethra include:

* Severe pain in the abdomen - Ask the patient where it hurts.

* Rigidity and tenderness to the abdomen - Palpate the abdominal area for rebound.

* Inability to urinate - Ask the patient if he or she has been able to void urine.

* Bloody discharge - Ask the patient or examine the genital area if necessary.

* Shock - The signs and symptoms of shock may be present. Evaluate the signs.

Before administering emergency care for urinary organ injuries, always take the patient's vital signs.

* Place the patient in a comfortable position.

* Continue to monitor the patient's vital signs.

* Arrange for transportation to a medical facility.

* Treat the patient for shock if the signs and symptoms for shock are present. If oxygen is available, administer oxygen as outlined in Appendix A.

* Ask the patient not to void, if possible.

Injuries to External Male Genitalia

Injuries to the external male genitalia can be extremely painful but are rarely life-threatening. Avulsion or tearing of the skin of the penis or scrotal sac can result from a number of mechanisms of injury. Some mechanisms, such as a kick in the groin, lacerations from sharp instruments, or when clothing gets caught in a power take-off, result in these types of injuries. When such injuries occur, cover the penis with sterile material and try to salvage any avulsed skin (Figure 9-7). If the penis is partially or completely amputated, immediate attention must be directed to control the bleeding. Direct pressure with a sterile dressing is usually effective. An effort should be made to recover the amputated part; it should be wrapped in a moist, sterile dressing, placed in a plastic bag, and transported in a cooled container.

If there is an impaled instrument or object in the urethra, do not manipulate or attempt to remove it; secure the organ as found. A diaper-type dressing will usually suffice.

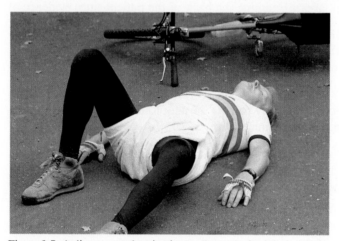

Figure 9-7. A diaper-type dressing is usually used with injuries to the male genitalia.

Injuries to the Female Genitalia

The uterus, ovaries, and Fallopian tubes are internal organs. They are subject to the same kind of injuries as other internal organs. Injuries to the internal female genitalia are rare because of their protection by the pelvis. If the pelvis is bruised or fractured, injury to the female genitalia should be suspected. The force involved that fractures the pelvis may injure the bladder, uterus, or Fallopian tubes. Many times childbirth causes injury to the surrounding vaginal tissue.

Injuries to the external female genitalia (vulva, clitoris, and lips) can involve many types of soft tissue injury and are very painful.

Emergency Care for Female Genitalia

As a First Responder, you will not be able to treat injuries to the internal female genitalia except for the management of shock. If open injuries exist, emergency care is like that for any other similar injury. Cover the area with a sterile multitrauma dressing and arrange for immediate transport to a medical facility, administer oxygen if it is available.

Injuries to the external female genitalia are painful and can involve many types of soft tissue injury. Emergency care involves use of compresses, direct pressure to control bleeding and use of diaper-type dressings to hold dressings in place. If an instrument or object is impaled in the vaginal opening, never attempt to move or remove it.

SUMMARY

Injuries to the chest may affect the injured person's ability to breathe or cause major blood loss within the chest cavity. Whenever the abdomen is injured, severe bleeding or inflammation can be caused by the spillage of stomach and intestinal contents into the abdominal cavity.

Patients having injuries in the abdomen or pelvic area should be transported to a medical facility. Care for soft tissue injury remains the same as with other areas of the body. Pain in the torso will usually reduce the patient's ability to breathe. Always remember to continually monitor these patients to assure sufficient air exchange.

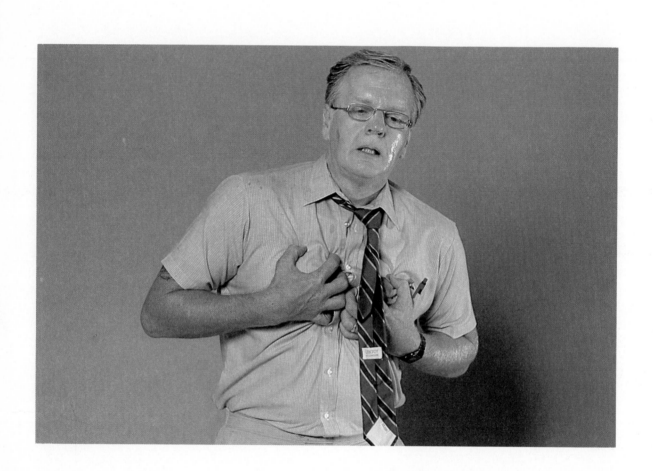

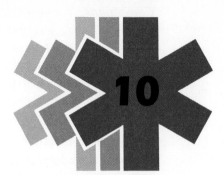

MEDICAL EMERGENCIES

KEY CONCEPTS AND SKILLS

By the end of this chapter, you will be able to:

✳ Recognize and describe the basic treatment for a patient exhibiting the signs and symptoms of a stroke.

✳ Recognize and describe the methods to protect the patient with either local or generalized seizures.

✳ Recognize and describe the proper treatment for a person displaying the signs and symptoms of the following:

Asthma
Bronchitis
Emphysema
Hypoventilation
Hyperventilation
Angina
Heart Attack
Congestive heart failure
Hypoglycemia
Diabetes (hyperglycemia)
Stroke (cerebrovascular accident – CVA)

KEY WORDS

Acetone – A colorless, fragrant liquid that is found in small amounts in the urine. In diabetics this acetone is found in larger quantities.

Angina Pectoris – Chest pain often related to exercise, emotional stress, or exposure to extreme cold.

Arteriosclerosis – Build up of fatty acids in the bloodstream. Cholesterol is one of these fats.

Asthma – Condition causing the air tubes of the body to constrict.

Breath Minute Volume – The normal amount of air exchanged per minute by the average adult. This normal amount is equal to about 6 quarts of air.

Bronchitis – An infection of the bronchial tubes causing a chronic, productive cough.

Carpopedal Spasms – Cramps of the hands and/or feet.

Cerebrovascular – Relating to the vascular system and blood supply of the brain.

Coma – A prolonged unconscious condition.

Congestive Heart Failure (CHF) – The heart's inability to pump effectively and maintain adequate blood flow.

Convulsions – A sudden and violent contraction and relaxation of a group of muscles.

Cyanosis – A bluish condition of the skin. Usually appears around the mouth, fingertips, ear lobes, and the lining of the eyelids. May extend to the face, hands, feet, ears, and even the entire body. Caused by reduced oxygen content in the patient's blood.

Diabetes – The failure of the body to produce enough insulin for proper sugar metabolism.

Edema – An abnormal displacement of fluid into tissues presented as swelling.

Elevated Temperature – A body temperature above the normal temperature of 98.6 °F (37 °C).

Emphysema – A chronic pulmonary condition characterized by the alveoli losing their elasticity.

Enzyme – A product that serves as a catalyst. It causes a reaction to take place without becoming involved or being changed in the process.

Epilepsy – A seizure condition for which the cause is not really known.

Extracellular – Occurring outside a cell or cell tissue or in the cavities between cell layers or groups of cells.

Heart Attack – Death of heart muscle due to occlusion of the blood vessels on the heart. Sometimes called an infarction.

Hypertension – High blood pressure. Normal blood pressure for an average adult is 120/80. Systolic pressure of 150 and diastolic pressure over 100 are considered hypertensive.

Hyperventilation – Rapid breathing. Any rate about 20 breaths/min. is considered hyperventilation, but 30 breaths/min. is really the start for this condition.

Hypoventilation – Insufficient air exchange due to slow or occluded breathing; a rate of less than 6 is considered hypoventilation.

Intercellular – Space within the cells.

Ischemia – A decreased blood supply to a body part or organ.

Metabolism – The chemical changes in living cells that provide energy for vital body processes and activities.

Occlusion – A blockage.

Reyes Syndrome – Swelling of the brain caused by infection. Usually occurs in children. This disorder is often fatal.

Seizure – See Convulsions.

Stroke – A cerebrovascular accident (CVA). A rupture or blockage of a blood vessel in the brain that may cause a patient to slip into a coma or die.

CEREBROVASCULAR ACCIDENT (STROKE)

As discussed in Chapter 8, the brain is protected by the skull which allows very little space for swelling. Certain portions of the brain control particular functions. For example, the midbrain regulates blood pressure, breathing, temperature, and all other basic functions. The remainder of the brain allows us to talk, walk, and sense the world around us. The control centers responsible for those less life-saving functions are located toward the surface of the brain (Figure 10-1).

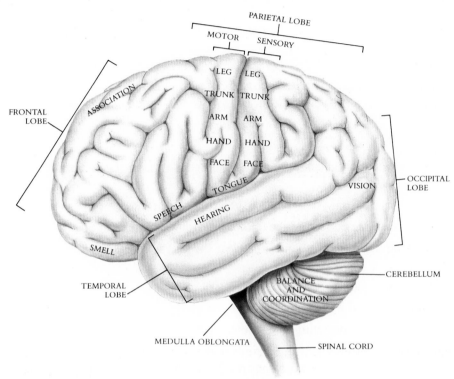

Figure 10-1. Functions located throughout the cerebral cortex. (From Raven, P.H. and Johnson, G.B.: Biology, St. Louis, 1986, The C.V. Mosby Company.)

Once a portion of the brain is injured, this segment may die. When brain cells die, they are not replaced. When portions of the brain die, the bodily functions controlled by that portion of the brain cease to function.

Any incident resulting in a loss or decrease of circulation to the brain may bring on a *cerebrovascular accident* (stroke). There are two types of stroke that primarily affect the brain. The first type occurs gradually as deposits block the blood supply to the brain. This gradual bleeding is called *arteriosclerosis* and is a normal process of aging. The buildup of fatty products like cholesterol block the flow of blood to the brain.

The second type of stroke occurs rapidly and is usually caused by the rupturing or sudden blocking of one of the important blood vessels to the brain tissue. Fatty deposits may break loose from the walls of an artery. When this deposit reaches an area in a blood vessel that is too small, it blocks the affected vessel. One of the end results of high blood pressure (also called the "silent killer") is the rupturing of one of the blood vessels of the brain. Blood leaks out into the surrounding brain tissue causing swelling and death to the brain cells.

The signs and symptoms of stroke are basically the same regardless of their cause. The signs include:

* Inability to speak or form words, e.g., slurred speech

* Paralysis (usually of one side of the body)

* Altered consciousness

    Memory loss
    Disorientation

* Headache

* Visual disturbances

* Seizures

A stroke may present with any of the above signs and symptoms.
Occlusive strokes may also occur suddenly or following a sudden headache.

EMERGENCY TREATMENT FOR STROKE

Care for a stroke victim should be administered in a gentle and caring manner. Make the patient as comfortable as possible.

* Protect the airway from foreign objects, the tongue and saliva.

* If possible, place the patient on the affected side and maintain an open airway.

* Constantly monitor breath sounds and clear the airway if any gurgling or snoring noises are heard.

* Keep the patient warm.

* Administer oxygen if it is available.

* Arrange careful transportation to a medical facility.

The major causes of seizures are trauma, infection, and high body temperature. The cause of the seizure may not be known. A head injury may result in seizure activity. Most seizures caused by fever are the result of an infection, but may also be the result of a tumor in the temperature control section of the brain. Epileptic seizures are caused by nerve disorders and require slightly different emergency treatment.

Temperature-Induced Seizures

Most seizures (convulsions) caused by elevated body temperature can usually be controlled. Aspirin or other antitemperature medicine should not be used. Studies indicate these drugs either mask or possibly preclude Reye's Syndrome. Reye's Syndrome is an often fatal disorder of brain swelling and pressure.

Temperature induced seizures (104 °F., 40 °C) in adults are usually caused by an infection involving the brain or a tumor in the area of the brain that controls body temperature. Temperature reduction is necessary to protect the patient from further brain damage. However, as in children, you should not use aspirin or other antitemperature medicine. Several other methods for reducing body temperature may be used for both children and adults:

* Remove as much clothing as possible.

* Bathe the patient in tepid water (86 °F, 30 °C).

* Do not cause the patient to shiver; this causes the body to hold more heat.

* Maintain an open airway on all patients with impaired consciousness as described in Chapter 4.

* Arrange transportation for the patient to a medical facility as soon as possible.

Epileptic Seizures

There are two primary types of epileptic seizures: major or mild.

Major seizures usually involve the patient's entire body, such as muscular contraction, respiratory impairment, and end in a period of altered consciousness. The patient may be unable to answer any questions for periods up to 4 hours following the seizure. A major seizure may cause the patient to fall and injure themselves. The only sign or symptom you may find is an unconscious patient who has fallen and is unable to answer any questions.

Mild seizures are sometimes not noticed by anyone, even the patient. They may range from a few seconds of blank staring to a minor twitching of specific body areas.

Treatment of an epileptic seizure is limited to the following:

✳ Protect the patient from bodily harm, e.g. falling down.

✳ Do not restrain the patient.

✳ Reduce body temperature if necessary.

✳ Maintain the airway of all unconscious patients in their post seizure state as described in Chapter 4.

✳ Do not question the patient immediately following the seizure.

✳ Look for a medic alert tag or similar card.

✳ Patients with major seizures should be seen in a medical facility as soon as possible.

RESPIRATORY EMERGENCIES

As discussed in Chapter 4, the respiratory system consists of three distinct sections:

1. Tubular section (dead space)

   ✳ Nose - heats, cools, moistens, dries, or otherwise climatizes and purifies the air to be received in the lungs.

   ✳ Mouth - secondary external organ for accepting air for the lungs. The mouth does not have the purifying or climatizing characteristics found in the nose.

   ✳ Larynx - voice box or "Adam's apple."

   ✳ Epiglottis - the flap protecting the opening to the lower airway.

   ✳ Trachea - a thick-walled tube connecting the voice box with bronchi.

   ✳ Bronchi - tubes that conduct air between the trachea and the alveoli (air sacs). These tubes continue to divide until each ends at a tiny air sac (alveolus).

2. Air exchange portion

   ✳ Alveoli (air sacs) - each lung contains millions of these tiny thin-walled sacs that look like clusters of grapes. These thin-walled sacs allow air (or specific components of air) to diffuse across their walls into and out of the bloodstream.

   ✳ Alveolar capillaries - very small blood vessels wrap around each alveolus, conducting blood in such a manner that each cell is forced to pass single file by the alveolus. They line up like tank cars to pass off waste or receive oxygen. A small amount of water also passes through this membrane. This water is then conducted out of the mouth and nose. This moisture (insensible water) causes vapor when one breathes out.

3. Internal respiration portion

✱ Red cells - blood cells responsible for transporting oxygen throughout the body. When oxygenated, these cells are bright red, giving arterial blood its characteristic red color. Venous or unoxygenated blood has a bluish cast.

✱ Plasma - the liquid portion of blood. Plasma is the transport medium. It moves the white and red blood cells in the blood stream to each cell.

There are several kinds of respiratory emergencies and treatment for each of them differ as do the causes. Major kinds of respiratory emergencies include:

✱ Hypoventilation - when the air exchange is less than that required to support normal bodily functions.

✱ Hyperventilation - when the exchange of air is rapid causing large amounts of carbon dioxide to be removed from the body.

✱ Asthma - caused by the constriction of the air conduction tubes to the lungs.

✱ Bronchitis - a chronic, productive cough that is usually caused by an infection of the patient's bronchial tubes.

✱ Emphysema - a chronic obstructive pulmonary condition that continues to worsen until the patient can no longer move enough air in and out of the lungs to support life.

Hypoventilation

An average adult patient, at rest, moves about 6 quarts of air every minute into their lungs. The volume increases or decreases with body needs. When hypoventilation occurs, the net result is a build-up of waste gases not only at the cellular level, but also within the entire body. This type of buildup can also be caused by insufficient oxygen in the air that is exchanged by the lungs.

Signs and symptoms of hypoventilation include:

✱ Slow or rapid breathing (less than 6 breaths/min or greater than 30 breaths/min).

✱ Extremely shallow breathing.

✱ Cyanosis (a blue color seen in the fingernails and mucosa).

The causes of hypoventilation include:

✱ Injury to the chest wall.

✱ Restriction of the trachea, bronchioles, or bronchi, e.g., asthma.

✱ Loss of elasticity of lung tissue (chronic obstructive pulmonary disease).

✱ Anatomical or foreign body (mechanical) obstruction of the upper airway.

✱ Atmosphere not conducive to good breathing as when toxic gases are present.

Perform the following 5 steps when caring for a patient suffering from hypoventilation:

1. Remove the patient from the toxic atmosphere.

   CAUTION: Toxic atmospheres are also dangerous to First Responders.

2. Clear the airway of any obstruction using the Heimlich maneuver as described in Chapter 4.
3. Perform rescue breathing as described in Chapter 4.
4. If oxygen is available, administer it to the patient as described in Appendix A.
5. Perform chest wall stabilization as shown in Figure 10-2.

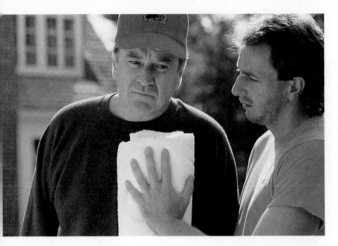

Figure 10-2. Chest wall stabilization.

Hyperventilation

Large amounts of carbon dioxide are removed from the body when a patient breathes rapidly. The normal drive to breathe is the result of the presence of high amounts of carbon dioxide in the blood stream. The body reverts to a secondary drive when too much carbon dioxide is exhaled. During this changeover from the primary to the secondary drive, the patient will continue to breathe faster and faster (40-50 respirations/min) until they become unconscious or stop breathing. This unconscious period may last for 3 or 4 minutes. After a balance is obtained, the patient will breathe normally again.

Between the onset of hyperventilation and unconsciousness, the patient will experience these classic signs and symptoms:

* Tingling around the mouth and nose.

* The nose turns fiery red. This condition is called the "clown's nose."

* Nasal flaring.

* Tingling of the hands and arms.

* Cramping of the hands and feet (carpopedal spasms).

* Extreme anxiety.

A person rarely dies from hyperventilation, but the condition may be caused by one or more extenuating circumstances. The major causes of hyperventilation include:

* Blood loss

* Diabetes

* Emotional crisis causing anxiety

A person cannot die from holding their breath, unless other more serious conditions mimic hyperventilation. The patient will not die from simply breathing rapidly.

If the patient is breathing rapidly following trauma or if any of the signs of internal bleeding are present, do not suspect hyperventilation. Rather, treat the patient for the appropriate trauma such as internal injuries. Loss of red blood cells causes a person to breathe faster to provide more oxygen to the cells. (Deep sighing breathing does not require rebreathing techniques.)

The following procedure explains treatment for hyperventilation. Using a small paper bag, mold the paper bag around the patient's mouth and nose so that no air leaks around the opening as shown in Figure 10-3. This will trap any carbon dioxide and re-establish the gas balance. In suspected or actual trauma patients, *administer* oxygen. *Do not* use the paper bag technique.

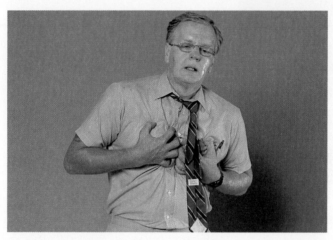

Figure 10-3. A hyperventilating patient.

When the balance of internal gases is restored, the patient will regain sensation in the hands, feet, and around the mouth. The breathing rate becomes slower. Most hyperventilation is initiated by an anxiety reaction. This reaction is usually caused by stress and relieved by rest and relaxation. If the balance of gases is not restored within 3-5 minutes, and the patient does not slow his or her breathing rate, treat the underlying cause. Anxiety-induced hyperventilation will correct itself within 5 minutes.

Asthma

Asthma is caused by constriction of the air conduction tubes to the lungs. It may be triggered by an allergic reaction to some stimulus or may be of psychogenic origin. Air cannot effectively pass through the air tubes when they are reduced in size by muscular spasm. Asthmatic spasms usually occur when the patient attempts to exhale. This condition causes the patient to trap waste gases at the alveolar level. They then struggle to push air out and usually become anxious. More children than adults have asthma and most outgrow the problem.

Signs and symptoms of asthma include:

✻ History of asthma in the patient's family

✻ Difficulty in breathing

✻ Wheezing

✻ Anxiety when the patient is breathing

✻ Fast heart rate

The following care should be provided for the asthma patient:

✻ Reassure the patient.

✻ Ask the patient if there is a history of asthma.

✻ Look, listen, and feel for air exchange if the patient is having difficulty in breathing.

✻ Listen for noisy breathing.

✻ Assist the patient in taking their medication. Many asthma patients trigger an attack by taking too much medication. When this occurs, additional medication will usually make the attack more severe. Most asthma medications work quickly and are short acting. Providing support is the most important step while initiating a call for medical help. Follow the local medical protocols when treating the asthmatic patient.

✻ Place the patient in a comfortable position.

NOTE: Asthmatic patients breathe better sitting upright.

Bronchitis

The patient suffering from bronchitis will have a chronic, productive cough, that is usually caused by the patient's smoking, exposure to industrial pollutants, or germs. Bronchitis is seldom a problem for the First Responder. Occasionally a person with this disorder coughs so violently that they exchange an insufficient amount of air.

The signs and symptoms of bronchitis include:

✻ Breathing difficulty

✻ Wheezing in inhalation and exhalation

✻ Productive cough (yellow and green mucus)

✻ History of smoking

Steps may be needed to assure adequate air exchange. Make the patient comfortable and activate the EMS system. If oxygen is needed and available, administer it as described in Appendix A. Place the patient in a comfortable position to assist more effective breathing.

Emphysema

Chronic obstructive pulmonary conditions continue to worsen until the patient can no longer move air in and out of the lungs to support life.

The primary stage of emphysema is evidenced by the following signs and symptoms:

✳ The patient appears pink and puffy looking

✳ The patient's chest is large and barrel shaped (Figure 10-4)

✳ The patient must puff to breathe

✳ There is a shortness of breath

✳ The patient has a history of smoking or has worked in an environment that produces toxic wastes, e.g., a coal mine or living in a city with poor air pollution control.

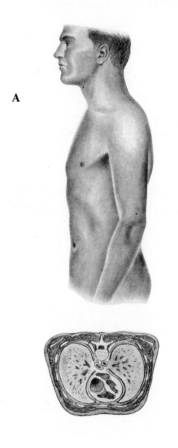
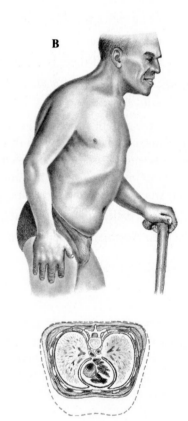

Figure 10-4. **A,** The normal chest. **B,** The chest of the patient with COPD. (From Seidel, H.M., et al.: Mosby's Guide to Physical Examination, St. Louis, 1987, The C.V. Mosby Company.)

An emphysema patient is sometimes referred to as a "pink puffer." As the condition continues to worsen, the body's breathing changes from measuring carbon dioxide in the blood to lack of oxygen. This elevated presence of carbon dioxide causes the patient to look pink and dusky in color.

A chronic condition of emphysema will continue to deteriorate over a period of months or years. The patient will experience extreme difficulty in exchanging sufficient amounts of air to support life. As this occurs, the patient begins to turn blue and swell from dependent edema. These patients slowly become known as "blue bloaters."

The following signs and symptoms appear in a patient in the final stages of emphysema:

* Cyanosis
* Barrel chest
* Extreme weight loss
* Shortness of breath, especially with exertion
* Cough
* Sitting up to breathe, leaning forward, and using the neck muscles to assist with breathing
* An oxygen source is usually present

If you administer oxygen, do so with extreme caution. Oxygen should never be withheld from the patient who needs breathing assistance. Lack of oxygen is the primary stimulus causing a patient with emphysema to exchange air. Any oxygen given to the patient may cause respiratory arrest. If this happens you must be ready to breathe for the patient.

Emphysema is a chronic condition for which there is no cure. Reassurance and comfort are the most important steps in caring for a patient with emphysema. Placing the patient in a sitting position to effectively support breathing will aid the patient.

CARDIOVASCULAR EMERGENCIES (HEART CONDITIONS)

Each cardiac cell receives blood from arteries originating from the aorta (Figures 10-5a and 10-5b). The two primary vessels (coronary arteries) are filled with blood when the heart is at rest (during diastole). Oxygen and nutrition are supplied to each cell from these arteries and waste products are

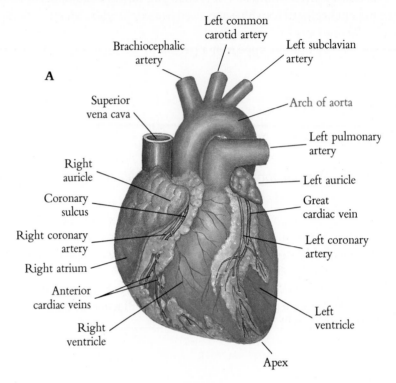

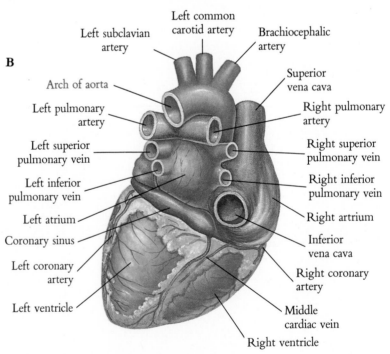

Figure 10-5. **A,** The anterior chest. **B,** The posterior chest. (From Seidel, H.M., et al.: Mosby's Guide to Physical Examination, St. Louis, 1987, The C.V. Mosby Company.)

moved by a matching system of veins. This unoxygenated blood then empties into the right atrium
upper chamber).

Heart tissue cannot store oxygen and is dependent on a constant supply of blood for nourishment
nd waste removal. Pain occurs at any site when it is deprived of oxygen. This lack of oxygenated
lood is referred to as ischemia. Occlusion, or narrowing, of the primary arteries are the two causes
hat reduce blood flow to heart tissue. The results of these two conditions will be discussed separately.

Chest Pain (Angina Pectoris)

Chest pain normally results from one of two conditions. Spasms of the blood vessels or fatty depos-
ts may build up in the walls of the arteries. Like rust in a pipe, these deposits reduce the flow of blood
o the heart cells (Figure 10-6). Tightness in the chest is usually initiated by stress and relieved with rest.
The patient complains of a heavy pressing sensation within the chest. This sensation may radiate to
he neck or arms.

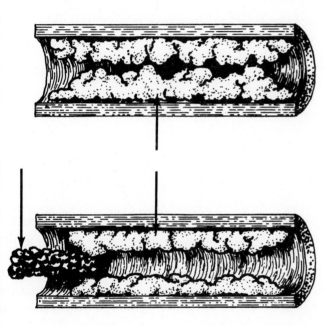

Figure 10-6. Coronary artery occlusion.

It is very difficult to differentiate angina from a heart attack. Angina does not cause lasting damage
o the heart muscle. A heart attack always damages heart cells. All chest pain patients should be seen
y a physician.

Many heart patients use a dilator drug. These drugs may include both the short-term drug nitro-
lycerine and the longer-acting Isordil. These drugs may be held under the tongue, placed on the body
or absorption through the skin, or taken by mouth. The tablets placed under the tongue appear to be
he fastest acting. These drugs dilate the arteries and allow more blood to reach the heart. They may
lso lower the patient's blood pressure. However, these drugs may cause the patient to have a head-
che since they also dilate the blood vessels in the head. This headache is usually gone within a few
ninutes. It is normally safe to give the patient additional dilator medication in the quickest acting
orm under the instruction of a doctor.

Care for the angina patient should consist of:

✳ Reassurance and comfort

✳ Assisting with the administration of dilator medication

✳ Keeping the patient still and quiet

✳ If necessary and available, administer oxygen as described in Appendix A.

All chest pain patients should be seen by a physician. Activate the EMS system. If the patient's condition is not relieved by two nitroglycerine tablets given 10 minutes apart, treat the person for heart attack as described in the following section. Local medical protocol must be followed.

Myocardial Infarction (MI) (Heart Attack)

When one or more of the coronary arteries becomes blocked, an area of heart muscle not receiving blood from the affected vessel dies. This involved muscle portion is said to be infarcted. Dead cells are never replaced. Just as scars form in other tissues of the body, scars form in the heart muscle. The heart muscle's ability to expand and contract is reduced. It is less effective.

The signs and symptoms of heart attack include:

✳ Chest pain - heavy, squeezing pressure unrelieved by any change in position, relief of stress, relaxation, or any other manipulation the patient may try; pain may radiate to other parts of the body; symptoms may often be confused with indigestion or heartburn.

✳ Shortness of breath.

✳ Weakness or tiredness.

✳ Sweating.

✳ Nausea and vomiting.

✳ Pallor.

✳ Irregular pulse (many persons die during the first few hours after a heart attack because of irregular beats.)

A patient may exhibit any or all of these signs during a heart attack. Some persons will even deny these signs and symptoms when they occur. The first sign of an attack may be sudden death (cardiac arrest). Many victims will display apprehension or fear of dying. "Silent" heart attacks occur in some people and do not cause recognizable signs or symptoms. Some people will exhibit the symptoms of indigestion. These symptoms include nausea, weakness, or dizziness. This variety of symptoms makes recognition of a heart attack difficult. If any doubt exists, the patient should be treated as a heart patient until a heart attack is ruled out. The skin color of a heart attack victim becomes like the pallor of fine china. This translucent color is usually significant.

> **CAUTION:** Biological death begins in 4-6 minutes after circulation and breathing cease. Basic life support must be administered immediately. The heart attack patient must be watched closely. Approximately 60% of heart attack patients die within the first 2 hours after the initiation of the attack. Sudden death or cardiac arrest may be the first sign that an infarct has occured.

Care and treatment of the heart attack victim includes:

✳ Provide basic life support if cardiac arrest occurs

✳ Have the patient sit still and comfortable

✳ Loosen the patient's clothing

✳ Do not allow the patient to assist in moving

✳ Monitor the patient's pulses every 5 minutes until help arrives

❋ Administer oxygen if available (Appendix A)

❋ Reassure the patient

❋ Activate the EMS system

Heart attack patients are more likely to live and return to useful work if they have received proper initial treatment. It is important to remember that you control the situation. If you act afraid, the patient will sense this feeling and become anxious. Remain calm.

Heart Failure

Since the heart has 2 chambers on each side, the circulation varies if the muscle on one side of the heart fails to function efficiently. When the muscle on the right side of the heart fails, the amount of blood being pumped into the lungs is reduced. The pressures rise within the heart's right chamber (atrium and ventricle) and back into the venous system of the body. This increase of pressure on the venous side causes the patient's body to swell (edema).

swell. This swelling may become severe in the daylight hours, but will recede during the night when the patient is sleeping in a prone position. This is *right-sided heart failure*.

Left-sided heart failure occurs when the muscles of the left side of the heart cannot efficiently move the blood to the body. The backup of blood occurs in the lungs when the left side fails. The result is usually pulmonary edema.

Both types of failure are usually caused by high blood pressure (hypertension) and may be secondary to a heart attack.

Right-Sided Congestive Heart Failure

The signs and symptoms of right-sided (congestive) heart failure include:

❋ Swollen ankles (dependent edema)

❋ Need to urinate several times a night

❋ Shortness of breath on exertion

As a First Responder you will usually not need to treat right-sided heart failure. Since it may be caused by a heart attack or emphysema, treat the patient for the cause. Occasionally the elderly patient will develop an irregular heart beat. This will cause the heart to lose its ability to pump effectively.

Persons with right-sided failure are given medicine to slow and strengthen their heart beat. The most common drug used for this purpose is *digitalis*. This drug is sometimes prescribed by one of the known trade names, *Lanoxin®* or *Digoxin®*. Assume any patient using these drugs is being treated to control heart failure.

Care for the patient with right-sided heart failure includes:

❋ Treating the cause (heart attack or emphysema)

❋ Loosening clothing (especially shoes)

❋ Administering oxygen (Appendix A)

❋ Activating the EMS system

Left-Sided Heart Failure (Pulmonary Edema)

High blood pressure or a heart attack affecting the left pumping chamber of the heart will cause left-sided heart failure. When pressure in the left ventricle rises, blood backs up into the lung capillaries. If this pressure reaches a sufficient level, plasma will spill over into the patient's air sacs (alveoli) causing the person to drown in their own fluids. Many other conditions can cause pulmonary edema, but the only one discussed in this chapter will be left-sided heart failure. This condition usually occurs rapidly and is often seen at night when the patient is sleeping.

The signs and symptoms of left-sided heart failure include:

* Patient's need to sleep sitting up using pillows or sitting up in chair.
* Complains of a smothering sensation when attempting to sleep lying down flat.
* Sudden onset of shortness of breath
* Wet, bubbly breath sounds
* Spitting up frothy, pink fluids
* Marked fear of dying
* Possible chest pains
* Possible high blood pressure
* Rapid pulse

Left-sided heart failure starts rapidly and is a serious emergency. The patient will literally drown in his or her own fluids without immediate rapid care.

Care for the left-sided heart failure patient includes:

* Providing basic life support if cardiac arrest occurs
* Sitting the patient up and attempting to make them comfortable
* Loosening any restrictive clothing
* Do not allow the patient to assist in moving themselves about
* Reassuring the patient
* Administering oxygen if available (See Appendix A)
* Activating the EMS system

> **NOTE: Left-sided heart failure is a serious emergency. The treatment is the same as that for a heart attack.**

DIABETES

Two primary conditions affect the diabetic patient: diabetic coma and insulin shock.

Diabetic coma occurs when the blood contains too much sugar (hyperglycemia).

Insulin shock occurs when the blood has too little sugar (hypoglycemia). Insulin is an enzyme produced in the pancreas. Insulin is essential for the cell to obtain sugar from the blood and use the sugar to produce energy.

Diabetic Coma (Hyperglycemia)

Diabetic coma occurs when the pancreas cannot produce enough insulin or when sufficient sites on the cell wall do not allow sufficient sugar into the cell. Each cell in the body needs insulin and sugar to produce the energy required for metabolism. Diabetic coma can be the result of three different causes:

1. Insufficient insulin available.
2. Two few receptor sites on the cell wall to allow enough sugar into the cell.
3. Too many complex starches eaten for the insulin present to process.

The onset of a diabetic coma is slow, usually occurring over several days or even weeks.

The signs and symptoms of a diabetic coma include:

* Confusion
* Sighing, deep respiration
* Warm, dry skin
* Headache
* Excessive thirst
* Loss of appetite
* Acetone breath (like the smell of fingernail polish)
* Excessive urine output
* Signs of infection, e.g., fever or wounds

Care for the diabetic coma include:

* Making the patient comfortable.
* If in doubt of coma or shock, administer sugar in the form of something to eat or drink (a candy bar or orange juice). This should only be done for a conscious patient. Watch the unconscious patient's airway closely.
* Activating the EMS system.
* Administering oxygen (See Appendix A).

Insulin, or a product causing the pancreas to secrete more insulin, are the only treatments for diabetic coma. Giving the diabetic coma patient sugar will not hurt them and may be life saving if hypoglycemia exists. Drugs causing the body to secrete more insulin are taken in pill form, while insulin must be injected into the body. As a First Responder you should try to recognize diabetic coma though the only care to be given is supportive until the patient can be taken to a medical facility.

Insulin Shock

Hypoglycemia (low blood sugar) occurs when the blood sugar level falls below the body's minimum requirement. This condition may be caused by any of the following:

* Overproducing of insulin in the pancreas
* An overdose of injected insulin
* Failure to eat properly
* The liver's inability to store a sufficient amount of sugar for reserve
* Overexercise

The body depends on insulin in relationship to sugar for proper production of cellular energy. Unlike diabetic coma, hypoglycemia occurs when too little sugar is present in the blood.

Any or all of the following signs and symptoms may be present in a hypoglycemic patient:

* Altered consciousness, perhaps bizarre behavior
* Combativeness, irritability
* Confusion
* Cold, clammy skin
* Weak and shaky feeling (uncoordinated)
* Extreme hunger
* Rapid weak pulse
* Visual disturbances
* Seizures

The hypoglycemic patient will do strange things when this emergency occurs. They have been known to take off all their clothes in public or to act as if they were intoxicated. Many patients have died in the drunk tank of jails because no one realized they had a medical condition and may not have been drinking alcohol. Restraint sometimes has to be used before the patient can be treated.

Administer care for the hypoglycemic patient as follows:

* Protect the patient from injury, restrain the patient if necessary.
* If the patient is conscious, administer sugar by mouth (use cola, orange juice, candy, etc.).

  CAUTION: The airway must be protected for all patients with altered consciousness, Do not allow the sugar to occlude the patient's airway.

  NOTE: One cannot always differentiate a diabetic coma from insulin shock. If you are in doubt, and the patient is conscious, treat them both alike by giving sugar or sweet products. The diabetic coma patient will not be harmed, but the insulin shock patient may have their life saved with rapid care.

SUMMARY

Medical emergencies are often harder for the First Responder to treat than trauma situations. The signs and symptoms are often not as obvious. The most important aspects of treatment include:

✻ Airway management

✻ Respiratory support

✻ Circulatory support

✻ Bleeding control

✻ Proper body positioning

✻ Body heat maintenance

The patient usually will be able to relate their symptoms. You must be able to recognize the specific signs of injury or disease. These signs and symptoms will then have to be categorized for severity. When in doubt always treat the patient for the worst possible condition. Support the patient, and assure their transportation to a medical facility.

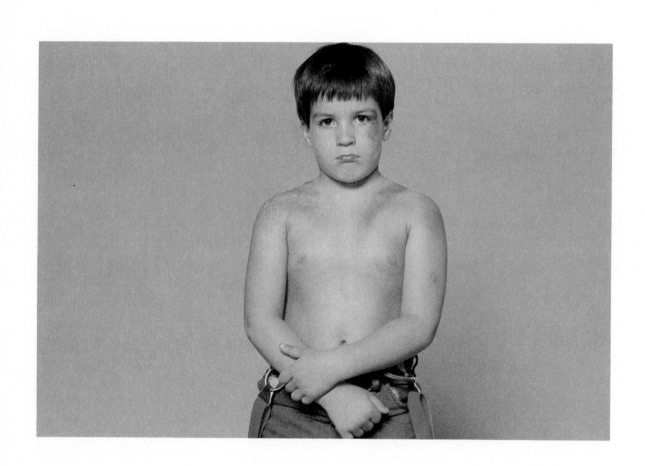

CRISES: PSYCHOLOGICAL RESPONSE TO CRISIS. ABUSE: CHILD, SPOUSAL AND ELDERLY; RAPE; DEALING WITH DEATH AND DYING

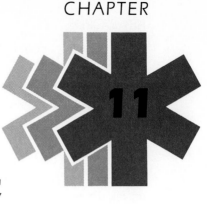

CHAPTER

11

KEY CONCEPTS AND SKILLS

By the end of this chapter, you will be able to:

✱ Describe the concepts of normal and abnormal behavior.

✱ Identify the following psychological and behavioral crises:
- Acute anxiety
- Phobias
- Depression
- Suicidal tendencies
- Rage
- Paranoia
- Disorganization or disorientation states

✱ Describe the factors identifying the potentially violent patient.

✱ Describe the emotional problems common to emergency medical situations.

✱ List the general questions that are helpful to assess a patient's state of mind.

✱ State the care procedures for victims of rape, child, spousal, or elderly abuse.

✱ Describe the concept of "active listening."

✱ Relate personal feelings dealing with death and dying.

✱ Differentiate between the usual and definitive signs of death.

✱ Identify the causes of death that may require the presence of the medical examiner.

✱ Describe the grief cycle.

✱ Describe the three general principles for patient management.

✱ Describe the specific principles for management.

KEY WORDS

Acute anxiety – Severe restlessness, shakiness, and the inability to concentrate or adjust to a recent stressful situation.

Behavioral crisis – Alteration of a person's response or inability to respond to his or her environment.

Child Abuse – The physical, sexual, or mental mistreatment of a young person between infancy and puberty.

Deep tendon reflex (DTR) – A brisk contraction of a muscle when its tendon is stimulated.

Delusions – False beliefs held by a person regardless of logic, fact, real experience, or environment that are inconsistent with the individual's own knowledge and experience.

Dementia – A progressive deteriorating mental state. May be caused by drug intoxication or a variety of organic diseases such as Alzheimer's diseases.

Dependent Lividity – The pooling of blood in areas of the body lower than the heart. Skin color becomes blotched and dark purple. This is a sign commonly seen following death.

Depression – A mental state characterized by dejection, a lack of hope, and absence of cheerfulness.

Deprivation – Mental isolation of an individual from normal emotional responses.

Diarrhea – The frequent passage of watery bowel movements.

Disorganization – Changes in a person's characteristics, causing the loss of most or all of a personality's distinctive features.

Disorientation – The inability to estimate direction or location, or to recognize time or people.

Disruptive functioning – The inability to adjust to a stressful situation, e.g., a mass casualty situation or the death of a loved one.

Emaciated – An excessive leaness caused by disease or a lack of nutrition.

Empathy – The ability to recognize and share insight into the feelings, emotions, and behavior of another person and their meaning and significance.

Incontinence – The inability to retain urine, semen, or feces due to the loss of sphincter control.

Insomnia – The inability to sleep, or sleep that is prematurely ended or interrupted by periods of wakefulness.

Malignant – Tending to become worse and produce death.

Malnourished – The lack of proper nutrition for the body or improper absorption and distribution of food.

Paranoia – A disorder characterized by fixed but growing delusions of persecution, harrassment, or mistreatment.

Phencyclidene hydrochloride (PCP) – A dangerous drug that causes extreme hallucinations and flashbacks that may cause the user to become violent.

Phenomena – Changes recognized by the senses that occur in an organ or vital function; objective symptoms.

Phobia – An abnormal fear. For example, claustrophobia is the fear of being in enclosed places.

Psychosomatic – Relating to the mind and body; indicating illnesses in which some portion of the cause is due to emotional causes.

Putrefaction – The decay of animal matter, especially protein associated with foul odors and poisonous byproducts.

Rage – Violent anger.

Reality – The awareness of external demands and adjusting to one's environment.

Reprisal – An act of revenge; regaining something given or causing pain in getting something back.

Rigor mortis – The rigidity of muscles that begins shortly after death.

SIDS – Sudden Infant Death Syndrome. The unexpected and sudden death of an infant that occurs during sleep. Also referred to as "crib death".

Socioeconomic strata – Various social and economic levels of society; for example, low, moderate, or high income families.

Suicidal tendency – A movement or action to take one's own life.

Symptomatic distress – The agony concerning a symptom.

Undernutrition – Lack of nutrition due to improper food intake or faulty absorption by the body.

Vindictive – Disposed to seek revenge; intended to cause anguish or harm to someone.

The clinical signs to assess respiration, heart action, blood pressure, and other vital life functions are usually easily determined and understood by the First Responder. Diagnostic assessment alerts the First Responder to life-threatening situations such as respiratory distress, massive internal hemorrhage, or cardiac arrest.

Mental crises are not as easy to recognize and diagnose. Except in the more extreme cases, indications of psychological or behavioral crises are not as easy to assess or manage. The First Responder cannot simply apply a gauze pad to a person that is having an acute anxiety attack. In fact, the situation is so complex that touching a patient may be hazardous, or a soft touch with your hand may help alleviate the situation.

Managing the person undergoing a behavioral crisis requires different skills. These skills involve carefully managing the patient and also dealing with patient/family/bystander relationships. In cases of behavioral emergencies, the skills of all responders may be pressed to the limit because of the often exaggerated and unpredictable responses of the patient and the time necessary for management. Besides the behavioral crisis, medical or traumatic complications may exist.

The normal care provided by a First Responder may be inefficient or ineffective. The behavioral crisis may be one of the few times a First Responder will have to exercise creative management of a situation.

Behavior is one of the most complex phenomena of human existence and may be defined as a reaction, adjustment, or response to the environment, both physical and psychological. In a behavioral crisis, a person's perception of reality may be changed or distorted. Events and things no longer exist in their usual frame of reference.

Behavioral crises take many forms, so the First Responder must have an understanding of the basic forms. It is not necessary to know a complex classification of psychiatric disorders — that is the responsibility of the mental health professional. However, the First Responder must recognize the major characteristics of psychological and behavioral crises.

Everyone has experienced some form of behavioral crisis. When that sinking feeling occurs in your stomach, when you feel sweaty, have palpitations, and are jumpy, when a loved one dies or you lose a patient, and you feel deeply saddened, you are in a crisis. Most people adjust to these circumstances. If a person does not adjust well, more unusual behavior patterns develop. As these modifications become more frequent and intense, a maladjustment pattern may become part of a person's behavior.

The following sections describe a variety of behavioral crises.

ACUTE ANXIETY

An acute anxiety attack is one of the most difficult psychological emergencies to describe. Acute anxiety is similar to fear but it is usually not related to any specific situation, location, or person. Many patients experiencing this reaction have difficulty identifying the cause.

Acute anxiety attacks occur when a person's capabilities (such as training or physiologic state) and the current demands overstimulate that person.

Some of the signs and symptoms that may help you assess this reaction are (Figure 11-1):

* Rapid pulse
* Rapid breathing
* Increased perspiration
* Dizziness
* Uneasy (queasy) feeling in the stomach
* Dryness of the mouth (rapid breathing)
* Tingling sensation in the hands and mouth
* Inability to swallow

Patients with acute anxiety are generally:

* Restless
* Fearful
* Tense
* Shaking

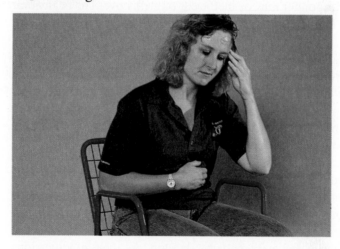

Figure 11-1. The anxious patient.

Anxious persons may be pondering, pacing, or complaining of bodily ills. They generally cannot concentrate. These patients often feel overwhelmed and their sense of time is extended — seconds seem like minutes, and minutes seem like hours.

A patient with an acute anxiety attack demands immediate care and treatment. It is not unusual for this patient's actions to cause others to become anxious. This patient may be pouting, screaming, or sitting in a cowering position. Unconsciousness is not uncommon if the anxiety attack is severe or prolonged.

Care for a patient with an anxiety attack by establishing rapport — showing warmth, genuineness, empathy — and trying to identify and clarify the focal problem.

PHOBIAS

A *phobia* is a fear of a situation or object. A phobia can be described as fear looking itself in the mirror. Phobias have been called the malignant psychological disease of the "what-ifs"; they generally result when a person directs anxiety toward a particular thing. It may be height, water, crowds, being in a closed place, animals, or any other object or situation imaginable.

A phobic patient will be (Figure 11-2):

❋ Anxious

❋ Reluctant

❋ Suspicious, depending on the particular phobia

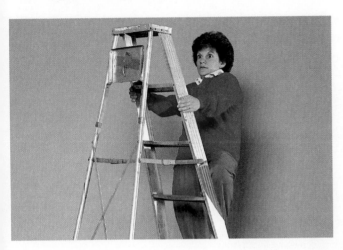

Figure 11-2. The phobic patient.

The phobic person may show an unnatural fear of what might be considered a normal activity such as walking down stairs.

Caring for this patient involves carefully explaining and rehearsing with the patient exactly what will be done and how it will be done. Explain to the patient that you understand. The primary goal is to calm these patients and assure them that you are there to help.

DEPRESSION

Depression is a mental state characterized by dejection, a lack of hope, and absence of cheerfulness. Depression takes two forms. Mild depression is the most common emotional disturbance in the United States. It is estimated that serious depression affects 1 in 5 persons sometime during their lives. The depressed patient may show some of the following symptoms (Figure 11-3):

* A general slowing down
* Sadness
* Hopelessness
* Extreme tenseness and irritability
* A tendency toward isolation from the environment
* Extreme agitation and unable to remain still
* Pacing, wringing the hands, or rocking may occur

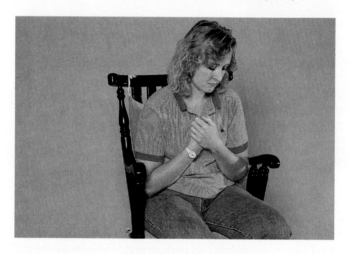

Figure 11-3. The depressed patient.

In desperation, this patient may strike his or her body against a hard object like a wall. In severe cases, the following symptoms may occur:

* Desire to be alone
* Depression often followed by insomnia
* Loss of appetite
* Loss of interest in sex
* Constipation
* Extreme feelings of worthlessness or guilt

Care for a patient who is depressed involves establishing contact and may require long and repeated efforts. It is important that only one responder be designated as the communicator. This allows the patient to place confidence and trust in one person. Care is directed to quietly talking to the patient. Ask questions to gain a common ground for communication. A goal of initial emergency care is support and help.

It is very important to determine if suicide is a danger. Some persons experiencing moderate and severe depression may consider suicide as the only "solution" to the pain. Separation from reality increases as depression worsens. There is a common fear that asking a depressed patient about suicide will cause him or her to think about or attempt to kill themselves. Experience has shown that patients are relieved when asked about their desire to die. Not asking can be a mistake!

SELF-DESTRUCTIVE PATIENT (POTENTIAL SUICIDE)

Consider suicide serious. A person threatening suicide is experiencing a crisis that appears unsolvable. Suicide is often a "cry for help." This patient is generally looking for someone who will listen (Figure 11-4).

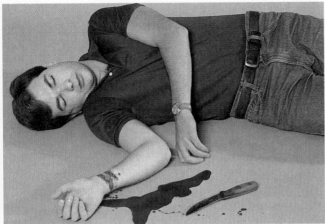

Figure 11-4. The self-destructive patient.

Assess the risk of suicide to determine the probability of success. These factors include:

* The seriousness of the intent

* The method

* The available means

* The specific plan

Trained personnel should remove dangerous objects from the patient. This must be done before "talking down" or other handling is attempted.

> **REMEMBER:** Consider the armed patient potentially homicidal as well as suicidal. Do not frighten or make the patient suspicious. Above all, do not jeopardize *your own life* or the lives of any members of your team. If a lethal weapon is involved, law enforcement intervention is needed.

Reaching a suicidal patient should be accomplished early, but do not attempt physical contact if the patient is conscious and wants to talk. Never stand directly in front of a door in case a weapon is fired. Leave all doors open behind you.

Special communication skills are required for dealing with a mental health crisis. These skills are even more important when you are involved with a potential suicide due to the imminent threat to life.

After the immediate danger has passed by talking down the patient, encourage him or her to discuss the situation. Ask, "What is wrong?" and, "Have you ever felt this way before?" Reassurance is needed to help this patient through *this* crisis. A responsible person should always be with a suicidal patient. Do not leave a suicidal patient alone.

Developing a relationship in a short time is important. Avoid using statements such as:

* "Oh, don't do that"

* "Don't pull the trigger"

* "Don't jump"

These statements challenge the patient and indicate that you may not understand.

A better response is, "I really hope you decide not to jump (or pull the trigger) because if you do, I won't have the opportunity to help you."

This statement indicates you want to assist in every possible way. *Do not dismiss* a seemingly minor event since it may be extremely important to the patient. The suicidal patient requires medical assessment.

> **REMEMBER:** NEVER LIE to a suicidal patient.

RAGE

Rage is an expression of violent anger. A person in a rage may create a disturbance, be hostile, or be physically aggressive and combative (Figure 11-5). These actions may be misdirected. The patient in a rage may be:

* Highly argumentative
* Insulting
* Challenging and armed for protection

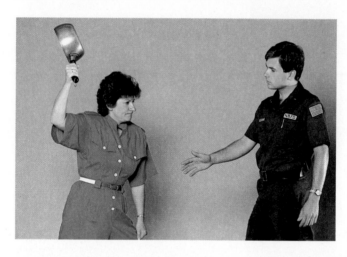

Figure 11-5. The raging patient.

The enraged person may bang on the wall and break or throw objects at the people trying to help. This patient is angry and ready to fight anyone. The patient in a rage will often resist attempts for assistance. These patients generally have sharply defined areas of "personal space." When this space is entered, the patient may feel threatened and react with fear of violence. Do not approach this patient "straight-on"; approach this patient at a 45-degree angle. Check to see if there is any object present at the patient's disposal that can harm you or bystanders. If so, call the law enforcement officials *immediately*.

It is important that First Responders identify themselves to reduce the patient's fear. The First Responder should be concise and honest when telling these patients what is expected. It is important that the First Responder not tower over the individual. Maintain eye contact but approach the patient in a nondefensive manner. Be careful to provide for means of exit.

PARANOIA

Paranoia is a disorder that is characterized by fixed but growing delusions of persecution. A paranoid person believes someone or something may be harmful. This patient is often (Figure 11-6):

* Overly distrustful
* Suspicious
* Seclusive
* Jealous
* Very uncooperative
* Hostile

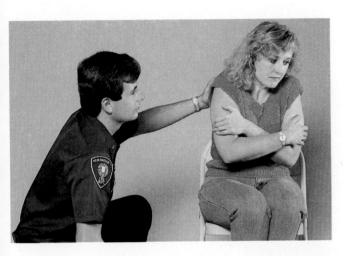

Figure 11-6. The paranoid patient.

Delusions may also be voiced. These patients feel singled out. They feel that someone is planning to harm them or that they are being spied on by "enemies." The First Responder must approach this patient carefully because a paranoid patient may feel that he or she is going to be harmed, and you are a suspect.

Again, First Responders must identify themselves and explain what they are trying to do.

REMEMBER: A paranoid patient's hostility and agitation may increase when a First Responder intrudes into his or her personal space, so be calm and friendly in your approach.

DISORGANIZED AND DISORIENTED PATIENTS

Disorganized and disoriented patients have lost some or all contact with reality. Normal lines of communication have broken down. These individuals may not be able to distinguish between voices, noises, sights, smells, or other perception, many of which are imagined. These patients may not be aware of their feelings toward other individuals and may be unable to distinguish what is really happening.

The disorganized patient loses the ability to distinguish between perception and fact. These patients often think that others can read their minds. They also think that if they wish for something hard enough, it will occur. Their world is often imaginary. They may be coherent or speak a "personal" language. Often these patients cannot understand why others misinterpret their current mode of speech.

Disorganization usually occurs slowly (Figure 11-7) and these individuals usually sense that something is wrong. They begin to lose contact with reality and are often aware that they are hallucinating or having delusions because their ability to function is impaired.

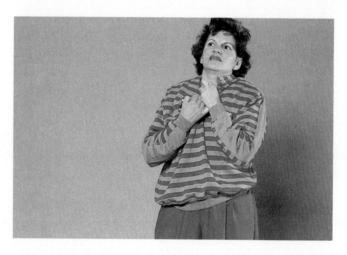

Figure 11-7. The disorganized patient.

As the disorganization becomes more complete and disorientation occurs, they lose the ability to distinguish between real and unreal; they often mistake fantasy for reality. Alzheimer's disease and dementia are examples of conditions that present as disorganized behaviors.

The disorganized or disoriented patient requires a structured but precise explanation of the care being rendered. This patient is unable to remain attentive; contact is often difficult. Repetition of simple, consistent, but firm, direction is necessary. Do not attempt to obtain a detailed history other than a name and address. Use simple statements to communicate with the disorganized patient. Ask simple questions and offer simple answers.

ASSESSING THE POTENTIAL VIOLENT PATIENT

First Responders encounter many violent patients. This may be due to:

✳ Drug overdose, for example, PCP

✳ Alcohol withdrawal

✳ Illness, such as hypoglycemia

✳ Head trauma

Four clues may help assess a patient's potential for violence. These are:

1. *Posture:* How is the patient sitting: is he or she sprawled limply in a chair? Is the patient relaxed or stiff and guarded? If the patient is sitting tensely, this may often be a sign preceding violent behavior (Figure 11-8a).

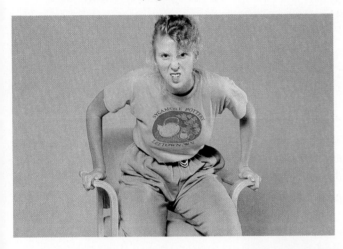

Figure 11-8a. Patient posture.

2. *Speech:* Is the patient's voice too loud or too soft? Is the voice level calm or strident? Very slow or very fast? Is the patient verbally threatening? The louder, more strident the voice and speech quality, the greater potential for violence (Figure 11-8b).

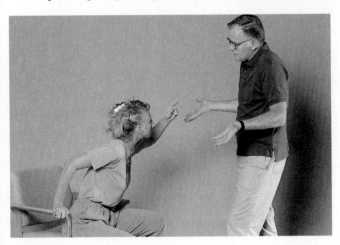

Figure 11-8b. Patient speech.

3. *Motor activity:* This may be the most important sign. What are the patient's movements? Are they coordinated, jerky, and awkward? Is the patient unable to sit still, or is he or she pacing about the room? Facial expression: are they flat, unexpressive, rageful, fearful, or elated (Figure 11-8c).

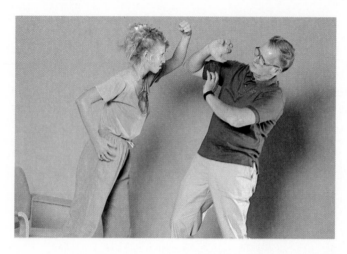

Figure 11-8c. Patient movement.

4. *History:* A past history of violent behavior is an important clue. If the family or patient states that he or she has been violent before, believe them (Figure 11-8d)! Information should be maintained by departments that can alert First Responders to such past occurrences.

These behaviors are all indicators of potential violence so be on the alert for them.

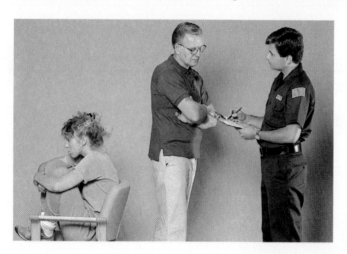

Figure 11-8d. Patient history.

THE EMOTIONAL EFFECT OF SUDDEN ILLNESS OR TRAUMA

An accident or sudden illness may affect everyone. Many individuals react by becoming disorganized, dazed, or overwhelmed by the situation. The aura of the emergency scene may cause many individuals to lose a sense of reality.

Typical concerns of patients are:

* Possibility of dying

* Pain and disability

* Loss or interruption of usual relationships or roles

* Nature and extent of care and further treatment

Some of the usual responses to injury or illness are:

* Psychological shock

* Disbelief

* Acute anxiety reaction

* Volatile emotional state

* Disrupted functioning

Trauma, as well as disease, can produce anxiety, disorientation, disorganization or paranoia. Head trauma, for example, can cause instant personality changes. Behavioral symptoms may be the only manifestation of physical condition. These symptoms may range from depression to violence.

The First Responder should recognize the signs and symptoms that accompany emotional crises:

* Anxiety, nervous behavior

* Shallow respiration

* Sharp chest pain

* Abdominal cramps

* Diarrhea

* Nausea or vomiting

Responding in the following manner will usually help the injured or seriously ill patient:

* Inform the patient who you are, what you or others are doing, and where the patient will be taken.

* Avoid negative comments about the patient's condition, like, "Oh, oh, he's going to…".

* Assure the patient that you will try to locate and notify the patient's family.

* At the scene (and during transportation, if you are involved) try to orient the patient to his or her surroundings.

* Be honest without shocking the patient, for example, "Yes, your injuries are serious, but here's what we're now doing . . . ".

* Provide hope, for example, "I'm not giving up on you, don't give up on me…". "I want to help you…will you help me?"

* Use discretion in relaying news to the patient about the death of a family member, passengers, victims, or others.

RAPE

Special management is required for any patient, either female or male, adult or child, who has been a victim of this violent crime. Your first duty is to assess the scene. Preserving evidence is important and will assist the law enforcement agency. Consider the following:

✱ Do not remove clothing and undergarments except as necessary to render care.

✱ Do not contaminate any involved areas by your examination.

✱ Do not permit the victim to shower or clean-up prior to medical exam or investigation by law enforcement officials.

✱ Do not intensively question the victim. Questioning should be done by a physician or others.

✱ Listen to the patient and cover him or her with a blanket.

Attending to the psychologic needs are important aspects of care. Due to your gender, you may not be the desired person to help.

Many law enforcement agencies have specially trained teams to deal with rape victims. The First Responder should ascertain the existence of such groups and activate them as soon as possible.

> **REMEMBER:** Alert the responding EMS agency of your findings. Notify the receiving hospital as well as the rape crisis team if one is available. It is advisable never to be alone with a patient in this condition. If you interview a rape victim, be sure to do so in the presence of other witnesses.

Carefully record any information the patient relates. If the patient has to urinate or defecate, collect the specimen and transport it with the patient.

CHILD ABUSE

Child abuse has existed since biblical times. However, it was not until the twentieth century that the battered child and spouse syndrome was recognized as a social and medical problem. States now have laws requiring the reporting of child abuse. Most of these laws provide immunity for those persons required to report such incidents. In some states it is a crime if you fail to report suspected abuse cases.

Most medical professionals are required to file reports of suspected abuse. First Responders should be familiar with statutory requirements existing in individual states. First Responders may not be required to file a report, but law enforcement officials and often firefighters must. Even if there is no statutory requirement for reporting, consult emergency department medical personnel or law enforcement officials to alert them of your suspicions.

It is estimated that there are 1.6 million children abused annually; of these 2,000 die. Two-thirds of the victims are under 3 years of age. In infants (1-6 months of age), abuse ranks as the second highest cause of death. Sudden Infant Death Syndrome (SIDS) is first. In children ages 1-8 child abuse is the second leading cause of death. Of the new cases of abuse reported each year, 5% will result in the death of a child. The death rate for a second occurrence can be as high as 50%.

Recognizing Abuse

The most serious cases of child abuse are easily recognized, but in mild or questionable cases diagnosis may be difficult. These cases are a great concern for the professional. Failure to recognize such cases may affect a state's ability to provide temporary or permanent caring in a safe environment for the child. Additionally, the opportunity to provide needed help to strengthen the family and make the home safe for the child may be missed.

Characteristics of the Abused Child The characteristics of the abused child are:

* Behavior inappropriate for age
* Excessive (or absence of) crying
* Exhibits fear (or absence) of adult authority
* Wary of physical contacts with adults
* Caters to the whims of adults
* Wears long pants or long sleeved garments
* Learning disabilities
* Habitual truancy or tardiness in school

The following are clinical signs of physical abuse and severe neglect:
Observe injuries inappropriate for the child's age and maturational level. Examples include:

* Fractures of the lower extremities in a child too young to walk.
* Burns caused by cigarettes (Figure 11-9a), which may show up as festering burn blisters, excavation marks from fresh burns, usually found on the palms, soles, and buttocks. The imprint left by a hot item such as a fireplace poker or iron (Figure 11-9b) may indicate abuse.

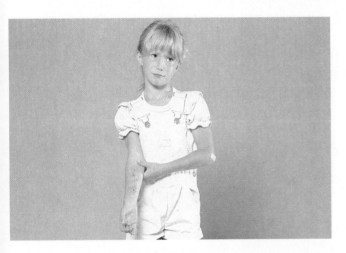

Figure 11-9a. Cigarette burns.

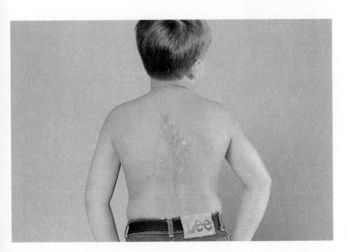

Figure 11-9b. Imprints caused by hot objects.

✱ Characteristic marks from slaps or bruises caused by a looped rope or electric cord (Figure 11-9c). For example, a gag tightly tied around a child's mouth as a punishment for crying will leave characteristic marks at the corners of the mouth.

✱ Watch for bruises or wounds in various stages of healing. This implies repeated exposure to trauma, especially if they are found in the head or neck region (Figure 11-9d).

✱ Malnourishment may also be accompanied by water deprivation. Observe for poor skin tone, abnormalities of the mouth and mucous membranes, abdominal distention, wasted buttocks, and untreated skin lesions. The malnourished child will look *emaciated*. This child's weight is usually below the average for children of their age.

✱ Be alert for signs of neglect. Look for evidence of more than "surface dirt," such as rarely changed diapers or ears, nose, and fingernails that are dirty due to neglect.

✱ Examine external openings and genitalia for unexplained tenderness or other evidence of trauma.

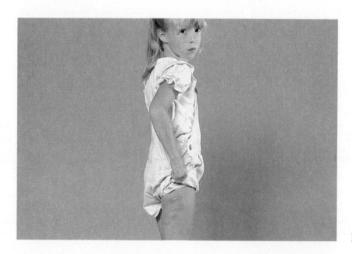

Figure 11-9c. Marks caused by an electric cord.

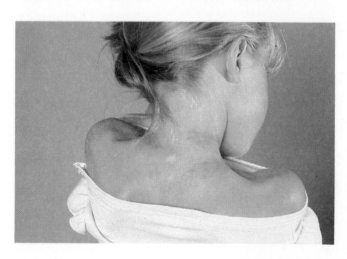

Figure 11-9d. Bruises.

Abusing Parents

Parents or other involved adults may lack emotional response and be noncommittal or unconcerned about the child's condition. They may be unconvincing about the child's injury. Contradictory explanations may be given if the parents are interviewed separately. Parents of abused children generally have unreasonable expectations and requirements for the child's age and developmental status. They may expect, for example, a young child to follow a rigid schedule for sleep and play that would ordinarily be typical for an older child. Abusing parents, who may have been abused themselves, are likely to believe that physical force is a reasonable way to control behavior.

Abusers Profile

The following list is a profile for child abusers:

* Not a homogeneous group: all socioeconomic strata have abusers
* Natural parents: 95% of the abusers
* Baby sitters: 4% of the abusers
* Mothers prone to physical abuse, neglect
* Fathers prone to sexual abuse
* Families in an isolated or military environment
* Military families living on a military base
* Families with financial problems
* Parents who are young and immature or that have problems
* Persons with a low tolerance for frustration
* Have a past history of abuse as children themselves

The Abused Child

Many abused children refuse to admit that abuse has occurred, especially when their parents are present. Questioning the child may produce fear of reprisal from the abusing parent. Abused children are often passive, accepting, and very frightened. They are normally not hateful or vindictive toward the abusing parent; in fact, as they grow older, they are likely to feel guilty about the parent's misbehavior and actively seek love and forgiveness from the abusing parent.

The First Responder should do the following if he or she suspects child abuse:

* Provide care for the injuries or trauma
* Identify possible child abuse
* Alert the appropriate authorities
* Recognize that it is important for the abused child to be seen by a physician

   REMEMBER: These acts alone will provide protection from abusive parents.

It is important that all First Responders findings be documented in writing and relayed to the receiving unit. The goal of management is to provide necessary care. This includes attention to primary life needs, caring for secondary injuries, and psychological support.

SPOUSE ABUSE

Fifty-two percent of all married women are thought to be victims of abuse or domestic violence. Abuse is found in all sectors of our society. Men are also abused, but the majority of victims are women. Most victims do not seek medical attention unless the injuries are life threatening. The battered spouse syndrome has some of the following characteristics:

* Repeated emergency room visits/EMS calls for "minor" injuries, and a history of being "accident prone"

* Soft tissue injuries: injuries to the back, stomach, breast area, and the head, especially where covered by hair (Figure 11-10a).

* Simple questionable explanations of injuries

* Psychosomatic complaints

* Pain, especially if chronic

* Suicidal gestures/attempts

* Depression

* Substance abuse

* Sexual abuse

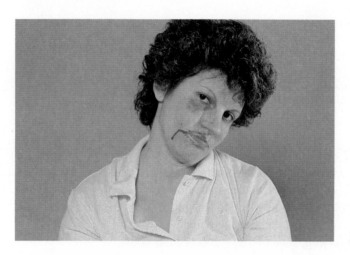

Figure 11-10a Spouse abuse.

Caring for the spouse abuse victim presents special problems for the First Responder. In addition to recognizing the presence of life-threatening problems, dealing with the emotional problems of the victim, the presence of children and possibly of the abuser himself, make this emergency care difficult.

The First Responders care for spouse abuse victims should:

* Support the airway, breathing, and circulation.

* Gather urgent medical information.

* Treat injuries.

* Provide psychologic and emotional support.

* Assure the safety of any children that are present.

* Contact the proper authorities

ELDERLY ABUSE

The elderly most vulnerable to abuse and neglect are those least capable of independent living. Many are frail and of advanced age (i.e., over 75), have chronic diseases, and are often physically and/or mentally impaired. The usual profile for elderly abuse is:

* The victim is over 65.
* Multiple chronic diseases or disorders present.
* The victim may have dementia.
* The victim may have insomnia and walk in his or her sleep and shout.
* Incontinence may be present.
* Dependent upon others.

Those who abuse or neglect usually fall within this profile:

* Household conflict, e.g., marriage problems.
* Marked fatigue.
* Unemployment.
* Financial difficulty.
* Substance abuse.
* History of being abused.

Assessment

Assessment of the abused and neglected elderly is not unlike those of other abused persons. Be alert if any of the following symptoms are found (Figure 11-10b).

* Bruises and welts on the body
* Cigarette, rope, twine, or chain burns.
* Lacerations and abrasions, particularly about the face.
* Head injuries: absence of hair or other indications of head beatings.
* Malnutrition.

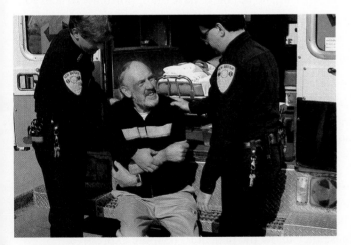

Figure 11-10b. Abuse of the elderly.

Emergency care is no different from that provided for similar cases. Basic life support must be provided before evaluating additional problems. Due to sensory loss and perhaps decreased mental alertness, it may take repeated questioning to get answers. A careful, respectful, and empathic approach is extremely helpful.

CRISIS MANAGEMENT - ACTIVE LISTENING

The First Responder must develop the skill of "active listening." Active listening helps to develop a rapport with a patient in a relatively short time (Figure 11-11).

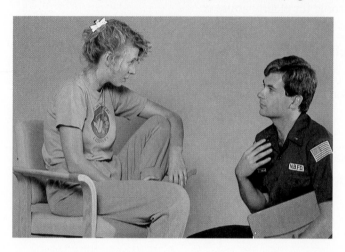

Figure 11-11. Active listening.

Active listening means being honest and open with the patient. Avoid any criticism, anger, or rejection. The First Responder should appear interested, self-assured, hopeful, and show *empathy* for the patient's situations.

Time is an essential factor and must be used to gain the individual's confidence. The patient may make statements such as:

✳ "No one cares about me."

✳ "Nobody gives a damn."

✳ "It's not worth going on; I'm going to jump."

✳ "I want to die."

An active listener responds with a statement such as:

✳ "Well, it sounds as though you are saying it's not worth going on, but I really hope you decide not to jump because if that is what you do, I will no be able to have the opportunity to help you."

This communicates that you are concerned and wish to help.

Assessment begins with open-ended statements such as:

✳ "What kind of problems have you been having?"

✳ "You seem to be down today."

✳ "You appear very angry."

These statements may lead to an open expression of feelings. When you make them, you must do so in a noncritical, nonjudgmental manner. Encourage the patient in this manner:

✳ Nod your head or say, "Uh-huh," "Yes," "I see," or "Go on."

✳ "Here's what I understand, am I correct?"

This technique is nondirective and helps continue communication. Avoid questions that can be answered simply "yes" or "no" except when assessing symptoms. Avoid "why" questions; instead try to use "how" and "what" questions because they allow the patient to be more expressive.

Provide support, reassurance, and demonstrate interest in the patient. Reassurance should be realistic and should not indicate that "everything is okay." It is not okay, otherwise you would not be there.

DEATH AND DYING

We rarely discuss death in our daily lives. Yet, in the public safety sector, death is encountered many times. Understanding the aspects of death is both personally and professionally important.

Death was once expected in American life. In earlier American history, when life expectancy was brief (compared to life expectancy today), death was more readily accepted. Most people had experienced the death of someone close to them. Today, as our life expectancy has dramatically increased, nearly two-thirds of all deaths occur among those 65 years and older. Nearly 60% of all deaths are attributed to heart disease and cancer. Today death occurs in a different setting. Death may occur suddenly or after a prolonged disease. The setting is often a long-term care facility, a hospice, or on the highway.

The First Responder may respond to the scene where death has occurred. Examples include:

✴ A traffic fatality (Figure 11-12a)

✴ A violent crime (Figure 11-12b)

✴ An industrial accident (Figure 11-12c)

✴ In someone's home (Figure 11-12d)

It is important that First Responders face their own feelings concerning life, identity, and death. One must be able to clarify and accept their own emotions. These emotions must be integrated with past and present experiences involving life and death.

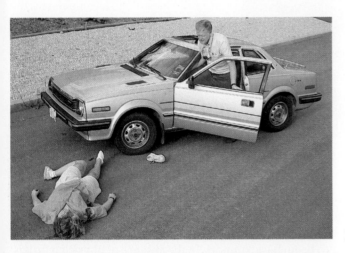

Figure 11-12a. Traffic fatality.

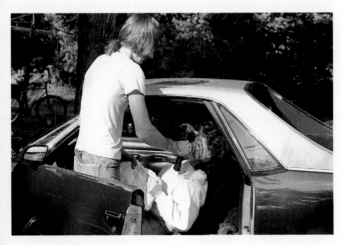

Figure 11-12b. Violent crime.

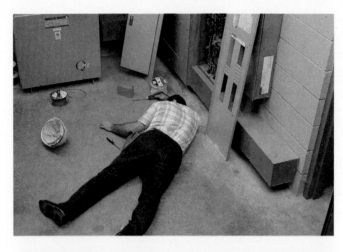

Figure 11-12c. Industrial accident.

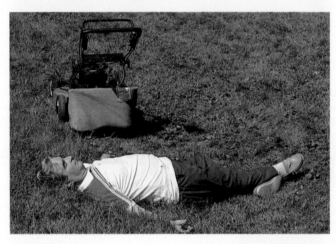

Figure 11-12d. In someone's home.

Signs of Death

What are the signs of death? For many years, death was believed to occur when breathing and heartbeat stopped. This definition has changed in many states' brain death statutes. The breathing/heartbeat check is an acceptable test for the First Responder when considering the initiation of basic life support. Questions often arise whether to begin basic support. In the absence of physician orders, (e.g., DNR: do not resuscitate) a general rule is:

❋ If the body is still warm and intact, initiate emergency care. An exception to this rule is cold temperature-related emergencies to be discussed in Chapter 14.

Here are some of the typical and obvious signs of death:

❋ Unresponsive to painful stimuli

❋ Lack of a pulse or heartbeat

❋ Absence of breath sounds

❋ No deep tendon or corneal reflexes

❋ Absence of eye movement

❋ No systolic blood pressure

❋ Dependent lividity

❋ Profound cyanosis

❋ Lowered or decreased body temperature

Definitive signs of death:

✽ Obvious mortal damage, e.g., body in various parts

✽ Rigor mortis

✽ Putrefaction

Medical Examiner's Cases

Involvement of the medical examiner depends upon the nature and scene of the death. In most states, when trauma is a factor or in suspected criminal or other unusual situations, the medical examiner is required.

If emergency care is initiated, keep careful notes of what was done or found. These records will be important for later investigation.

✽ Mark, if you can, the location of the body with chalk or special crayons (Figure 11-13).

✽ Note the anatomical position: prone, supine, sitting, etc.

✽ Note how the scene of death appeared to you. You may be the only qualified person to relate this data.

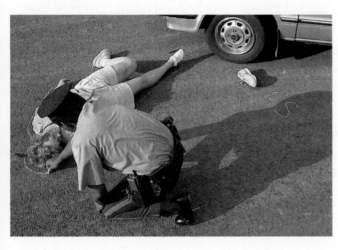

Figure 11-13. Marking the location of the body.

The following are considered medical examiner's cases:

✽ Dead on arrival (DOAs)

✽ Deaths without previous medical care

✽ Self-destruction (suicides)

✽ Violent deaths

✽ Poisoning - known or suspected

✽ Death resulting from accidents - direct or indirect

✽ Suspicion of a criminal act

Coping with Death

Grief is expected when a loved one or a close friend dies. Understanding the ways people cope with death will help the First Responder provide initial support. Responses to the death of loved one may not develop until days or months after, e.g., around holidays.

Normal grief reactions include:

* Symptomatic distress
* Preoccupation with the dead person
* Guilt and self-blame
* Irritability
* Social withdrawal
* Behavioral crisis

Persons also experience a fairly well-defined cycle of grief. These stages are:

* Denial: A response to the overwhelming fact of the death. For example, "No, that just can't be true," or "No, he's not dead; you're not telling me the truth," are typical of denial.

* Anger: Bad news is projected into the environment and displaced in all directions. "Why me?" is a common reaction, This phase is marked by lashing out against others. Someone must be blamed.

* Bargaining. For example, Why now, he just retired? Can't he stay longer?

* Begin to accept the change that death has brought

* Depression

* Acceptance

* Integration and resolution of the death

Grieving does not necessarily unfold in an exact order; some steps are bypassed or take place in a different order. Some persons regress; they go back and forth as events occur in which the dead person played a prominent part.

SUMMARY

When dealing with a behavioral or psychological crisis, the First Responder's responsibility is to reduce the impact of the stressful situation. Prepare to cope with the crisis. Always attempt to reduce life-threatening incidents or lessen psychological damage by rendering initial care.

Remember 4 general principles:

1. Protect yourself
2. Contain the crisis
3. Render appropriate emergency care
4. Arrange transport to a definitive medical care facility

These simple principles will help:

✳ Prepare to spend time with the patient.

✳ Be calm and direct.

✳ Identify yourself.

✳ Assess the patient at the scene.

✳ Interview the patient alone if possible, except in cases of rape.

✳ Sit down to interview the patient.

✳ Listen to the patient.

✳ Be interested.

✳ Maintain a nonjudgmental attitude.

✳ Provide honest reassurance.

✳ Present a definite plan of action.

✳ Encourage purposeful movement.

✳ Assume you can talk with any patient.

The following will help assess the patient's condition:

✳ Is the patient easily distracted?

✳ Are the patient's responses appropriate for the time, place, and situation?

✳ Is the patient alert and able to communicate coherently?

✳ Is the patient's memory intact?

✳ What is the patient's mood?

✳ Does the patient seem abnormally depressed, elated, or agitated?

✳ Does the patient seem to be fearful or worried?

✳ Is there disordered thought, delusion, or hallucination?

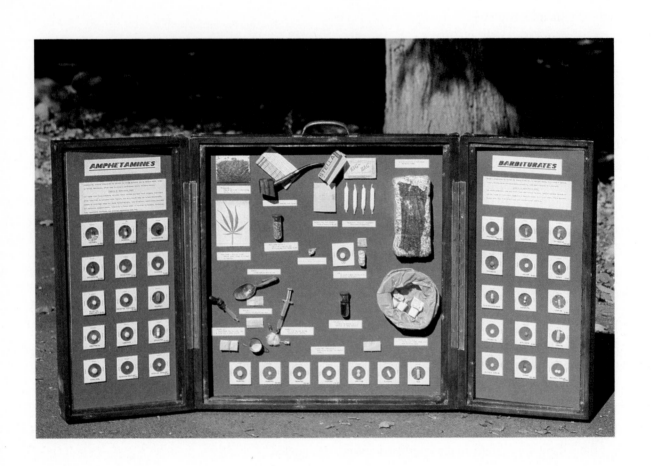

POISONS, BITES, STINGS, ALCOHOL AND DRUGS

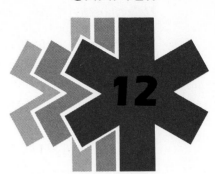

12

KEY CONCEPTS AND SKILLS

By the end of this chapter, you will be able to:

✻ Identify and describe the appropriate initial care for the poisoned, drugged, or intoxicated patient.

✻ List the classes of arthropods that can cause harmful and painful bites.

✻ Describe the signs, symptoms, and emergency care for persons injected with poisonous substances from insect bites and stings.

✻ List four poisonous snakes common to the United States.

✻ Describe the signs, symptoms, and physical findings of the various snake bites.

✻ Describe the emergency care for snake bites and stings.

KEY WORDS

Absorbed – Taken in or sucked up.

Adsorbent – Holding a substance in suspension or solution.

Activated charcoal – A type of absorbent used for certain types of injested poisoning.

Anorexia – Lack of appetite that results in being unable to eat. May be caused by poorly prepared food or unattractive food or various psychological causes.

Antivenin – Substance that neutralizes the venom of snakes and insect bites.

Arthropods – Largest phylum of animal life that includes spiders, insects, and beetles.

Caustic – Corrosive and burning substances that will destroy living tissue. Examples include silver nitrate, potassium hydroxide, and Drano®.

Corrosive – The eating or wearing away of a substance or tissue by a destructive agent. Examples include hydrochloric acid, sulfuric acid, battery acid.

Delirium tremens (DTs) – A psychic disorder involving visual and auditory hallucinations. This condition is found in habitual and excessive users of alcohol.

Depressant – A drug that decreases a bodily function or nerve activity.

Dilutent – A substance that makes a mixture or solution weaker, e.g., water or milk used to dilute an injested poison.

Elliptical – Oval-shaped.

Envenomization – Poisoning caused by an animal bite; for example, a snake or scorpion bite.

Erythema – An abnormal redness of the skin due to capillary inflammation.

Euphoria – A feeling or state of good health; an exaggerated feeling of well-being; mild elation.

Hallucinogen – A drug, chemical, or agent that excites the central nervous system. Hallucinogens may cause hallucinations, mood changes, anxiety, sensory distortion, increased pulse and temperature, and dilation of the pupils. Examples are LSD, mescaline, and PCP.

Hemotoxic – Having a poisonous effect on the blood.

Inhale – To breathe in.

Injected – Forcing a fluid into the body, e.g., using a syringe, or venom forced into the body via a snake's fangs.

Millimeter – One thousandth of a meter.

Narcotic – A drug that produces sleep, stupor, or unresponsiveness. Examples are opium, codeine, morphine, and heroin.

Necrosis – Localized tissue death that occurs in cells due to disease or injury. This dead tissue or bone is surrounded by healthy tissue or bones.

Neurotoxic – Having a poisonous effect on the nerves.

Overdose – Too great a dose of a therapeutic or illegal substance; a toxic amount of a drug.

Poison – A substance which, when taken into the body by ingestion, inhalation, injection, or absorption, interferes with normal body functions.

Post-seizure behavior – A reduced functioning of activity; to be sleepy or comatose.

Salivation – The act of secreting saliva.

Stimulant – Any substance that increases the rate of activity of a body system.

Vasoconstriction – A narrowing of the blood vessels.

Venous tourniquet – A device placed around an extremity to reduce the venous return of circulating blood; used in treating cases of poisonous snake bites.

Vertigo – Dizziness. A sensation of moving around in space or having objects move about the person.

POISON

A poison is any substance that causes harm or even death to any cell in the body. Poison can be ingested (swallowed), inhaled, injected, or absorbed. The following sections describe poisoning and how to handle emergency situations.

Ingested Poisons

Signs of ingested poisons vary according to the substance swallowed. The following signs and symptoms are common in victims that have swallowed poison:

* Constriction or dilation of the pupils
* Altered consciousness
* Excessive sweating or salivation
* Extremely slow, fast, or irregular pulse rate
* Nausea or vomiting
* Diarrhea
* Epigastric pain
* Extremely fast or slow breathing
* Irregular respiration
* Coughing
* Distinctive odor (depending on the poison)
* Burns, odors, or stains around and in the mouth (if a corrosive substance was ingested)
* Presence of containers that are used to store medications or other hazardous substances

Emergency care of the person who has ingested poison includes:

✻ Identification of the poison. There are usually telltale signs of the ingested poison such as the product's container or distinctive odor.

✻ Calling the Poison Control Center (or emergency department) to determine:

  Components of the product considered toxic
  Amount of the product considered toxic
  How the product may be diluted
  Signs and symptoms caused by the product

✻ Determining the amount taken and the time when the poison was swallowed.

✻ Diluting the poison, do not give too much of the dilutent or you may cause the patient to vomit.

✻ Administering 1 or 2 glasses of milk or water. Give the patient an amount of fluid relative to the amount of poison ingested.

✻ If the person does vomit, collect and keep a portion of the vomitus, if possible, for transfer to the hospital with the patient. This can be analyzed to show how much and which product was injested.

✻ Administering an adsorbent, such as activated charcoal. One tablespoon well-mixed in a glass of water to form a slurry. Administer this mixture at the direction of the Poison Control Center.

Inhaled Poison

Some gases that are found in everyday use are toxic. These gases include:

✻ Carbon monoxide

✻ Ammonium gas

✻ Chlorine gas

✻ Smoke (mixture of toxic and air-occlusive gases)

✻ Cyanide gas

✻ Propane

Most of these products, with the exception of carbon monoxide (CO), can be recognized by their distinctive odors. Suspect CO poisoning if the patient is found in an area where the products of incomplete combustion are found, e.g. an unventilated garage with a motor vehicle running. Very few symptoms or signs may be recognized with CO inhalation. The First Responder may determine dyspnea exists. The skin may appear dusky. This patient can rapidly go into respiratory arrest.

Some gaseous products are extremely dangerous because they do irreparable harm by scarring the respiratory tract. The First Responder can only move these patients from the source, place them upwind, and arrange transportation to a medical facility as rapidly as possible.

REMEMBER: Protect yourself first if poisonous gases are suspected.

Treatment for persons who have inhaled poison involves:

✻ Moving the patient outside and upwind of the area in which the exposure occurred.

✻ Administer oxygen, if available, to dissipate the gas (see Appendix A).

✻ Administer CPR, if necessary.

✻ Use care when performing rescue breathing; residues of the poison may be present in the patient's mouth.

Absorbed Poison

Many poisons can cause major cellular damage of the body when they come in contact with the skin. The skin will normally not allow water to enter the body, but some oily products can be absorbed and enter the body. The following skin contaminants may be washed with soap and water. Use large quantities of water when washing the affected areas.

* Cyanides
* Caustics
* Hydrocarbons (petroleum distillates)
* Pesticides

The treatment for absorbed poisons includes:

* Protect yourself from the product.
* Remove the patient from the source.
* Ensure the airway.
* Administer CPR, if necessary.
* Administer oxygen if available (see Appendix A).
* Wash the affected area with large amounts of water to reduce absorption. (Some products like dry lime should be brushed off the skin first.)

Pay special attention to hairy areas and skin creases.

* Do not let the patient stand in the washwater. Additional poison may be absorbed through the feet.
* Treat for shock, if necessary.
* Arrange transportation to a medical facility.

    REMEMBER: When the First Responder arrives, the poison may have been absorbed in sufficient quantity to produce signs or symptoms. Washing (10-15 minutes) will prevent further absorption, but will not reduce the amount of poison already in the body. The skin may be tinted or colored by the presence of some poisons.

DRUGS

Patients with drug problems, either legal or illegal substances, may experience drug intoxication, overdose, or withdrawal. Table 12-1 shows the effects of the major drug groups narcotics, depressants, stimulants, cannabis (marijuana), and hallucinogens.

Hallucinogens can cause hyperactivity, belligerence, and auditory or visual hallucinations. These patients may be soft-spoken and use short sentences. Patients who have overdosed may show symptoms of agitation, disorganization, paranoia, or depression.

If restraint is indicated, do so cautiously; most states require law enforcement authority to restrain the patient. Loud, forceful speaking may agitate these patients.

TABLE 12-1 Drugs and Their Effects

A drug can be defined as any non-nutritonal chemical substance that can be absorbed into the body. The word "drug" is commonly used to mean either a medicine or something taken (usually voluntarily) to produce a temporary (usually pleasurable) effect. Sometimes, the two categories overlap. Morphine may be prescribed as a medical treatment for relief of pain. Self-administered by an otherwise healthy person, it gives a tempory sense of well-being. Some drugs, including morphine and nicotine are strongly addictive and harmful. Such apparently innocent substances as tea and coffee may be addictive (or more accurately the caffeine that they provide may be addictive) and also capable of harming some people. The following list of drugs commonly used by addicts does not include caffeine, alcohol, nicotine, or tranquilizers, which are discussed elsewhere.

Type of drug	What it does	Outward signs of use	Some long-term effects
Amphetamines, often called pep pills, uppers, or diet pills.	Speeds up physical and mental processes, produces extreme energy and unusual excitement.	Weight loss, dilated pupils, insomnia, diarrhea, trembling.	Paranoia and violent behavior. Possible death from overdose.
Barbiturates, often called downers.	Produces extreme lethargy and drowsiness.	Blurred and confused speech, lack of coordination and balance.	Disruption of normal sleeping pattern; dangerously double vision; possible death from overdose, especially in conjunction with alcohol. Often ulcers at injection site.
Cannabis, including marijuana and hashish, often called pot, grass, and hash.	Relaxes the mind and body, heightens perception, and causes mood swings.	Red eyes, dilated pupils, lack of physical coordination, lethargy, sometimes hallucinations, and cardiac irregularities.	Long-term physical effects include brain, heart, lung and reproductive system damage. Decreased motivation.
Cocaine, often called coke, snow, crack.	Stimulates nervous system and produces heightened sensations and sometimes hallucinations, and cardiac irregularities.	Dilated pupils, trembling, apparent intoxication, cardiac arrest.	Ulceration of nasal passages if drug is "sniffed"; generalized itching, which can produce open sores.
Opiates, including opium, morphine, heroin and methadone.	Relieves physical and mental pain, and produces temporary euphoria.	Weight loss, lethargy, mood swings, sweating, slurred speech, sore eyes.	Loss of appetite leading to malnutrition; extreme susceptibility to infection; absence of periods in women, possible death from overdose.
Psychedelic drugs, including lysergic acid (LSD) and mescaline.	Upredictable. Usually produces hallucinations which may be pleasant or frightening.	Dilated pupils, sweating, trembling, sometimes fever and chills.	Possible irresponsible behavior, although apparently not addictive, a single drug-taking episode may cause long-term psychological upset.
Volatile substances such as unhaled fumes of glue, cleaning fluids, and "poppers."	Produces hallucinations, giddiness, temporary euphoria, and sometimes unconsciousness.	Obvious confusion, dilated pupils, flushed face.	Risk of brain, liver, or kidney damage; possible suffocation from inhalation.

Drug Classifications

Drugs are usually classified according to the following groups:

Stimulants (uppers)

❋ Central nervous system stimulants, including:
Amphetamines
Caffeine
Antiasthmatics (bronchodilators)
Vasoconstrictors
Cocaine

❋ Signs and symptoms of overdose, including:
Excitement
Restlessness
Talkativeness
Irritability
Respiratory failure

Depressants (downers)

❋ Central nervous system depressants, including:
Marijuana
Opiates
Tranquilizers
Barbiturates
Specific solvents (gasoline, alcohol)

❋ Signs and symptoms of overdose, including:
Drowsiness
Slow pupil reaction
Slow pulses
Slow or inadequate respiration

Hallucinogens

❋ Mind-altering drugs, including:
LSD (lysergic acid diethylamide)
Mescaline
Mushrooms
Peyote
Phencyclidine hydrochloride (PCP)

❋ Signs and symptoms of overdose, including:
Panic behavior
Mood changes
Hallucinations

Many drugs can be adsorbed (held in suspension) and can be removed from the body if they are recognized in time.

ALCOHOL

Alcohol is a depressant affecting coordination, reaction time, vision and judgment. In large quantities, e.g., chugging a pint of whiskey, alcohol can cause death. Other life threatening medical emergencies may mimic alcohol intoxication. These include:

* Hypoglycemia
* Head injury
* Toxicity
* Post epileptic seizure

Treat intoxicated patients in the same manner as any other sick or injured person. An added medicolegal responsibility exists due to the patients' decreased mental ability. Signs and symptoms of alcohol overdose include:

* Unsteadiness
* Odor of alcohol on the breath
* Flushed facial appearance
* Slurred speech
* Disorientation
* Nausea and vomiting
* An altered level of consciousness

To treat an alcohol overdose:

* Monitor the airway. Be prepared for the patient to vomit; the gag reflex may be reduced, which makes aspiration more likely.
* Monitor breathing as alcohol slows respiration.
* Administer oxygen, if available (see Appendix A).

Alcohol Withdrawal

An alcoholic person without a drink within a reasonable time may experience delirium tremens (DTs). A high percentage of these patients will die unless treated.

The signs of acute withdrawal include:

* Hallucinations
* Confusion
* Restlessness
* Tremors of extremities

Care for this patient by protecting him or her from further injury and monitoring the ABCs.

Place any patient with altered consciousness on their side with their head hyperextended to prevent aspiration of vomitus.

REMEMBER: Take all containers near the patient to the hospital.

SNAKE BITES

When deaths caused by bites and stings are analyzed, the killer is almost always anaphylactic shock. Very few snakebite victims die. More people are killed annually in the United States by bee and wasp stings than from snakebites.

Snakes

There are approximately 120 species of snake in the United States of which about 30 are poisonous. While about 45,000 bites are reported per year, fewer than 15 deaths are reported. The mortality rate from snakebite is very low. Snakebites occur more frequently in the southern states, and at least 90 percent of all snakebites occur between March and October. Because snakes prefer night activity, a high proportion of bites occur between 3 PM and 9 PM; one-half of these involve children and teenagers.

Snakes travel short distances in search of prey. They are usually not attackers. Snakes move very slowly but during a strike, a snake can move very fast—about 8 feet/second.

> **REMEMBER:** If a snake is present during an emergency situation, try to avoid it or hold it to the ground with a long stick. *Do not handle* a live snake unless you are trained in such handling.

There are two primary types of poisonous snakes:

✴ Neurotoxic, e.g.,

    Coral snake

    Cobra

✴ Hemotoxic (pit vipers), e.g.,

    Rattlesnake

    Water moccasin (cottonmouth)

    Copperhead

You can recognize a poisonous snake by looking at the markings, eyes, head, and anal plates as shown in Figure 12-1.

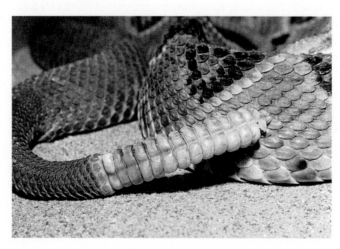

Figure 12-1. The anal plates of the rattlesnake. (Photo by Tom Stack/Tom Stack & Associates)

Coral Snakes

The most common neurotoxic snake found is the coral snake (Figures 12-2 and 12-3). A few of the offshore sea snakes found in and around tropical waters are also neurotoxic.

The coral snake:

* ✳ Is red, black, and yellow with a black snout featuring a yellow or yellowish-white head ring.

* ✳ Has a slender body and reaches up to 40 inches (101 cm) in length.

* ✳ Has short, unhinged solid fangs.

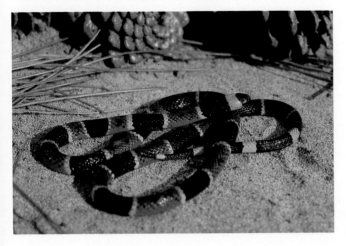

Figure 12-2. The coral snake. (Photo by Bob McKeever/Tom Stack & Associates)

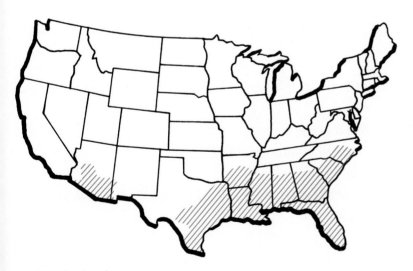

Coral snake
(Elapidae family)

Figure 12-3. Location of the coral snake throughout the United States.

Most people are bitten while playing with the coral snake or reaching down into a bushy area where it is hiding. Because this snake's fangs are solid, venom slides down into the puncture or scratch wound. The coral snake does not strike like a pit viper, i.e., using the fangs to inject venom, but rather chews through the skin. Venom may not be introduced into the bitten area if the snake is quickly brushed away. Because the coral and scarlet king snakes have simialar color, the following chart shows differences between them.

Principal Identification Characteristics

Coral Snakes	Scarlet King Snakes
Poisonous	Nonpoisonous
Black nose	Red nose
Red, yellow, and black	Red, yellow, and black
Yellow bands touch black bands	Yellow bands do not touch black bands

A rule to follow to differentiate the coral from the scarlet king snake is, "Red on yellow, kill a fellow; black on yellow, mellow fellow."

The signs and symptoms of a coral snake bite are:

* The onset of poisoning takes 1-12 hours
* Minimal pain and swelling
* Mood change: euphoria, anxiety, or depression
* Drowsiness
* Increased salivation
* Partial muscle paralysis of the eyelids, throat, chest, and muscles
* Seizures
* Coma

Using a constricting band to treat the bite from a neurotoxic snake does very little; consult local medical advice.

Treatment of a neurotoxic snakebite consists of:

* Keeping the extremity bitten dependent (lower than the heart).
* Keeping the patient still and comfortable.
* Washing the wound well with soap and water, since venom may be left on the skin or clothes.
* Monitoring the patient's vital signs.
* Treat for shock.
* Arranging for transport to a medical facility.

Pit Vipers (Rattlesnakes, Water Moccasins or Cottonmouths, and Copperheads)

Most pit vipers have 2 fangs that resemble hollow needles in the front of the upper lip. Those hollow openings reach from poisonous pouches on either side of the head to the tip of the fangs (Figure 12-4). The snake injects poison through these hollow openings.

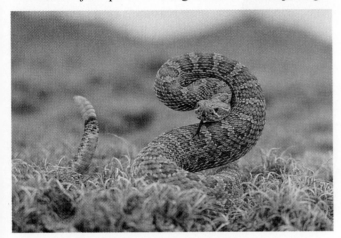

Figure 12-4. A pit viper. (Photo by John Cancalosi/Tom Stack & Associates)

The identifying features of pit vipers are:

✱ There is a facial pit between the eyes and nostril

✱ They have a triangular head with a hinged jaw

✱ The hollow upper jaw fangs fold up against the roof of the mouth

✱ The eyes are elliptical (cat-like)

✱ The scales form a single row on the undersurface of tail

The signs and symptoms of pit viper bite and envenomization are:

✱ The onset of poisoning is immediate and worsens in up to 8 hours; envenomization may take as long as 36 hours.

✱ Severe burning and pain around fang marks.

✱ Swelling around the site of the bite (and beyond in severe envenomizations).

✱ Rapid pulse.

✱ Lowered blood pressure (hypotension).

✱ Blurred vision.

✱ Nausea.

✱ Vomiting.

✱ Excessive sweating.

✱ The skin may turn blue from ruptured blood vessels.

✱ Faintness and dizziness.

Treat all bites in the same manner. Many factors can affect the amount of poison received by a person including:

✱ Amount of toxin in the snake's pouches

✱ Size and age of the patient

✱ Location of the bite on the patient

Adults are usually bitten either on the arms or legs. Children have a greater tendency to pick up the snakes and sometimes are bitten on either the face or trunk.

Rattlesnakes (Figure 12-5) are found throughout most of the United States (Figure 12-6). The pigmy rattlesnake and its larger cousin, the timber rattler, are highly poisonous. Rattlesnakes are not territorial and usually bite only in self-defense or when frightened.

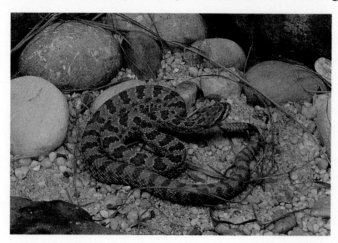

Figure 12-5. A rattlesnake. (Photo by David M. Dennis/Tom Stack & Associates)

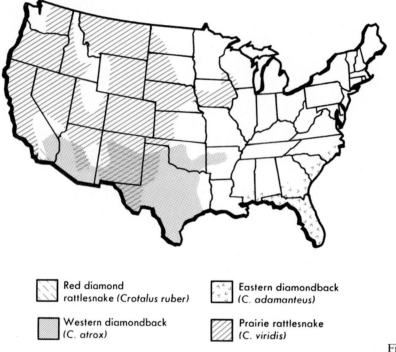

Red diamond rattlesnake (*Crotalus ruber*)

Western diamondback (*C. atrox*)

Eastern diamondback (*C. adamanteus*)

Prairie rattlesnake (*C. viridis*)

Figure 12-6. Locations of rattlesnakes throughout the United States.

Water moccasins (Figure 12-7a) and copperheads (Figure 12-7b) are hemotoxic like rattlesnakes. The snakes are territorial (Figure 12-8) and may be aggressive in protecting a given area.

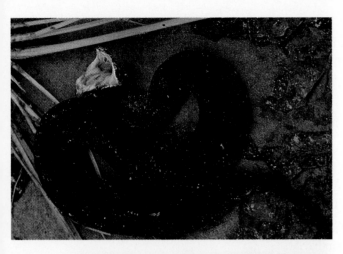

Figure 12-7a. The water moccasin. (Photo by John Cancalosi/Tom Stack & Associates)

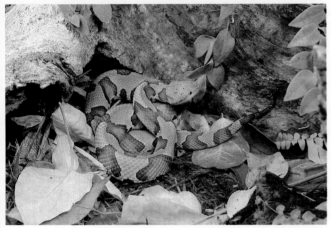

Figure 12-7b. The copperhead. (Photo by David M. Dennis/Tom Stack & Associates)

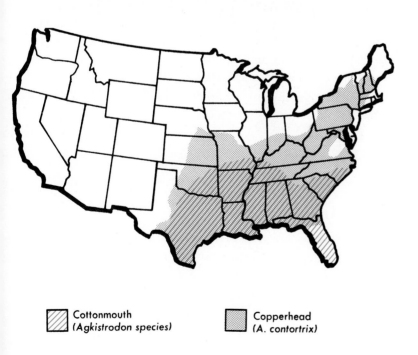

Cottonmouth
(*Agkistrodon species*)

Copperhead
(*A. contortrix*)

Figure 12-8. Territories of snakes.

Treatment

A high percentage of all snakebites do not result in envenomization of the patient. If the patient can be placed in a medical facility within 1 hour, only the following care is necessary:

* Calm and reassure the patient.
* Identify the snake.
* Keep the bitten area level or dependent (below the level) to the heart; if the bite is on an extremity, immobilize it with a splint.
* Treat for shock.
* Clean the site of the bite with soap and water.
* Remove any rings, bracelets, or other constricting items.
* Arrange for EMS transport of the patient to a medical facility.
* Give oxygen, if available (see Appendix A).

Everyone seems to panic when someone is bitten by a pit viper. If the patient cannot be treated at a medical facility within an hour, take the following steps:

* Remain calm!
* Seat and keep the patient calm.
* Keep the bitten area dependent.
* Check the bite. Redness and swelling are present almost instantly if envenomization has occurred.

    NOTE: Venous tourniquets and incision with suction are of little value. Promptly transporting the patient to an emergency facility for antivenin treatment is more important.

If medical advice in your area deems this practice acceptable, do the following:

* Within the first 5 minutes, place constricting bands approximately 2 inches (5 cm) above and below the bite. Do not seal off pulses to the extremity or venous blood flow.
* If the bite is on an extremity and more than 4 or 5 hours will elapse before hospitalization, you may make minor incisions with a clean blade to allow you to suck the venom in the area. This should be done under a physician's instruction and within 30 minutes after the bite. Do not cut more than ¼ inch (5 mm) to avoid cutting through tendons, arteries, or veins. Avoid sucking with your mouth, if at all possible. Commercial snakebite kits have suction devices.
* If the patient can be placed in a medical facility in 4 or 5 hours, none of these efforts are needed.
* Immobilize the extremity.
* Treat for shock.

SPIDER BITES

More deaths occur annually from spider bites and insect stings than from snakebites. There are approximately 20,000 species of spiders and scorpions (arachnids). Most of these insects are venomous. Spiders are active both in the daytime and at night. The venom of some spiders, milliliter for milliliter, is more potent than that of pit vipers. Two poisonous varieties are the black widow (Latrodectus mactans) spider (Figure 12-9a) and the brown recluse (Loxosceles recluse) spider (Figure 12-9b).

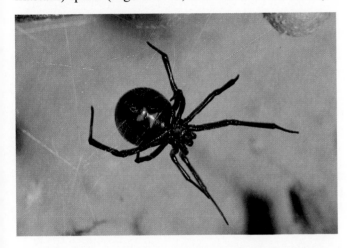

Figure 12-9a. The black widow. (Photo by Rod Planck/Tom Stack & Associates)

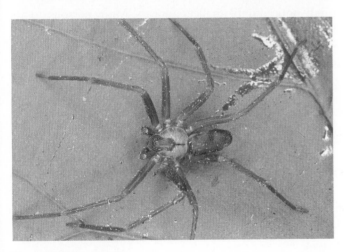

Figure 12-9b. The brown recluse spider. (Photo by Ann Moreton/Tom Stack & Associates)

Black Widow Spider

Few deaths have been reported from black widow spider bites. The bite is moderately painful, but local inflammation is minor although some swelling and redness may occur at the site. The more severe symptoms are caused by the systemic response to the toxin. Within 4 hours after the bite, the patient will suffer:

* Abdominal cramps
* Nausea
* Vomiting
* Sweating episodes

These symptoms will continue for approximately 24 hours but rarely cause permanent damage. Physical signs of the black widow spider bite are:

* Two small fang marks approximately 1 mm apart
* Little local swelling.

The body's reaction is neurologic. Signs and symptoms of a black widow bite are:

* Pain in the shoulders, back, and abdomen
* Headache
* Dizziness
* Swelling (edema of the eyelids and conjunctiva)
* Skin rash and itching
* Respiratory distress
* Perspiration
* Elevated skin temperature in the area of bite
* Weakness

In severe cases the signs and symptoms are:

* Hypertension
* Cardiac abnormalities

Severe cases cannot be treated in the field except by applying cold water or ice to the puncture site. Support the patient's vital functions and arrange EMS transport to a medical facility. If antivenin is available, it must be administered by a physician.

Brown Recluse Spider

The bite of the brown recluse spider is rarely noticed until an ulcer appears. Many persons do not know they have been bitten. The toxic substance injected by this spider is norepinephrine, which causes the small blood vessels around the site to occlude.

Signs and symptoms of a brown recluse spider bite include:

* Minor initial pain at the site, which is often overlooked.
* Nausea and vomiting
* Fever and chills
* Hypertension
* A blister and localized pain appear after approximately 2 hours; a reddened (erythematous) ring is observed.
* After 3 or 4 days as the ring becomes larger, and tissue death (necrosis) occurs; the blister breaks, leaving an ulcer.
* Formation of a black scar within 1 week
* Severe pain sometimes involving the entire limb
* Secondary infection of the site

REMEMBER: Children and the elderly are more severely affected by these bites.

Support vital functions and arrange EMS transport to a medical facility.

Scorpions

Only a few of the several hundred species of scorpions are poisonous (Figure 12-10). The sculptured scorpion (Centruroides sculpturatus) found in the southwestern United States and Mexico is the only species that is dangerous to humans.

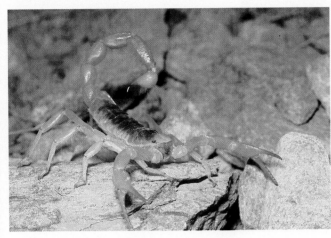

Figure 12-10. Only a few of several hundred species of scorpions are poisonous. (Photo by Joe McDonald/Tom Stack & Associates)

Scorpions live in arid regions and are night creatures. They are most active from April to August and are found under the bark of eucalyptus and cottonwood trees, on the undersides of objects, and sometimes in houses.

The signs and symptoms for a scorpion bite include:

✳ Severe pain, tingling, and a burning sensation around the site

✳ Excessive salivation and perspiration

✳ Difficulty in swallowing

✳ Nausea and vomiting

✳ Restlessness

✳ Cardiac irregularities, including cardiac arrest

Relieve pain with cold application to the wound site and immobilize if an extremity is involved. Be prepared to administer CPR-BLS. Arrange EMS transportation of the patient to a medical facility. Antivenin is available for scorpion bites.

Centipedes and Millipedes

Some of the larger species of centipedes can inflict a painful bite that may cause swelling and redness. Symptoms rarely last more than 48 hours. The bite of all centipedes is poisonous. Millipedes do not bite, but when handled may discharge a toxic secretion that will irritate the skin.

The signs and symptoms of a centipede or millipede bite include:

✳ Local pain

✳ Secondary infection 2-3 days after the bite

An ice cube will help reduce the pain of a centipede bite. The toxic secretions of a millipede should be washed from the skin with soap and water.

BUG AND BEETLE BITES

Several species of bugs and beetles are harmful to humans. Examples are the assassin bug (Traitoma protracta) beetle (Figure 12-11) and meloid beetles.

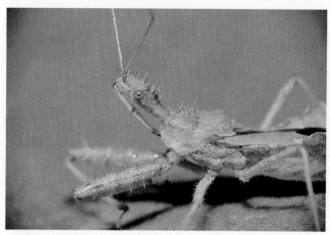

Figure 12-11. The assassin bug. (Photo by Rod Planck/Tom Stack & Associates)

The signs and symptoms of these bites include:

❋ Allergic reaction

❋ Anorexia (loss of appetite)

❋ Nausea

❋ Chills

❋ Fainting

❋ Itching

❋ Blisters

Relief of allergic reactions usually require medical attention. Apply cold packs to help reduce pain.

BEES

Many people are allergic to bee stings (Figure 12-12) and will develop an anaphylactic reaction. (See Chapter 6 for a review of anaphylactic shock.)

People who are highly allergic often carry a kit containing epinephrine (adrenalin), which must be injected immediately.

REMEMBER: The signs and symptoms of anaphylactic shock are:

❋ Generalized itching and redness

❋ Swelling of the face and tongue

❋ Breathing difficulty

❋ Weak pulse

❋ Anxiety

If the patient has a drug kit with epinephrine, inject the drug as directed by local medical protocol.

MAMMAL BITES

Report dog and cat bites to police; in some areas this report is required by law.

The primary care for a bite from any warm-blooded animal is careful washing of the wound with soap and water. Ensure that a domestic animal's rabies injections are up to date. If they are not or the animal cannot be found, urge the patient to go to a medical facility for follow-up care. Human bites are more likely to cause infection than animal bites.

Assure that anyone bitten by another human is seen at a medical facility if the skin is broken.

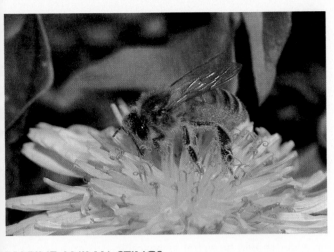

Figure 12-12. The bee. (Photo by John Shaw/ Tom Stack & Associates)

MARINE ANIMAL STINGS
Jellyfish, Sea Anemones, and Coral (Figure 12-13)

The signs and symptoms of a jellyfish sting include:

* Severe pain and possible paralysis
* Vasoconstriction
* Blisters
* Itching
* Nausea
* Headache
* Muscle spasm, especially in the back and abdomen
* Perspiration
* Vertigo
* Dyspnea

Emergency care for jellyfish stings includes:

* Rub the affected area with sand.
* Sprinkle or douse the affected area with alcohol.
* Next, sprinkle the affected area with meat tenderizer, (This inactivates the stinging substance).
* Cover the affected area with talcum powder.

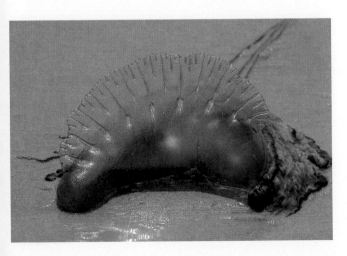

Figure 12-13. The portuguese Man o'war. (Photo by Wendy Shattil and Robert Rozinski/Tom Stack & Associates)

Starfish and Sea Urchins Stings (Figure 12-14)

The signs and symptoms of starfish and sea urchin wounds include:

* Puncture wounds (from spines)
* Intense pain, aching
* Swelling (early)
* Redness
* Nausea
* Respiratory distress with possible paralysis
* Tingling of the lips and face (late)
* Loss of muscle tone

Inactivate the toxin from the puncture wound by soaking the affected area in hot water for approximately 30 minutes. The temperature of the water should be as hot as bearable.

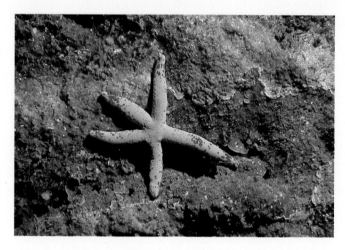

Figure 12-14. The starfish. (Photo by Brian Parker/Tom Stack & Associates)

Poisonous Fish Stings

There are approximately 500 known species of poisonous fish. Toxicity may vary from season to season. Some poisons are released or activated when the fish is eaten.

The signs and symptoms of wounds inflicted by fish vary greatly, including:

* Life-threatening conditions involving neurologic, cardiac, and respiratory problems
* Nausea
* Vomiting
* Headache

REMEMBER: Most of these patients should be seen at a medical facility.

tingray (Figure 12-15)

The signs and symptoms of stingray stings include:

* Severe pain

* Respiratory distress

* Seizures

* Lacerations up to 7 ¾ inches (20 cm)

* Nausea, vomiting, and abdominal pain

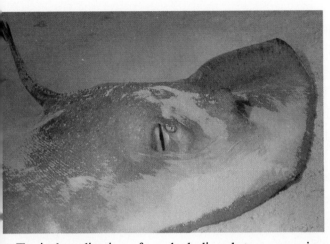

Figure 12-15. A stingray. (Photo by Dave Woodward/Tom Stack & Associates)

Topical application of an alcoholic substance may inactivate the venom. After inactivation, dry sand, flour, or baking soda may be dusted on and scraped off with the residue.

Placing the affected limb in hot water may reduce pain and inactivate the venom.

Scorpion Fish (sculpin, stu-fish, zebra fish)

The signs and symptoms of a scorpion fish would include:

* Severe pain

* Swelling

* Shock

* Cyanosis

Emergency care for most of these envenomizations includes:

* Washing with salt water

* Placing the extremity in water as warm as bearable for 30-90 minutes or until pain subsides. Be careful not to use water that is so hot that it will scald the patient.

NOTE: Removal of the integumentary sheath requires surgery.

SUMMARY

Patients who have ingested poisons should be treated in the following manner:

* Identify the poison.
* Ascertain the amount taken and the time.
* Dilute the poison whenever possible.
* Protect the patient's airway.
* Do not allow the patients to hurt themselves.
* Reassure the patient.
* Be alert for shock or allergic reactions.
* Monitor the level of consciousness.
* Evaluate for further illness or injury.
* Preserve evidence.
* Arrange EMS transport to a hospital.
* Provide basic life support if needed.

Treatment for inhaled poison involves the following:

* Remove the patient from the source of the poison.
* Administer oxygen, if available (see Appendix A).
* Provide basic life support, if necessary.

Treatment for absorbed poisons includes:

* Remove the patient from the source.
* Wash the skin with a large amount of water.

Most bites and stings can be treated by thorough cleansing of the wound site. Be alert to those which cause anaphylaxis. Stay calm and treat the patient for any life-threatening condition. Arrange EMS transport to a medical facility.

PREGNANCY, CHILDBIRTH, AND NEWBORN CARE

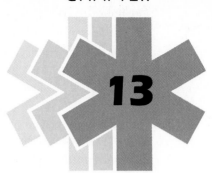

KEY CONCEPTS AND SKILLS

By the end of this chapter, you will be able to:

❋ List the parts of the female genital system.

❋ Define pregnancy.

❋ List procedures necessary to assist in the normal delivery of a baby.

❋ Describe a prolapsed cord.

❋ Describe baby presentations.

❋ Describe needed care for the newborn baby.

❋ Describe necessary care for:

      Excessive bleeding for both the baby and the mother

      Miscarriage

      Shock

KEY WORDS

Abortion – The termination of pregnancy before the fetus is developed enough to be expected to live if born.

Amniotic sac – A thin-walled bag that contains the fetus and amniotic fluid during pregnancy.

Breech birth – Presentation of feet, knees, or buttocks instead of the head in childbirth.

Cesarean section – Removal of the fetus by means of an incision into the uterus, usually by way of the abdominal wall.

Eclampsia – Major toxemia of pregnancy accompanied by high blood pressure, convulsions, and coma.

Ectopic pregnancy – An abnormal pregnancy in which the implantation of the fertilized ovum occurs outside the uterine cavity.

Fallopian tubes – Tubes or ducts that extend laterally from the lateral angle of the uterus and terminate near the ovary.

Fetus – An unborn offspring in the uterus from the third month to birth.

Labor – The process beginning with dilation of the cervix, delivery of the fetus, and expulsion of the placenta.

Menstrual period – The recurring cycle in which the decidual layer of the endometrium is shed then regrows. The cycle reoccurs every 28 days.

Mucous plug – Mucus that accumulates in the cervical canal during pregnancy.

Neurovascular – Relating to both the nervous and vascular system.

Orthostatic hypotension – Hypotension that occurs when a person is in an erect (upright) position.

Os – The opening of the cervix.

Ovaries – The ovaries produce ovum (egg) and hormones such as estrogen. Two pair of female organs found on each side of the lower abdomen beside the uterus.

Parturition – The process of giving birth.

Pedal edema – A condition in which the ankle and foot tissues contain an excessive amount of tissue fluid.

Perineum – The external region between the vulva and anus in a female or between the scrotum and anus in a male.

Pre-eclampsia – Toxemia of pregnancy characterized by increasing hypertension, headaches, and edema of the lower extremities.

Pregnancy – Gestation period; the condition of carrying a developing fetus in the uterus; in humans the duration is approximately 280 days.

Premature birth – Birth before full term (9 months) of development.

Prolapsed cord – The premature expulsion of the umbilical cord.

Trimesters – Period of about 3 months. The human pregnancy is divided into 3 trimesters.

Toxemia – Serious condition during pregnancy where there is edema of the legs, puffiness of face, headache, dizziness, convulsions, high temperature, rapid pulse, and high blood pressure.

Uterus – The womb; a pear-shaped, hollow organ in which the normal implantation of the fertilized egg occurs and the fetus develops.

Vagina – The tube that forms the passageway between the uterous and the vulva.

ANATOMY OF THE FEMALE REPRODUCTIVE SYSTEM

The female reproductive organs consist of (Figure 13-1):

❋ Ovaries

❋ Fallopian tubes

❋ Uterus

❋ Vagina

❋ Lubricating glands

The organs are discussed in detail in the following sections.

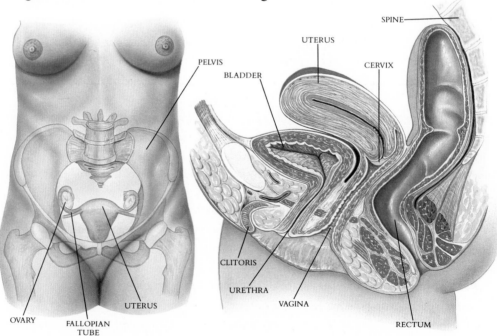

Figure 13-1. The female reproductive organs. (From Raven, P.H. and Johnson, G.B.: Biology, St. Louis, 1968, The C.V. Mosby Co.)

Ovaries

The ovaries are a pair of organs, found on each side of the lower abdomen beside the uterus. An ovary is often described as having the size and the shape of an almond. The ovaries perform two vital functions:

1. They produce, mature, and release the egg (ova) approximately every 28 days.
2. They secrete hormones.

Fallopian Tubes

The Fallopian tubes are also know as oviducts. They are the passageway through which the egg reaches the uterus. The Fallopian tubes contract in the direction of the uterus transporting the egg to the uterine cavity.

The Uterus

The uterus (womb) is the organ in which the fetus develops and from which menstruation occurs. There are two superior openings that are the connecting tubes to the ovaries. An opening in the inferior end is the *cervical os*. The lower-most portion of the uterus is the *cervix*. The lining of the interior portion of the uterus is the *endometrium*. The *placenta* will implant on the walls of the endometrium and provide support for the developing fetus. The fetus exists as a "parasite" attached to the mother's uterus until it is time to be delivered. When the baby is ready for delivery, the uterus, a muscular organ, begins rhythmical contractions. This rhythmic contracting is called *labor.*

The Vagina

The vagina (birth canal) connects the uterus with the outside of the body. It consists of smooth muscle lined with mucous membranes and is rough in texture. This organ has the ability to greatly extend during delivery but may also tear and bleed. The cervical os penetrates the superior portion of the vagina while the muscles and lubricating glands protect the lower vaginal opening.

Perineum

The perineum is shown in Figure 13-2. Hair and a protective pad of fat help protect the vaginal opening. The urethra is just anterior to the vaginal opening.

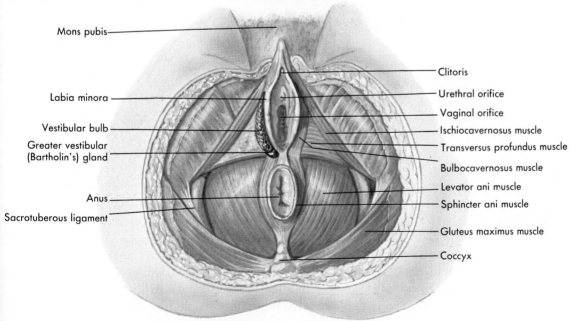

Figure 13-2. The perineum. (From Mosby's medical and Nursing Dictionary, 2nd edition, St. Louis, 1986, The C.V. Mosby Co.)

The signs and symptoms of pregnancy include:

✳ A menstrual period missed by more than 10 days (this may not be absolute)

✳ Fainting, syncope

✳ Noticeable breast changes (an increase in size of breast and changes in the nipples)

✳ Abdominal distention

The average pregnancy lasts less than 300 days and produces a newborn approximately 20 inches (50 cm) long weighing normally about 7 pounds (3.2 kg.).

FETAL DEVELOPMENT

The contact between the egg and the male sperm, or conception, usually occurs in a Fallopian tube. The newly fertilized embryo moves from the Fallopian tube to the uterus. During the next 7-9 days it will continue to rapidly grow (Figure 13-3). Upon reaching the uterus, it will be protected by a thin, filmy sac, filled with water, which is the amniotic sac. This membrane and solution will be the baby's home for the remaining period of the pregnancy. The sac and its contents will attach to the endometrium or inner lining of the wall of the uterus. At term there will be approximately 4 pints (2L) of fluid in the sac.

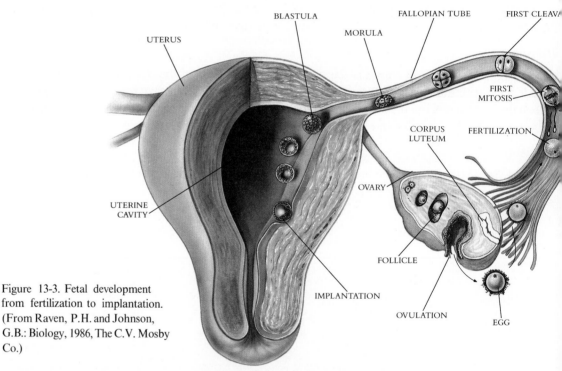

Figure 13-3. Fetal development from fertilization to implantation. (From Raven, P.H. and Johnson, G.B.: Biology, 1986, The C.V. Mosby Co.)

Twins may share or have two different placentas. If two implantations occur (fraternal twins) (Figure 13-4), each fetus will be protected by its own amniotic sac. More than one child may develop within a single protective sac. Identical twins usually share a single amniotic sac.

The new baby should have a heart beat by the end of the fourteenth week, but the beating may not be loud enough to be heard with a fetoscope until the twentieth week. From about the twentieth week until delivery, the mother will be able to feel the baby moving around within her. Most states now require a death certificate for any fetus aborted after the twentieth week (fifth month).

Though the baby is reasonably well protected by the mother and the protective sac, jolting or forceful movements should be avoided. Falls or other accidents may injure both the developing fetus or the mother. All expecting mothers should be evaluated by a physician if involved in an accident.

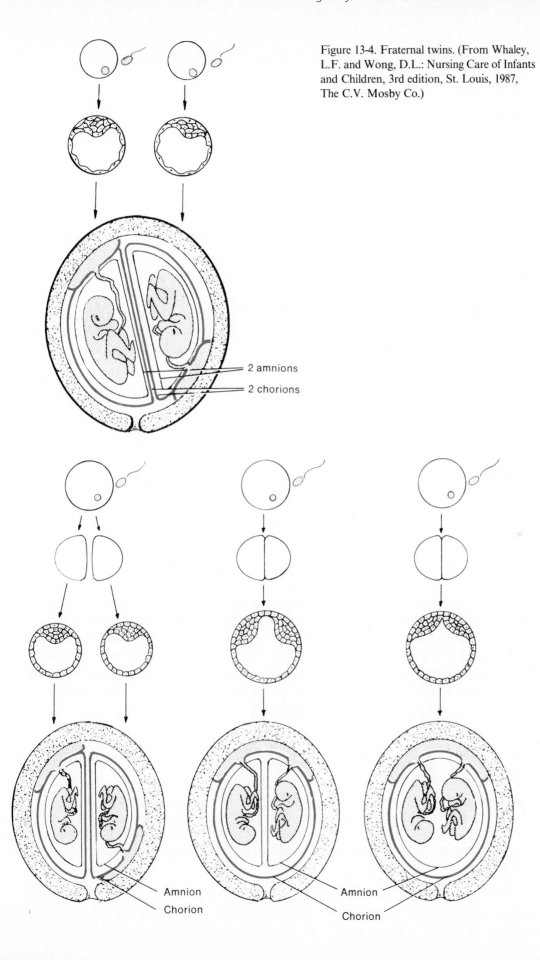

2 amnions
2 chorions

Amnion
Chorion

Amnion
Chorion

Figure 13-4. Fraternal twins. (From Whaley, L.F. and Wong, D.L.: Nursing Care of Infants and Children, 3rd edition, St. Louis, 1987, The C.V. Mosby Co.)

Many diseases interfere with fetal development. A few of these include:

* Measles
* Syphilis
* Herpes
* Scarlet fever
* Sore throat (Streptococcal)
* AIDS

Development of the new fetus may be hampered by drugs, smoking, or alcohol.

The mother should use caution during the period of pregnancy. Results of contact with these harmful sources may not be found until the child is born and some will have effects during the child's entire life.

PREGNANCY

Pregnancy is divided into three periods of 3 months or trimesters. Each trimester presents an opportunity for the First Responder to better recognize complications occurring to both the mother and the developing child.

* First trimester complications include:
    Ectopic pregnancy
    Bleeding
    Miscarriage (abortion)
* Second trimester complications include:
    Bleeding
    Traumatic injury to baby or mother
* Third trimester complications include:
    Bleeding
    Difficult delivery
    Traumatic injury to baby or mother

When a developing egg implants anywhere other than the uterus the pregnancy is ectopic. Ectopic means in another place. This other place may be in the mother's abdomen or the egg may become caught in the Fallopian tube. The location of this fetus will alter the signs and symptoms. For instance, a tubular pregnancy may present a sudden shock of unknown origin in a female of child-bearing age. The Fallopian tube may rupture when the fetus develops within the small confines of a tube. The following signs and symptoms, occurring during the first trimester, may indicate an ectopic pregnancy:

* Missing of one or more menstrual periods, the mother may not have noticed the missing period
* Abdominal pain (may refer to the shoulders)
* Mild vaginal bleeding
* Changes in blood pressure when the mother sits or stands upright (orthostatic changes)
* Unexplained shock

One must remember to ask questions and listen when evaluating all patients. Most pregnant persons will tell you what is happening to them. Some cannot accept the gravity of their being pregnant and will be unable to communicate their problems to the First Responder. All abnormal bleeding, shock of unknown origin, and vaginal or referred pain in child-bearing aged females should be fully evaluated for etopic pregnancy.

Emergency treatment involves recognition of the problem and:

* Treat for shock.
* Evaluate for hypotension. If the patient becomes dizzy or loses consciousness when sitting up or standing, suspect insufficient blood supply as a major cause.
* Administer oxygen if available (see Appendix A).
* Arrange transport by the EMSS since this may be a dire emergency.

MISCARRIAGE (ABORTION)

The terms miscarriage and abortion are used interchangeably. Any disrupting of pregnancy prior to normal delivery by unnatural means is an abortion. Induced or therapeutic abortions may be purposeful if the mother and her physician agree to the necessity for ending the pregnancy.

Spontaneous abortion is one of the most common causes of vaginal bleeding during the first trimester. If the patient suspects pregnancy any sudden vaginal bleeding should be considered an abortion until the patient is evaluated by a physician. All pregnancies terminated within the first 20 weeks, whether purposeful or spontaneous, are abortions and the patient should receive further evaluation. Infection or uncontrollable bleeding can occur after an abortion.

The signs and symptoms for an abortion include:

* Clots or other tissue passing from the vagina
* Vaginal bleeding
* Abdominal cramping
* Abdominal distention
* Nausea and/or vomiting
* Fever 100 °F (38 °C) or higher

Emergency care includes:

* Control bleeding. Place the patient in shock position. Cover the vagina with a sanitary pad or other absorbent material.
* Treat for shock.
* Help patient assume a position of comfort.
* Collect, protect, and transport any tissue or clots expelled from the vagina.
* Evaluate for hypotension.
* Administer oxygen if available (see Appendix A).
* Activate the EMSS.

BLEEDING (SECOND AND THIRD TRIMESTER)

Any bleeding during the second or third trimester may be an ominous sign. The causes for bleeding during these periods are life threatening to both the expectant mother and the child. In approximately 1 out of every 75 pregnancies, the placenta may separate from the uterine wall prior to the time for the baby to be delivered. This separation may or may not cause obvious bleeding from the vagina. The presence of blood is related to the attachment of the placenta and the baby's position. Large amounts of blood can be trapped in the uterus with the baby and not be expelled from the mother's vagina.

Occasionally the placenta will attach to the wall of the uterus at the cervical opening. In about 1 out of 200 pregnancies this tissue will separate from the uterine wall before time for the baby to be delivered (Figure 13-5). This separation at the opening usually occurs during the third trimester and most always is accompanied by visible blood from the vagina. Do not examine by feeling within the vagina. The loss of blood from either of the major causes may reduce the amount of oxygen the mother can provide for the baby and otherwise harm either the developing child or mother.

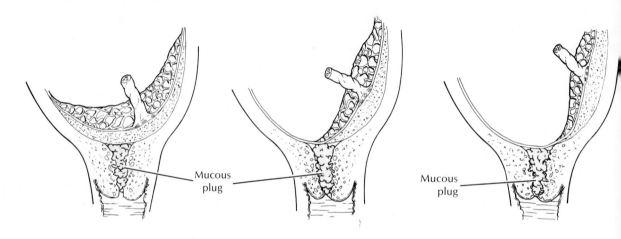

Figure 13-5. Placenta previa. (From Bobak, I.M. and Jensen, M.D.: Maternity and Gynecologic Care, 3rd edition, St. Louis, 1985, The C.V. Mosby Co.)

The signs and symptoms of sudden bleeding during the second or third trimester include:

❋ History of spotting or vaginal bleeding during pregnancy

❋ Vaginal bleeding (with or without pain)

❋ Pain (continuous and severe)

❋ Orthostatic hypotension (shock)

Care for the patient with any of the presenting signs or symptoms listed above during the second or third trimester of pregnancy includes:

❋ Pad the vaginal opening with sufficient quantities of absorbent pads or other suitable compresses.

❋ Place the patient on her side in shock position (head lower than buttocks).

❋ Maintain body heat.

❋ Administer oxygen if available (see Appendix A).

❋ Activate the EMSS.

REMEMBER! BOTH CONDITIONS ARE DIRE EMERGENCIES

TOXEMIA (PRE-ECLAMPSIA AND ECLAMPSIA)

Protein shifts with the body accompanied by high blood pressure result in toxemia of pregnancy. This problem usually does not appear until after the twentieth week of pregnancy.

The signs and symptoms of toxemia include:

* Sudden gain in mother's body weight
* Swollen ankles (pedal edema)
* Bloated feeling
* Elevated blood pressure (hypertension)
* Visual disturbances (light hurts the mother's eyes)
* Shakiness
* Pain
* Seizures

If the toxemia patient is found before seizures occur, she should be seen preferably by the physician supervising her prenatal care. If the supervising physician is not available she should be evaluated in a medical facility. If seizures occur, they should be treated as any seizure, but the mother must be seen at a medical facility immediately since the convulsions may cause injury or even death to the mother or developing child.

MOTOR VEHICLE ACCIDENT

Fetal death resulting from motor vehicle accidents may occur if the mother dies. The fetus is reasonably well protected, and unless the mother is severely injured, the developing child will usually not be harmed. However, a pregnant person involved in any jolting accident should be evaluated by a physician. Unless there are signs of pain, shock, vaginal bleeding, or the mother states a change in the way the baby feels, the patient does not require emergency transport, but the First Responder should still arrange transportation to a medical facility for all pregnant persons involved in accidents.

If the accident is severe enough to kill the mother, the developing baby can often be saved. The fetus can be supported with basic life support (BLS) administered to the mother while rapidly transporting the patient to the closest medical facility.

CHILDBIRTH

There are few emergency deliveries; most are simply unexpected. Unexpected deliveries should be handled carefully and calmly. Many person are jeopardized by rapid, unsafe transport when calm, cautious delivery is needed. If birth is imminent, safe delivery of the child should be completed by the First Responder unless a life-threatening situation exists. One should assure the mother is not presenting any signs of difficulty with the delivery. These include:

* Shock
* External vaginal bleeding (severe)
* Prematurity

Make every attempt to assure privacy for the mother during this time. Always keep a member of the family or at least another female with the delivering mother to help should problems arise. If any signs of complications are present, the mother and child should be transported to the closest emergency facility immediately.

Normal Delivery

Normal delivery may occur from the seventh to the ninth month. The mother has very little actual control over the delivery. She may reduce the required time by consciously helping push the baby through the birth canal using her strong abdominal muscles when spontaneous contractions occur. Since labor is very demanding, she should rest as much as possible between active contractions.

Labor is divided into three stages:

* STAGE ONE - From the first contraction of labor until the cervix is fully dilated, inches (10 cm)

* STAGE TWO - The end of cervical dilation until the baby is delivered

* STAGE THREE - The placenta delivers

FIRST STAGE

The length of the first stage of labor varies with the number of previous children delivered by the mother, lapse of time since the last delivery and the mother's age. A first child usually requires up to 10 hours for complete delivery. In subsequent deliveries the first stage of labor is normally shorter.

The following signs signal the beginnings of the first stage:

* Regular contractions occur, increase in intensity, and continue at closer intervals.

* The mucous plug from the opening of the cervix is expelled ("bloody show").

* The amniotic sac protecting the fetus breaks, emptying the amniotic fluid out of the vagina ("water breaking").

The entire first stage is involuntary. Help the mother understand and relax. She should not attempt to bear down with each contraction since she will need to save energy to help during the second stage (actual delivery). The first stage continues until the pains are 2-3 minutes apart and the head of the baby begins to appear from the vagina (crowning) (Figure 13-6).

During the first stage, the mother should be carefully transported to the hospital of her choice.

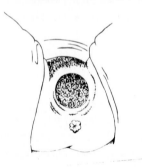

Figure 13-6. Crowning. (From Bobak, I.M. and Jensen, M.D.: Maternity and Gynecologic Care, 3rd edition, St. Louis, 1985, The C.V. Mosby Co.)

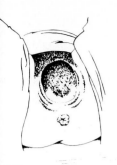 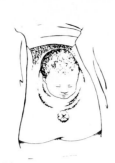 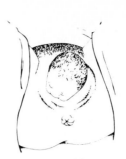 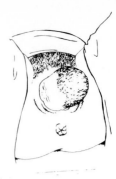

Figure 13-7. The process of birth. (From Bobak, I.M. and Jensen, M.D.: Maternity and Gynecologic Care, 3rd edition, St. Louis, 1985, The C.V. Mosby Co.)

SECOND STAGE

When crowning (the presenting part) occurs, the mother's vaginal opening is expanded by the baby's head and birth is imminent. The First Responder should prepare to deliver the baby and protect both the mother and new child (Figure 13-7).

✳ Place the mother on her back or side. Secure as much privacy as possible.

✳ If the mother is having respiratory difficulty, administer oxygen (see Appendix A).

✳ If in a car, have the mother place one of her legs over the back of the seat and one on the floor of the car. The child can then be delivered with the mother on her side or back.

✳ Do not insert your fingers into the vagina.

✳ As the baby's head presents, place gentle pressure with your fingers spread on the head to prevent sudden injury when the head is delivered. Use care where pressure is applied to the newborn's head since many soft areas (fontanels) are present between the islands of bone found in the newly developing skull. Use the flat of your hand. Be careful to assure gentle control of the head as the baby is delivered.

✳ After the head has been delivered, contractions usually recede for a few seconds than start again. The upper shoulder usually delivers next. Gentle downward pressure on the baby's head will help deliver the upper shoulder. Then gently raise the head to assist in the delivery of the lower shoulder. Protect the child's neck and feel to assure the cord is not wrapped around the neck. Do not pull on the cord.

✳ If the cord is around the neck, gently slip it up and over the baby's head or over the baby's shoulders.

✳ If the bag of water is still covering the baby, carefully tear it away to allow the baby to breath. Care should be taken to protect the new baby.

✳ Using a clean cloth, wipe away any mucus from around the mouth and nose. Remember, babies at birth breathe primarily through their nose.

✳ Assure all fluids are drained or cleaned from the baby's mouth and nose. If you have a bulb syringe, use it to suction fluids and mucus from the nose and mouth. Be sure to squeeze the bulb first before inserting it into the mouth or nose.

✳ The baby will be easily expelled. Support the baby since a newborn is slippery and easily dropped.

✳ If the baby does not breathe immediately (within 30 seconds), gently stimulate by wriggling the foot or stroking the chest toward the head (keep the child's head lower than the body). This will help in cleaning out mucus and other secretions.

✳ If spontaneous breathing does not occur, give mouth to mouth/nose resuscitation.

✳ Take the infant's pulse. The heart rate should be greater than 100 beats/min. The pulse can be best taken at the brachial artery on the baby's arm.

✳ Temperature control for the baby is very important. Wrap the baby up as quickly as possible to prevent loss of body heat.

✳ Place the baby at suckle on the mother's breast since this will help control vaginal bleeding and assist to expel the placenta.

✳ Do not raise the baby above the mother's stomach while the umbilical cord is intact, because this will cause the baby's blood to flow back toward the placenta and may cause shock. Remember, babies have very little blood volume (about 1.6 ounces) at birth.

THIRD STAGE

The third stage lasts from the delivery of the baby until the placenta is expelled. The placenta will deliver faster if the mother's abdomen is gently massaged. However, do not pull on the umbilical cord since a tear can cause serious bleeding. Prior to the delivery of the placenta, the cord may be tied. This will protect the baby and the mother from bleeding. Allow 10 inches from the baby, and make two secure ties a few inches apart (Figure 13-8). Shoelaces or any other suitable material can be used. If local procedures allow you to, cut the cord between the ties. Ensure bleeding is not occurring from either end of the cord. The entire blood volume of the infant may be no more than 1.6 ounces (50ml), and bleeding from the cord is potentially serious for both the mother and child. The cord does not need to be cut; it may be left intact until the mother and baby arrive at the hospital.

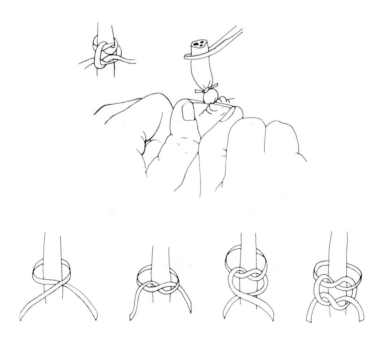

Figure 13-8. Tying the umbilical cord. (From Bobak, I.M. and Jensen, M.D.: Maternity and Gynecologic Care, 3rd edition, St. Louis, 1985, The C.V. Mosby Co.)

COMPLICATIONS

Prolasped Cord

Occasionally the umbilical cord will precede the baby out of the vaginal opening. Any pressure on the cord may prevent nutrition and oxygen from flowing to the baby. The cord is really the baby's life-line. Many times the cord will procede the baby through the cervical os. When this occurs, the cord will be pressed between the baby's head and the opening of the cervix. This can quickly reduce the amount of oxygen present for the baby's use. One can feel a pulse in the cord since 1 artery and 2 veins are present. Prolapse is a dire emergency.

Treatment for a prolapsed cord is as the follows:

* Check the cord to see if it is pulsating; if so, the baby is still alive.
* Place the mother in a head-down position and try to keep all weight off the cord. Pillows, blankets, or other bulky items may be used to help elevate the buttocks.
* Keep the cord moist.
* If available, oxygen should be administered (see Appendix A).
* Arrange rapid transportation to the nearest medical facility.
* You may need to place a finger on the cord to protect it and allow blood flow.

Unusual Presentations

Unusual presentations occur when the buttocks or extremities present at the vaginal opening instead of the baby's head. Very little can be done when a foot or arm present first except to arrange EMSS transportation to the nearest medical facility. A breech delivery (buttocks appear first) can be completed if the baby's head is not too large to clear the pelvic opening.

Remember the following when helping another deliver a breech baby:

* When the baby's buttocks or legs appear, they may need gentle manipulation that First Responder's can do to help them clear the vaginal opening.
* If the head does not deliver within 3 minutes, place your gloved finger in the vagina and form an airway tunnel for the baby to breathe. When the baby's chest delivers and expands, air or water will rush into the baby's lungs.
* Attempt to clear the baby's head by gently bending the baby's chin down on its chest. Remember the neck is easily damaged. *Do not* pull the baby!
* Initiate rapid transportation to the nearest medical facility while protecting the air tunnel. This may allow the child to breathe.
* Keep the baby warm.
* Follow local medical protocols if and when they exist.

Premature Birth

Any infant delivered prior to the eighth month or who weighs less than 5 pounds (2.4 kg) and measures less than 18 inches is considered premature.

REMEMBER: These infants lose heat rapidly and should be carefully dried and wrapped in a blanket. Monitor breathing and maintain body heat while arranging for EMSS transportation to a medical facility. If oxygen is administered, do not continue for longer than 20 minutes and limit the concentration to 40%. Make a tent over the baby's head using newspaper, aluminum foil, etc. and flow the oxygen into the tent in a slow gentle stream. Direct the flow of oxygen toward the top of the tent. *Do not direct the flow toward the infant's face or eyes.*

Multiple Births

After a baby is delivered, labor pains should cease. If they do not, expect a multiple birth. Most twins are born within minutes of each other.

Aftercare of the Mother

After the delivery, continue to observe and monitor the baby. The mother should also be closely observed for any adverse reactions. The uterus should be checked by palpating the abdomen to assure that it remains firm and there is no excessive bleeding coming from the vagina. Excessive bleeding would be in excess of 250ml (8 fluid ounces). If the uterus becomes limp, gently massage it by rubbing the mother's abdomen until it becomes firm. Its firm shape approximates a ripe grapefruit in size.

Clean the vaginal area with a clean, moist cloth; with another clean, moist cloth clean the perineal area and remove any fluids or fecal material that may have been expelled. If the perineum has been torn during delivery, apply direct pressure on the laceration with a sterile gauze pad or clean cloth. If bleeding is severe, elevate the mother's hips and legs and treat for shock.

Cover the vaginal opening with a clean sanitary napkin or other clean, large bulky cloth. Replace the used sheets and blankets with clean ones.

Cleanse the mother's face and hands with a damp cloth and keep her warm.

If she is thirsty, fluids can be given, unless she is nauseous or is experiencing other difficulties. Usually, the mother is very thirsty following delivery.

Comfort the mother as she will appreciate soothing words from you following this tremendous physical and emotional experience.

PEDIATRIC TRAUMA

The principles relating to the care of adult trauma also apply to children. Body size, vital capacities, or age require a different emphasis when rendering emergency care to children. Children do not understand their surroundings and are afraid when sick or injured. Care should be taken to explain to them what is happening. Let them express themselves. Keep the child and the patient together, if at all possible.

Airway

Children 6 months of age or younger breathe through their noses. Injury to the face. especially the nose can produce serious problems with the child's ability to breathe. Blood, teeth, tissue, vomit, or other substances can block nasal passages. The mouth is too small and the tongue is larger in relationship to the mouth. Obstruction by a swollen tongue can, for example, be a major cause of an airway obstruction.

Treatment includes:

* Open the airway. Use the chin-lift/jaw-thrust.
* Stabilize the neck. Think cervical fracture.
* Maintain body heat.

Shock

Shock is indicated by a rapid pulse, cool extremities, and a blood pressure (systolic) of less than 70mm. An easy rule to recall blood pressure limits for a child is:

✳ 80mm pulse twice the age in years; thus, a 2 year-old should have a systolic pressure of approximately 84mm.

Recalling the approximate level of vital limits for children may be helpful.

	Pulse	B/P (Systolic)	Breathing
	Upper Limit	Lower Limit	Upper Limits
Infant	160	80	40
Preschooler	140	90	30
Adolescent	120	100	20

Temperature Regulation

Children, due to the relationship of surface to body mass have difficulty in regulating body temperature. This variation is more critical during times of stress. They do not tolerate extremes in atmospheric temperature. They tend to lose body heat more quickly than adults. This is due partially to thinner skin and less body fat. Care should always be taken to maintain a normal body temperature of 98.6 °F (37 °C).

Head Injury

Children's heads are larger than adults in proportion to the child's body. This disparity causes many more potential injuries to the heads of children than adults. Most bleeding can be controlled by gentle direct pressure. *Do not* control bleeding and drainage from the eyes, ears, or nose unless you are sure no cerebral spinal fluid is present in the flow. Always treat for a neck injury when a child's head is hurt.

Extremity Trauma

Care for injuries to the pediatric patient are similar to those of adults. One exception involves injuries near the joints. Neurovascular injury is more prevalent in children who injure their bodies near the joining of two bones. Growth deformities may occur since the growth plates for bones are found near joints.

SUMMARY

Childbirth is a natural happening. The First Responder's responsibility is to support the mother and baby. The mother delivers the baby; the First Responder assists. Always be prepared for the unusual happening.

Trauma to infants and children always requires special attention. Remember, they are not just little people. You may need to be more aggressive when treating children.

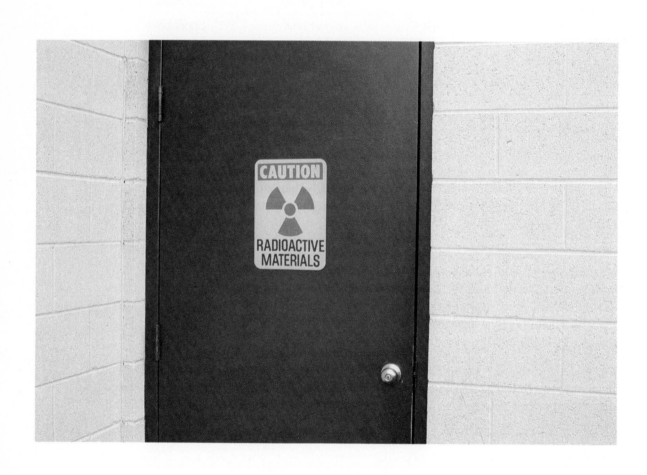

14

ENVIRONMENTAL EMERGENCIES

KEY WORDS

Acid – A substance that is characteristically sour in taste and neutralizes basic substances. Acids turn litmus paper red in color, and produces hydrogen ions when reacting with certain metals; a sour substance; also a slang name for LSD.

Alkali – substance with the chemical characteristics of a base that has the property of combining with an acid to form a salt, or with fatty acids to form a soap. Alkalis turn litmus paper blue in color.

Amnesia – Loss of memory caused by brain damage or emotional trauma. Often applied to episodes during which the patient forgets his or her identity.

Barbiturates – A group of organic compounds derived from barbituric acid that act as depressants on the central nervous system. Two examples are phenobarbital and secobarbital.

Conduction – The process of transmitting a nerve impluse.

Contraindication – A symptom of circumstance that prohibits the use of a drug or treatment that would normally be used, for example, a patient may have an allergic reaction to penicillin.

Convection – The transfer of heat through heated liquids or gases.

Core temperature – The body's temperature in deep structures such as the liver or heart.

Dehydration – Extreme loss of water from the body tissues. This condition occurs when the output of water from the body exceeds the water taken in.

Dermis – The inner, thicker layer of skin.

Diaphoresis – Profuse sweating.

Diving reflex – A protective reflex that closes off the trachea when water stimulates the laryngeal structure or face. This reflex is found in the newborn, but diminishes with maturity.

Epidermis – The outer layer of skin.

Evaporation – The change of a solid or liquid form to a gaseous form; the loss in volume due to conversion of a solid or liquid into a vapor.

First degree burn – Minor burns with damage that is limited to the outer layer of the skin.

Fourth degree burn – Deep burns affecting the muscle and bone resulting in structure damage.

Frostbite – An injury caused by freezing or the effect of freezing of a body.

Heat Cramps – Painful spasms of the muscles caused by overwork in a hot environment without replenishing salt and fluid.

Heat edema – A condition usually found in the elderly that visit tropical climates. The signs are swollen ankles and feet.

Heat exhaustion – An acute reaction to heat exposure marked by weakness, dizziness, cool and clammy skin, dilated pupils, and nausea.

Heat illness – Conditions such as heat edema, heat cramps, and heat exhaustion that result from exposure to excessive heat.

Heat stroke – A serious life-threatening condition in which the body's temperature is 105 °F (40.6 °C) or higher; the medical term is hyperpyrexia.

Heat syncope – Fainting caused by exposure to high temperatures.

High frequency current – Electrical energy that is transferred as heat. Measured in megahertz.

Hypothermia – A condition in which the body temperature is below a normal 95 °F (35 °C).

Integument – The skin, consisting of the dermis (upper layer) and epidermis (lower layers).

Ion – An atom, group of atoms or molecule that has gained an electrical charge through the gain or loss of an electron or electrons.

Ionizing – Breaking up compounds (acids, bases, salts) into their basic ions.

Listlessness – A condition characterized by apathy or indifference.

Megahertz – A unit of frequency equal to 1,000,000 cycles a second.

Metabolic activity – The building up, breaking down, and dying of living cells.

Near drowner – One who has almost drowned, usually under water for 20-30 minutes.

Obesity – An abnormal amount of fat on the body.

Phenothiazines – An organic compound used to make tranquilizers and antihistamines.

RAD – Radiation absorbed dose. A unit that measures the amount of radiation absorbed by human tissue.

Radiation – Energy that is given off in the form of waves or particles in all directions from a common center.

Roentgen – A unit to measure the amount of ionizing radiation; expressed as R.

Rule of nines – A method used to estimate the percentage of body surface area (BSA). Particularly useful in judging the amount of skin that has been burned. The head and both upper extremities each represent 9% of body surface; the trunk, front, and back each 18% each lower extremity 18% and the perineum 1%.

Second degree burn – Burns in which damage extends through the upper layer of skin and into the lower layers. These burns are not serious enough to prevent the growth of new skin.

Sepsis – Infection or contamination resulting from the presences of microorganisms or their poisonous products in the blood stream.

Soot – A substance produced by the incomplete burning of organic materials; observe for soot in burns, particularly inhalation burns.

Tachycardia – Abnormal, rapid heart action.

Third degree burn – Burns in which both the upper and lower layers of the skin are destroyed with damage extending into tissues below the skin.

Ventricular fibrillation – A heart condition fibrillation that results in rapid, shaky, and futile contractions of the ventricles.

Zero force current – Direct current (DC).

HEAT ILLNESS

Heat found naturally in our environment can drastically affect how the body functions. In addition, man-made materials and our contact with them can also produce unhealthy effects. For example, being in a highly heated drying room of a factory or near a nuclear reactor with leaking radiation exposes humans to life-threatening conditions or causes general deterioration of the body.

The body's sensitivity to heat depends on such factors as age, size, and state of health. The old and very young are particularly sensitive to changes in temperature because their regulatory mechanisms are not very adaptable. Prescribed drugs, alcohol, and other substances may also affect the body's temperature regulating mechanisms. Alcoholics are also prone to problems involving temperature regulation — both heat illness and hypothermia. Infection and heart disease may also bring on heat illness.

Climate is also a factor (Figure 14-1). Extreme heat, for example, together with high humidity makes most people uncomfortable and often irritable.

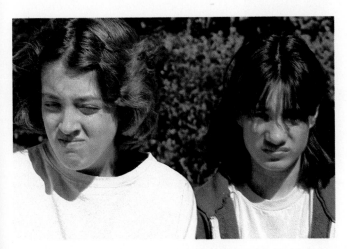

Figure 14-1. A hot, outdoor environment.

Exertion can also affect the body's heat regulatory mechanism. Individuals not accustomed to either rapid changes in temperature or the the stress of physical activity may suffer from heat-induced illness. Physical stress can affect conditioned athletes as well. For example, heat stroke is the second most common cause of death among high school football players. Factors that affect the body's response to heat include:

* Age.
* General health.
* Neurological changes.
* Frequent use of drugs because of their effect on perspiration.
* Metabolic activity.
* Thermal regulation.
* Obesity.
* Fatigue.

Heat illness ranges from minor changes in body function to life-threatening heat stroke. When the body's temperature reaches 102°-104°F, (39° 40°C), heat-related problems should be suspected. A temperature of 107.6°F (42°C) indicates a serious disorder. Heat stroke, the most serious of heat disorders, must be considered when the body's temperature is over 104°F.

The following sections describe a variety of heat-related conditions, how to recognize the signs and symptoms, and how to care for patients suffering from these conditions.

Heat Edema

Heat edema occurs most frequently in elderly people that are visiting tropical and semitropical locales (Figure 14-2). The signs are swollen feet and ankles. This condition results from the dilation of blood vessels in the skin and muscles. The edema is not a serious problem; simple elevation, the use of support hose, and a cooler environment should provide adequate emergency care.

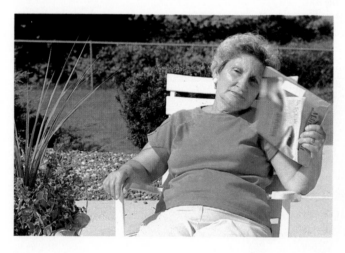

Figure 14-2. An elderly person with heat illness.

Heat Syncope

Heat syncope (fainting) may occur in those persons exposed to rising temperature, especially persons who are unaccustomed to high temperatures (Figure 14-3). Heat syncope frequently occurs during parades, drills, or when a person stands for a long period of time. Heat syncope is caused by blood pooling in the feet and legs. This condition more commonly occurs when perspiring reduces fluid volume.

Treat heat syncope in the following manner (Figure 14-4):

* Place the victim in a supine position.
* Give the victim a fluid and salt replacement (1 teaspoon salt in a glass of water or commercial electrolyte drinks such as Gatorade® or Thirst Quencher®).

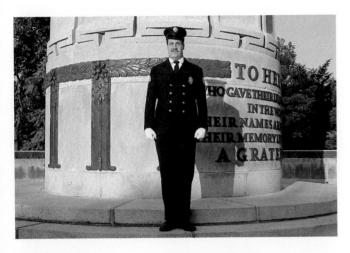

Figure 14-3. Heat syncope may occur when a person stands for long periods of time.

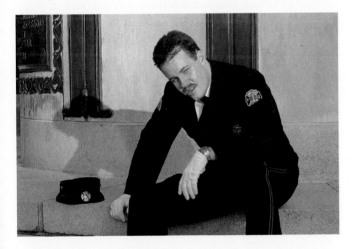

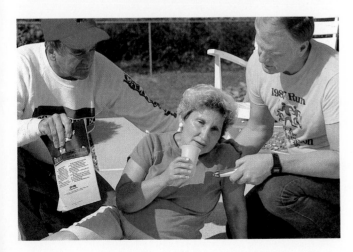

Figure 14-4. Treatment of heat syncope.

Heat Cramps

Heat cramps can result from the loss of water and salts, particularly sodium. The onset is rapid and occurs during strenuous physical activity in temperatures of 100 °F (38 °C) or higher. Individuals not used to the high heat usually are affected.

The normal signs and symptoms of heat cramps include:

✳ Severe pain, frequently in the arms and legs.

✳ Abdominal cramps.

✳ The cramp may feel like a knot.

✳ The "bellies" of the muscles are hot, with a temperature of 105 °F (40.6 °C) or higher.

✳ The skin is pale and wet.

Treat the patient with heat cramps in the following manner:

✳ Place the patient in a cool place.

✳ Place the patient in s supine position.

✳ Give the patient cool water with salt (1 teaspoon in 8 ounces of water) solution.

✳ *Do not* use hot packs.

✳ *Do not* massage the area of the cramp.

Heat Exhaustion

Heat exhaustion is caused by water depletion. Profuse perspiration (diaphoresis), loss of fluids (dehydration), vomiting, diarrhea, and heavy alcohol intake are factors that influence the onset of heat exhaustion.

The signs and symptoms of heat exhaustion include:

✳ Temperature may be normal to subnormal or the body temperature may be elevated 102 °-104 °F (39 °-40 °C).

✳ Normal blood pressure.

✳ Rapid pulse rate (100/min).

✳ Apprehensiveness.

✳ Cold, damp, and ashen skin.

✳ Nausea.

✳ Headache.

✳ Dizziness.

✳ Vision problems.

✳ Mild cramps.

✳ Irritability

Treat the patient with heat exhaustion in the following manner:

✳ Place the patient in a supine position.

✳ Place the patient in a cool environment.

✳ Loosen the patient's clothing.

✳ Give the patient, if he or she is conscious, cool water with salt (1 teaspoon in 8 ounces of water).

Heat exhaustion can rapidly progress into heat stroke.

Heat Stroke

Heat stroke (hyperpyrexia) is a serious condition requiring immediate care in a medical facility. If left untreated, heat stroke progresses to convulsions, coma, and death. Heat stroke is a massive disturbance of the body's heat regulating mechanism. It develops after strenuous activity or prolonged exposure to extremely hot, humid conditions. The elderly or very young are often affected most. More cases of heat stroke can be expected during a prolonged heat wave.

REMEMBER: Heat stroke is the most serious and life-threatening of the heat illnesses.

The predisposing factors to heat stroke are:

* Age, either very old or very young.
* Substandard housing or substandard ventilation.
* Lack of perspiration.
* Cardiovascular diseases.
* Lack of proper fluid balance.
* A history of prior heat illness.

The signs and symptoms of heat stroke include:

* High temperature 104.9° 105.8 °F (40.5° 41 °C); a temperature of 107.6 °F (42 °C) can cause irreversible damage to the brain, liver, and kidneys.
* Sudden onset.
* A pulse rate of 160 or higher.
* Rapid respirations (20-30/min).
* Blood pressure slightly elevated (widened pulse pressure).
* Pupils: early — contracted; late — dilated.
* Headache.
* Weakness.
* Dizziness.
* Loss of appetite.
* Nausea.
* Skin: red, hot, dry, and flushed with a lack of perspiration.
  NOTE: In well-trained athletes, the skin may not be hot and dry!
* Anxiety and listlessness.
* Possible twitching and muscle cramps

Table 14-1 compares the signs and symptoms of heat exhaustion and heat stroke.

TABLE 14-1 Comparison Of Signs and Symptoms For Heat Exhaustion and Heat Stroke.

	Heat Exhaustion	Heat stroke
Face:	Pale	Red and flushed
Skin:	Moist	Red, hot, and dry
Sweating:	Profuse	None
Temperature:	Normal	Extremely high
Pulse:	Weak and rapid	Strong and rapid
Unconscious:	Not usual	Usual

Use the following emergency care procedure to reduce the patient's temperature:

✳ Maintain the airway.

✳ Initiate cooling immediately.

✳ Remove all clothing. Wet a sheet in water and cover the patient.

✳ Place the patient in an air-conditioned environment or use fans to help cool the body.

✳ Arrange for transport to a medical facility immediately.

✳ Administer oxygen, if available (see Appendix A).

✳ Do not use topical rubbing (isopropyl) alcohol because of toxic effect from absorption through the skin; this is especially true in children.

COLD INJURY

Hypothermia

Hypothermia is the general cooling of the body. Energy sources are low and the core temperature becomes abnormally low: 95.0 °F (34.5 °C). Hypothermia is serious and often fatal. At 86 °F (36 °C) the brain can survive without perfusion for about 10 minutes. When the core temperature drops to 82.4 °F (28 °C), the patient is in grave danger. Persons have survived a hypothermic accident with a temperature of 64.4 °F (18 °C). In hypothermic cases, no one should be considered dead until they are warm and dead.

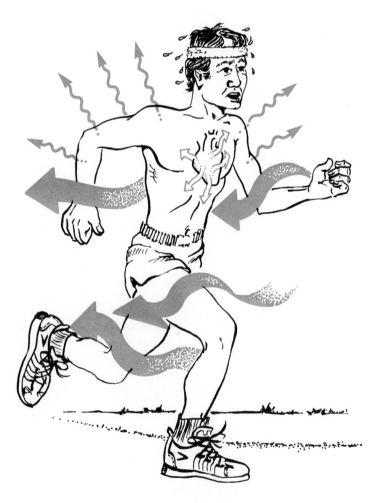

Figure 14-5. The body loses heat through these mechanisms.

The body loses heat through the following mechanisms (Figure 14-5):

✳ Radiation:heat loss from unprotected body parts.

✳ Conduction:transfer of heat from direct contact with a cold surface or object.

✳ Convection: transfer of heat by air or water.

✳ Evaporation: perspiration.

The causes of hypothermia are:

✳ Accidental: environmental, cold water immersion.

✳ Metabolic: endocrine disorders, low blood sugar (hypoglycemia).

✳ Central nervous system disorders: a brain tumor, cerebrovascular disease, head trauma, spinal cord trauma.

✳ Drug induced: alcohol, barbiturates, phenothiazines (e.g., Compazine®, Mellaril®, Thorazine).

✳ Burns.

✳ Malnutrition.

✳ Blood poisoning (sepsis).

Ventricular fibrillation is a chief threat in hypothermia. Careful movement of the patient is important as the heart is very unstable. Jostling the patient may cause the heart to fibrillate and fail.

As in heat illness, those most prone to hypothermia are:

✳ The old and very young.

✳ Alcoholics.

✳ Patients with medical conditions such as cardiovascular disease or diabetes.

Exhaustion, hunger, drunkenness, drug use, and high altitudes are also factors.

The signs and symptoms of hypothermia include:

✳ Lack of coordination.

✳ Shivering. (May be absent.)

✳ Semiconsciousness or unconsciousness, progressing to coma.

✳ Slow, irregular pulse.

✳ Core temperature below 95 °F (35 °C).

✳ Cardiac arrest

Table 14-2 describes the levels of hypothermia.

Table 14-2 Levels of Hypothermia

| Temperature | | Condition |
°F	°C	
99.6	37.6	Normal rectal temperature
98.6	37	Normal oral temperature
96.8	36	Increased metabolic rate
95.0	35	Shivering
93.2	34	Amnesia, difficult speech
91.4	33	Severe hypothermia
90.0	32.2	Shivering stops
89.6	32	Pupils dilated; altered level of consciousness
87.8	31	Blood pressure difficult to obtain
86	30	Progressive loss of consciousness, increased muscle rigidity,
85.2	29	Slower pulse and respiration
82.4	28	Cardiac problems develop
80.6	27	Voluntary motion lost along with pupillary light reflexes; the patient may appear dead
78.8	26	Patient seldom conscious

REMEMBER: Conventional thermometers only measure temperatures above 94.0 °F (34.4 °C) (Figure 14-6).

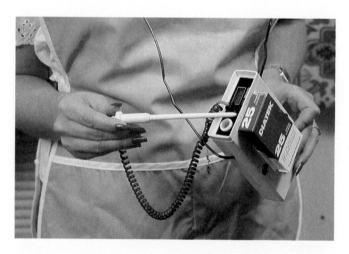

Figure 14-6. Conventional thermometers only measure temperatures above 94.0 °F (34.4 °C).

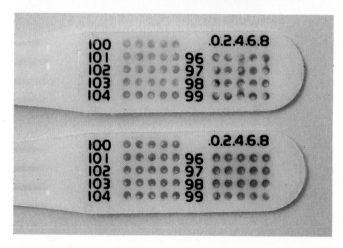

Treat the patient with hypothermia in the following manner:

✸ Ensure the patient's airway; in accidents, immobilize the spine.

✸ Begin the basic life support if necessary.

✸ Remove wet clothing and keep the body dry (Figure 14-7a).

✸ Rewarm the patient with blankets and warm packs (Figure 14-7b).

✸ Place the patient next to another person with normal body heat or place the patient between two persons in a sleeping bag.

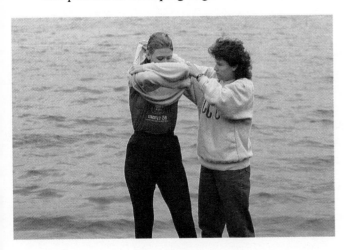

Figure 14-7a. Remove wet clothing and keep the body dry.

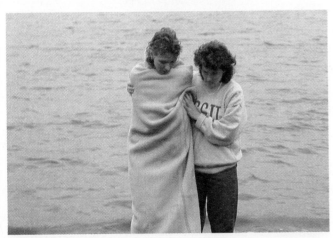

Figure 14-7b. Rewarm the patient with blankets and warm packs.

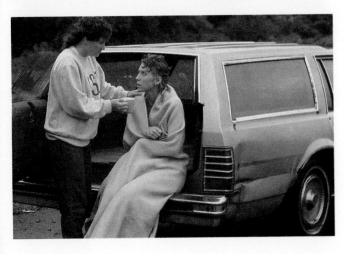

Figure 14-7c. Give hot liquids by mouth.

Handle the patient gently as the heart may fibrillate when the patient is handled.

Give hot liquids by mouth (Figure 14-7c). Warm fruit juice or diluted bullion is a good choice but avoid coffee, tea, or hot chocolate. Patients with decreased levels of consciousness or no gag reflex should be given nothing by mouth. Do not give a patient alcoholic beverages or allow the patient to move about.

Oxygen, if administered, should be warmed through a heated bubbler; oxygen concentration should not exceed 30-40%.

Frostbite

Frostbite occurs when body tissue freezes. Frostbite victims usually suffer from hypothermia.

As ice crystals form, in or between the cells, cell membranes rupture causing dehydration. The frostbitten areas are those most exposed: the fingertips, ears, nose, and lower extremities, particularly the feet and toes. Incidents of scrotal and penile frostbite in joggers has also been reported.

The onset of frostbite is generally painless so most people are unaware that the injury is occurring. Injury, fatigue, disease, poor nutrition, and alcohol or drug use will mask the early warning signs. Persons with dark pigmentation, especially blacks and those with previous cold injuries, are more susceptible to frostbite.

The early warnings of frostbite are (Figure 14-8a):

✳ Loss of flexibility in the extremities

✳ Dull ache in the early stages

Advanced frostbite produces (Figure 14-8b):

✳ Cold, gray (cyanotic), or mottled blue-white skin; the skin may also be white, yellow-white, or waxy

✳ Hard and inflexible skin and muscle

   REMEMBER: Advanced frostbite is painless.

Treat the patient with frostbite in the following manner:

✳ Rapid rewarming with warm water is essential. The water temperature should be 104°106°F (37.1°41.1°C).

   NOTE: Do not place the extremity over a fire or on a hot radiator. Excessive heat can cause extensive tissue damage.

✳ As rewarming occurs, the tissue should turn pink and become painful; this is a positive sign that the tissue is returning to a normal condition. The patient may complain of burning, prickling, or numbness.

✳ Pad and splint the frostbitten area to protect the tissue from further injury.

✳ If blisters develop, do not disturb or break them.

✳ Do not let victims smoke since nicotine causes constriction of the small blood vessels in the extremities. (A preventative measure is not to smoke while out in the cold weather for long periods of time.)

✳ Do not rub the frostbitten area with snow or ice; this will only add to the injury (Figure 14-9).

✳ Do not attempt rapid thawing if there is any chance of refreezing.

✳ Do not give the patient alcoholic beverages.

   REMEMBER: When frostbite and severe hypothermia coexists, delay rapid rewarming of extremities until the patient's core temperature nears a normal temperature of 98.6°F (37°C).

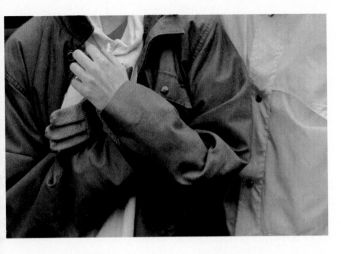

Figure 14-8a. Early warnings of frostbite.

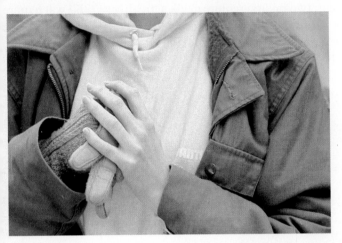

Figure 14-8b. Advanced frostbite.

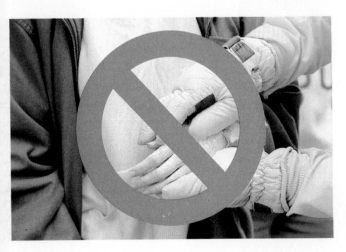

Figure 14-9. Do not rub the frostbitten area with snow.

BURNS

Body tissue can be burned by many environmental agents. These agents include:

* Thermal agents (hot water or fire) (Figure 14-10a).
* Chemicals (corrosives or phenols).
* Electricity (Figure 14-10b).
* Radiation (sunburn) (Figure 14-10c).
* Ionizing radiation (Figure 14-10d).
* Friction (rub burns) (Figure 14-10e).

Fire accounts for 66% of all burns, hot liquids for 27% and electricity for 1%. Most burns (81%) occur at home; 16% occur in vehicles; the rest occur on the job.

The tissues directly involved in burn injuries suffer the most damage. The effect of the burns on the body's overall function, rather than the local effect, is generally the reason patients die from burn injuries.

Nine million people are burned each year; two million require medical treatment. 50% will require hospital care, and of these 12% will die. Consider the following: a person can lose one lung, one kidney, or 90% of the liver and survive. A person with a full-thickness burn (a third degree burn) covering 10% of the body surface area (BSA) may not survive.

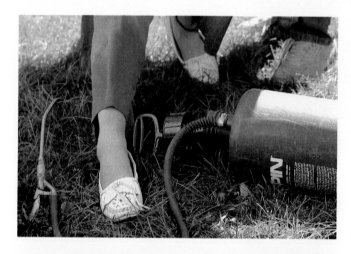

Figure 14-10a. Burns caused by a thermal agent

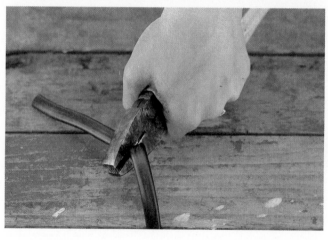

Figure 14-10b. Burn caused by electricity.

The skin (integument) is the body's largest organ. It is the chief protector of the body from infection, fluid loss, or temperature variation. The skin also serves as a medium for sensation and excreting wastes. Damage to the skin is a medical emergency.

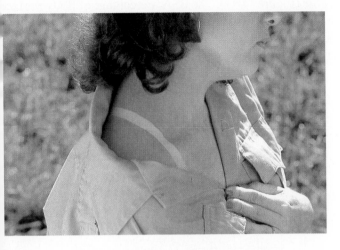

Figure 14-10c. Burn caused by radiation.

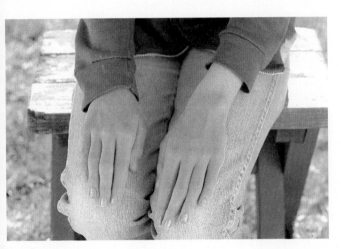

Figure 14-10d. Burn caused by ionizing radiation.

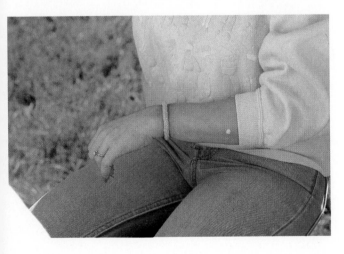

Figure 14-10e. Burn caused by friction.

The Rule of Nines

One important aspect of the First Responder's care in burn cases is estimating the percentage of the involved body surface. The more body surface involved in the burn, the greater the chance of death. The "rule of nines" is accurate for this purpose (Figure 14-11). The BSA (Percentage of Body Surface Area) of the average-sized adult male weighing 154 pounds (70kg) is about 18.5 square feet.

Table 14-3 describes the body areas and the percentages of body area covered by the rule of nines. An easy measure to remember is that one side of the hand (the palm and fingers) usually equal 1% of the adult body surface.

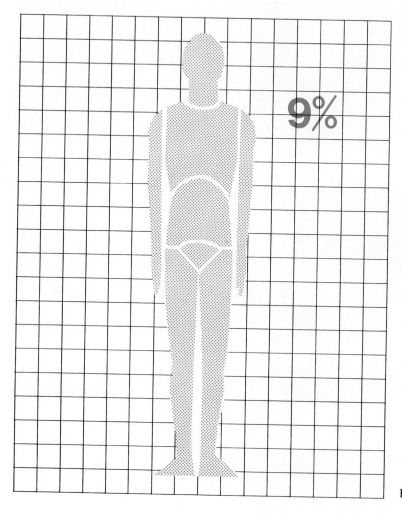

Figure 14-11. The rule of nines.

Table 14-3 Body Areas and Percentages Covered by the Rule of Nines

Body Area	Percentage of Body Area
Head, neck, face	9
Right arm, forearm, hand (front and back)	9
Left arm, forearm, hand (front and back)	9
Thorax (front)	9
Thorax (back)	9
Abdomen, lower ribs to groin	9
Back, lower ribs to buttocks	9
Right thigh, leg, and foot (front)	9
Right thigh, leg, and foot (back)	9
Left thigh, leg, and foot (front)	9
Left thigh, leg, and foot (back)	9
Genitalia	1
	100

Classification of Burns

Many classification systems exist for evaluating the nature of a burn. (Figure 14-12). The following system is one that is commonly used:

FIRST-DEGREE BURNS:

Involvement:	Epidermis.
Appearance:	Red.
Pain:	Painful.
Possible Source:	Sunburn or low-intensity flashes.

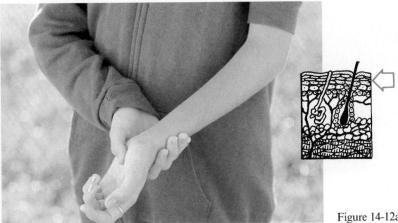

Figure 14-12a. First-degree burns.

SECOND-DEGREE BURNS:

Involvement:	Intermediate skin level; the dermis.
Appearance:	Blisters.
Pain:	Painful to the touch and sensitive to cold air.
Possible Source:	Scalds and flash flames.

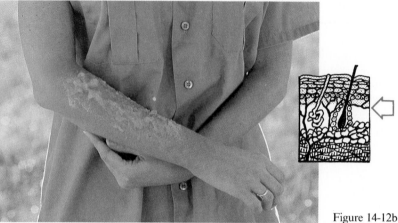

Figure 14-12b. Second-degree burns.

THIRD-DEGREE BURNS:

Involvement:	Deep dermal level with skin loss.
Appearance:	Dry, the skin may be white or charred and sometimes appear dull gray.
Pain:	Absent; surrounding areas may be painful because they are burns of a lesser degree.
Possible Source:	Fire.

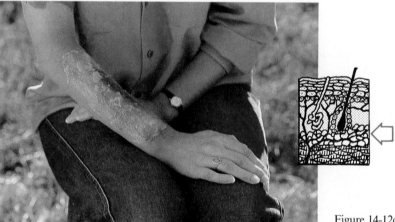

Figure 14-12c. Third-degree burns.

FOURTH-DEGREE BURNS:

Involvement:	Deep tissue, muscle, fat, bone, and cartilage.
Appearance:	Similar to third-degree burns; sometimes only the entry point is visible; look for entry and exit points.
Pain:	Absent.
Possible Source:	Usually electrical.

Burn injuries are divided into the following three categories:

Major burn injury includes:

✻ Second-degree burns of more than 30% of BSA in adults and more than 20% in children.

✻ All third-degree burns of 10% of BSA.

✻ All fourth-degree burns.

✻ All burns involving the hands, face, eyes, ears, feet, or genital area.

✻ All inhalation injuries.

✻ All electrical burns.

✻ Associated trauma of a major nature.

✻ Poor risk patients, for example, the elderly and young, those with cardiac disorders, diabetes, asthma, or kidney disorders.

Moderate-burn injury includes:

✻ Third-degree burns of 2-10% of BSA.

✻ Second-degree burns of 15-30% of BSA in adults and 20% in children; these injuries do not involve the eyes, ears, face, hands, feet or genital area.

✻ First-degree burns of 50% of BSA.

Minor burn injury includes:

✻ Third-degree burns of less than 2% of BSA.

✻ Second-degree burns of less than 15% of BSA in adults and 10% in children; these injuries do not involve the eyes, ears, face, hands, feet or genital area.

✻ First-degree burns of less than 60% of BSA

The Care of Burns

The care of burns includes:

❋ Stopping the burning process by extinguishing with lots of water or removing burning clothing (Figure 14-13). If the area is small, cool the affected area with water or compresses to stop continuing thermal injury. Many natural or synthetic fibers continue to smolder or retain heat.

❋ Maintaining ventilation: ensure a patient's airway. Administer oxygen, preferably humidified, if available (see Appendix A).

❋ Starting basic life support if necessary.

❋ Estimating the extent of burns.

❋ Arranging for transport of the patient to a medical facility if any of the following conditions are present:

> Burns over more than 15% BSA.
> Third-degree burns over more than 2% BSA.
> The patient is under 5 or over 60 years of age.
> Airway injury is present.
> Electrical injury is involved.
> Major trauma is associated with the burn.
> There is a preexisting disease or medical condition.
> Burns involving the face, hands, feet, or genital area.
> Suspected child abuse.

❋ Covering burns with dry, nonsticking sterile dressings or a burn sheet (plastic wrap).

❋ Not using cool fluids or ice for major burns, These will cause loss of body heat.

❋ Limiting the motion of burned areas in the extremities by using slings or padded splints.

❋ Applying no ointments (Figure 14-14).

Care for the minor and moderate burns is the same as for major burns. Cold water or saline flushing can be initiated for pain relief if second-degree burns cover 10% or less of the BSA. Continue this treatment for 10-15 minutes. Do not use ice. Obtain a brief medical history; and specifically ask the patient about any allergies.

Inhalation Injury

Be alert for burn injury to the respiratory tract. Assure that no upper airway obstruction is present. The signs of inhalation injury include:

❋ Soot in and around the mouth and nose.

❋ Singed eyebrows and nasal hair (Figure 14-15).

❋ Hoarseness.

❋ Facial burns.

❋ Impaired mental state.

❋ Confinement in a burning environment or involvement in an explosion incident.

If the epiglottis swells and the person is unable to swallow, total upper airway obstruction is imminent.

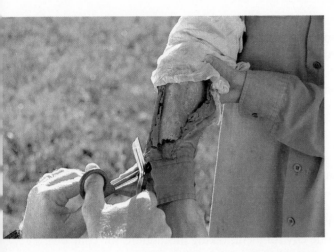

Figure 14-13. Stopping the burn process by extinguishing with lots of water or removing burning clothing.

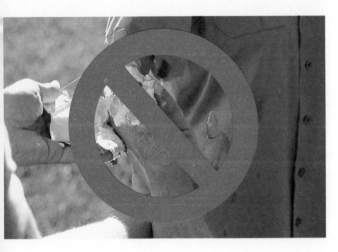

Figure 14-14. Apply no ointments.

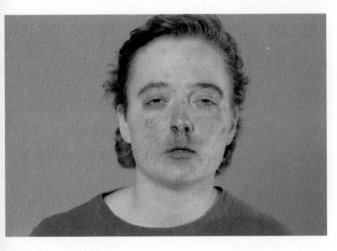

Figure 14-15. Sign of an inhalation injury.

Carbon Monoxide Poisoning

When combustion is incomplete, carbon monoxide (CO) is present, because it is a byproduct of combustion. CO poisoning is difficult to detect because the cherry-red mottled color of the skin and mucosa is usually absent.

The signs and symptoms of CO poisoning are:

* Cherry red mucous membranes.
* Unconsciousness.
* Irritability.
* History of prolonged smoke inhalation.
* Skin may appear dusky.

The care of carbon monoxide poisoning includes:

* Removing the person from the unsafe environment, taking precautions for your own safety.
* Starting basic life support, as necessary.
* Administering high-flow oxygen, if available (see Appendix A).

Chemical Burns

Treat for all chemical burns using the following technique:

* Flush the burn with large amounts of water. The method for flushing chemicals from the eyes is shown in Figure 14-16.

If the eyes are involved, continue washing for at least 20 minutes or until the EMS team arrives.

* Some chemicals are dry and require brushing before flushing.
* Alkali burns are more serious than acid burns because of their deeper penetration. These burns require longer flushing.
* Remove all contaminated clothing; be careful not to contaminate yourself!
* Do not attempt to neutralize any acid or alkali burn.

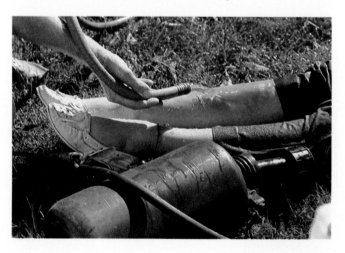

Figure 14-16. Flush the burn with large amounts of water.

Electrical Burns

Electrical burns are more serious than they may first appear. The form and extent of the burns are related to the amount of electrical current, the duration of the current, tissue pathway involved, and the frequency of the current.

High-frequency current (megahertz) transfers the energy to tissue as heat. The major effect of low-frequency (AC) (60 Hz) current is stimulation of skeletal, cardiac, smooth muscle, and nerve tissue with widespread destruction.

Intense heat (more than 20,000 °C) can be produced by high-frequency current that will dry up the tissue along the path of conduction. Electrical burns are usually more extensive that they appear because of the pathway of the current. Fluid is lost because of this widespread destruction. Acid-based imbalance and kidney failure are common in these burns.

Direct current (DC) if applied intermittently causes stimulation or produces heat if applied continuously. Pacemakers and defibrillators use direct current.

The following table describes various amounts of current and their effect on the body.

Table 14-4 Electrical Current and Its Effect on the Body

Amount of Current	Result
1/1000 amp (1 milliamp)	At the threshold of sensation
4-10 milliamps	Sensed as pain
30 milliamps	May cause unconsciousness
50-60 milliamps	May cause ventricular fibrillation

REMEMBER: 50 milliamps is less than 5% of the current required to energize a 100 watt light bulb.

Treat electrical burns in the following manner:

✳ *If the area is safe,* remove the victim from the source of the electrical current. Only a person trained and properly equipped (such as a power company employee) should attempt rescue. Cut off the source of electricity if possible by throwing a circuit breaker or disconnecting the device.

✳ Ensure an open airway.

✳ Start basic life support as necessary. Electrocuted victims may require extended basic life support.

✳ Administer oxygen, if available (see Appendix A).

✳ Care for associated trauma such as burns or fractures.

RADIATION EXPOSURE

Exposure to unsafe levels of radiation can occur, for example, as a result of an accident at a nuclear energy facility or an accident involving a vehicle transporting nuclear materials (Figure 14-17). Persons who routinely work with radioactive materials wear a badge designed to indicate total exposure to radiation over a certain period of time.

Radiation is measured in roentgens (abbreviated R). The radiation absorbed dose *(rad)* is a measure of the amount of energy absorbed by tissues.

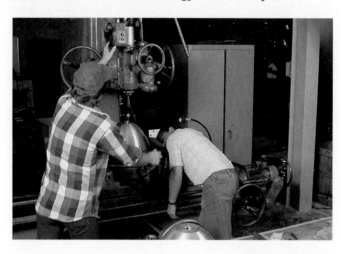

Figure 14-17. An accident scene involving nuclear materials.

The acute effects caused by short-term radiation are:

✳ 200-400 *rads* (whole body dose): nausea, vomiting, and loss of hair;

✳ 400-600 rads (whole body dose): gastrointestinal tract damage. Half of the people exposed to this amount will die within 30 days.

✳ 2000 rads or more (whole body dose) over a short period causes death within hours.

The signs and symptoms of radiation exposure include:

✳ Nausea

✳ Vomitting

✳ Dehydration

✳ Diarrhea

✳ Loss of appetite

✳ High fever

✳ A feeling of discomfort (malaise)

✳ Fast heart rate (tachycardia)

The First Responder's care of the persons exposed to radiation is limited. *Notify state police or the environmental protection agency immediately.* Restrict access to the incident area. Do not eat, smoke, or drink in the incident area. Specialists in radiation medicine will be needed.

Care for victims of radiation exposure in the following manner:

✳ *Protect yourself; do not enter a radiation zone* (Figure 14-18); observe the wind direction - stay upwind.

✳ *Establish a protective zone.* It is possible that you may be contaminated by a radioactive source.

✳ Flush the contaminated skin with large amounts of soap and water.

✳ Administer oxygen, if available (see Appendix A) and if other injuries are present.

✳ Give the patient fluids, especially salty solutions. Mix 1 teaspoon each of table salt and baking soda in 1 quart of water. Allow the patient to drink as much of this solution as practical.

✳ Care of the thermal effect from the flash burn is the same as for other burns.

✳ These patients need help from persons trained in dealing with radiation illness.

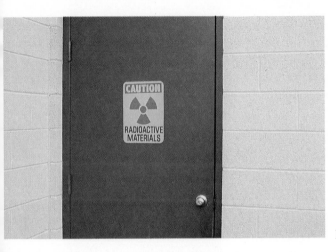

Figure 14-18. Do not enter a radiation zone.

NEAR-DROWNING

Near-drowning occurs when the process of drowning is interrupted or reversed. The term "near-drowner" is used to describe anyone who survives a "drowning" for more than 24 hours — hopefully with full body functions. The 1986 guidelines of the American Heart Association advise that resuscitation efforts should be initiated, even if an individual has been under water for a documented 20-30 minutes or more.

Several factors are worth noting in drowning cases:

✳ A diving reflex, more active in children than adults, causes breathing to cease and is triggered when one is immersed in cold water. The reflex shunts blood to the heart and brain.

✳ The heart rate slows, allowing the heart to continue pumping for up to 10 minutes after submersion.

Immersion in cold water slows the body's rate of activity (metabolism).

Treat near-drowning victims in the following manner:

✳ Start immediate basic life support as soon as possible. A cold heart is difficult to start, so do not give up too soon. There have been cases of successful resuscitation after 6 hours.

✳ Restore the body's temperature with blankets.

✳ Administer oxygen, if available (see Appendix A).

SUMMARY

Variation of environmental temperature and the body's ability to cope expose one to injury o
illness.

The environmental conditions in this chapter include:

* Heat edema

* Heat syncope

* Heat cramps

* Heat exhaustion

* Heat stroke

* Hypothermia

* Frostbite

The goal when treating heat or cold injuries is to normalize the injured persons body temperature
The skills required range from moving the person into a warm place or increasing the core body temperature.

Over nine million persons are burned each year. The First Responder should be prepared to recog
nize those burns considered critical. They include:

* Degree of burn

* Percent of body involved

* Area of body involved

* Causative agent of burn

The primary emergency care for burns involves treating for pain, maintaining sterility of the burr
area, and effective life support for breathing and blood pressure. Man-made chemicals and nuclea
devices add to the growing list of elements in the environment that can cause harm or death.

Rapid intervention by the First Responder often lessens the disastrous results. However, keep ir
mind that the initial responsibility is to protect yourself. Do not attempt an unsafe rescue.

GAINING ACCESS TO VICTIMS AND TRANSFER PROCEDURES

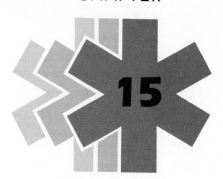

15

KEY CONCEPTS AND SKILLS

By the end of this chapter, you will be able to:

✳ Describe the procedure for gaining access to persons trapped in a vehicle after an accident:

When the vehicle is closed but upright.
When the vehicle is closed but overturned.
When the patient is pinned beneath the vehicle.
When vehicles are in contact with electrical hazards.
When vehicles involve hazardous materials.

✳ Describe the situations in which a person should not be moved.

✳ Describe the proper method to use when the victim must be moved.

✳ Describe the proper lifting of a patient who does not have a spinal injury.

✳ Describe an extremity lift.

✳ Describe the proper retrieval of a person in water.

KEY WORDS

Arc – To complete an electrical form or current. Electrical current moves through a conducting object or open air to seek a ground to complete its form.

Blanket drag – A procedure using a blanket to remove a patient from an accident scene.

CHEMTREC – Chemical Transportation Emergency Center. The national hazardous materials clearinghouse for 24 hour information. The toll free number is 1-800-424-9300.

Collar drag – A procedure using the patient's collar to drag the patient from the accident scene.

Cribbing – Wedging used to protect First Responders and others from becoming trapped under heavy objects.

Department of Transportation placards – Warning cards placed on all four sides of vehicles transporting hazardous materials across state lines. A placard is also attached to each shipping container containing hazardous materials.

Disentanglement – Remove a patient from an accident scene.

Extremity lift – A lifting procedure using the patient's legs and arms.

Firefighter carry – A lifting procedure performed by placing the patient over the shoulders of rescuer.

Gaining access – The first entrance to a vehicle or place.

Gas vapor cloud – A vapor caused by a fire, explosion, or the leak of a dangerous chemical.

Hazardous materials – Substances that are harmful or toxic to the cells of the body if they come in contact with the body in sufficient quantities.

Nonemergency move – A move that does not endanger a patient.

Packaging – Preparing a patient for transport.

Safety glass – A strong glass found in vehicle windshields with a heavy plastic protective lamination between two separate pieces of glass. This glass will crack but not shatter.

Tempered glass – Glass that is hardened with a metal alloy that causes it to shatter when broken. This glass is usually found in the side windows of all vehicles.

Walking assist – Removing patients from an accident scene by helping them to walk away.

Wind direction – The direction in which wind is moving.

Five of the most important aspects of accident assistance include:

1. Surveying the scene for hazards.
2. Containing those hazards.
3. Gaining safe access to the injured.
4. Providing assistance to the injured.
5. Contacting the EMSS for assistance.

The First Responder should first look for any containers involved in the accident. Gasoline or any other chemical container should have a distinctive look. They can be recognized by their size, shape, or construction. Some are even color coded to make them more recognizable. The U.S. Department of Transportation, (DOT) has a placard system to identify fire hazards, medical dangers, explosion dangers, and dangerous content mixtures found in containers of hazardous materials (Figure 15-1).

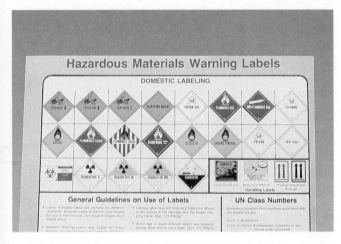

Figure 15-1. DOT hazardous materials sign.

This label will quickly provide the name and the dangers of the product. An important tool in the First Responder's kit may be a pair of binoculars to help read these labels from a safe distance.

Summon help as quickly as possible when an accident occurs. If no one else is present, find the nearest telephone and call for additional help. If you have access to a radio, use it. Know the channel used to monitor CB emergency calls in your area. Do not attempt anything you are untrained or unequipped to do. You may cause further injury.

THE PRELIMINARY SURVEY

The First Responder must resist the urge to rush into a situation without making a quick, overall survey of the scene. Many persons have sustained unnecessary injuries from failure to look before acting. If you are accidentally injured in the process of reaching the patient, you become an additional victim (Figure 15-2).

* Location of accident.
* Gas vapor cloud.
* Hazardous chemical placards or containers.
* DOT Labels on vehicles or containers.
* Liquid or powder spills.
* Wind direction, water, terrain and other weather hazards.
* Electrical sources.
* Ignition sources.
* Unstable overhead objects.
* Objects blocking the view of the accident scene.
* The number and type of vehicles involved.
* Approximate number of persons injured

Figure 15-2. What should the First Responder look for here?

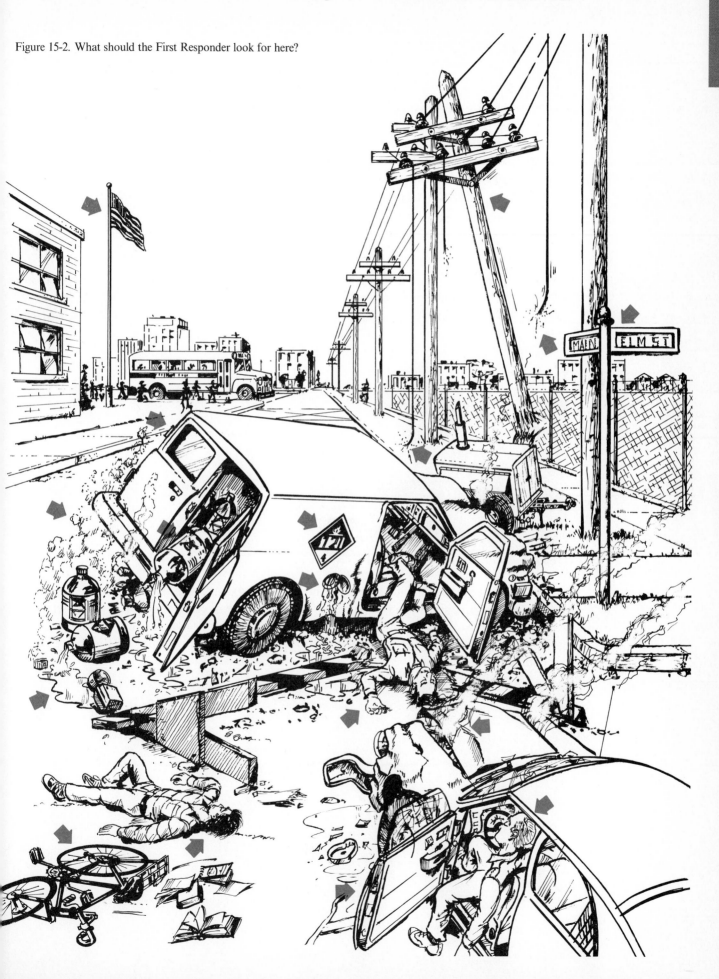

VEHICLE PLACEMENT

When arriving at an accident scene always attempt to park in a safe place. Do not block open traffic lanes unless absolutely necessary. Leave room for other needed responders to park so they can do their jobs efficiently. Make a quick overall survey of the scene before you do anything. If a law enforcement officer is present, ask them for directions. Always park upwind at a safe distance from the accident site, especially when hazardous materials are involved. Be sure to wear bright colored clothing and turn your emergency flashers on when parking near an accident site. This will warn other responders and will also help them to more quickly locate the scene.

Do not park in the roadway near the accident site except in the following cases:

❋ To warn oncoming traffic when their vision of the scene is blocked.

❋ To protect injured persons in the right-of-way.

❋ To protect yourself or others in the right-of-way.

When only one lane is available (Figure 15-3), place your vehicle on the shoulder of the road. Do not block traffic or other emergency vehicles from reaching the scene. An open lane may be improvised along the shoulder, or a parking lot may be used to divert traffic away from the accident site.

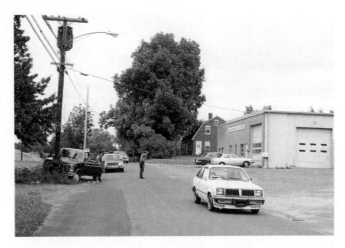

Figure 15-3. One-lane available.

If the accident occurs on a four-lane highway (Figure 15-4), park in the affected lane past the site of the accident. In some situations your vehicle may have to be parked before the accident to serve as a warning marker. Follow local practices. The presence of hazardous materials may not allow you to park in this location. If this occurs, find a safe place that will not cause problems for you or others responding to the accident.

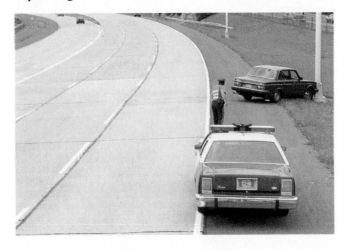

Figure 15-4. Four-lane highway.

Parking is usually simple on an expressway with service roads and medians (Figure 15-5). Remember to not block traffic flow and place your vehicle where you do not have to continue to cross flowing traffic.

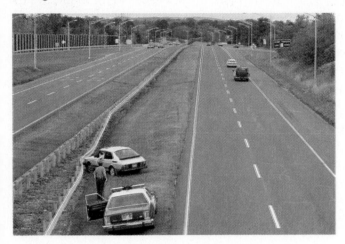

Figure 15-5. An expressway with service roads and medians.

There are five types of primary intersections:

1. One lane entering two lanes.

2. Two lanes entering two lanes.

3. Two lanes entering four lanes.

4. Four lanes entering four lanes.

5. Dual or multiple lanes entering dual or multiple lanes without medians (Figure 15-6).

Find a safe parking place out of traffic unless your vehicle is needed for protection of the scene.

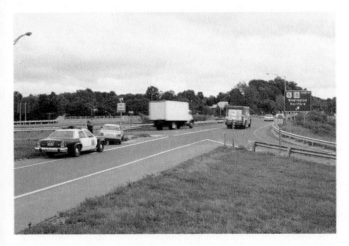

Figure 15-6. Dual or multiple lanes entering dual or multiple lane without medians.

CONTAINMENT OF HAZARDS

Preventing others from entering a potentially dangerous scene can reduce further injuries. Before you enter a possibly dangerous environment, measure the costs. If you can be more effective by protecting others from harm do so until the properly equipped responder can be summoned. Survey the scene with an eye toward preventing hazards that could complicate rescue. The following list describes these hazards and methods to control them:

✳ If a vehicle contains hazardous materials, park a safe distance upwind (with the wind at the responder's back) from the incident. Contact the agency in the area responsible for containment of hazardous scenes.

✳ Carefully look around if you notice downed electrical wires and call the power company if lines or poles have been knocked down. Locate the two poles before and after the broken wires. Draw an imaginary circle around the perimeter and park outside the circle (Figures 15-7a and 15-7b).

You can immobilize a downed wire that is throwing sparks by placing a spare tire on them to hold them in place (Figure 15-8). If you cannot perform this task safely, do not enter or allow others to enter the arc area of the wire. Require those involved in the accident to stay in place until the wire can be secured. Call the power company.

✳ Most fire hazards can be controlled by reducing the ignition sources. An automobile fire will usually occur at the time of impact. If it does not flash on impact:

Turn off all ignitions.
Disconnect battery ground cables.
Do not allow smoking on the scene.
Do not use tools that cause sparks.

Most scenes require a good overview, thinking of hazards, and knowing when not to enter the affected area. *Do not* attempt to enter the area unless all dangers are understood, correct protective clothing is present, and those entering are properly trained to control the hazard.

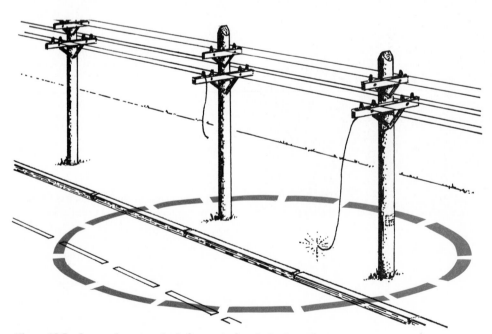

Figure 15-7a. Locate the two poles before and after the broken wires.

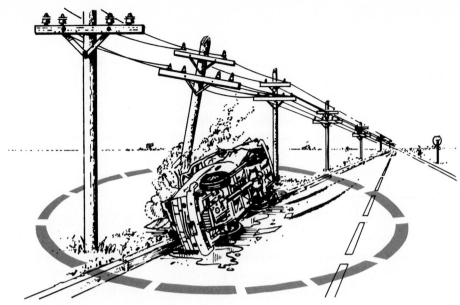

Figure 15-7b. Imagine a circle around the perimeter.

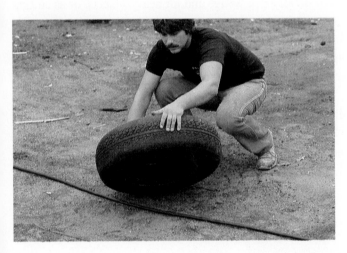

Figure 15-8. You can immobilize a downed wire that is throwing sparks by placing a spare tire on the wire.

GAINING ACCESS TO PATIENTS

Tools and Equipment

Special tools are not needed by the First Responder to gain access to accident victims. Each vehicle arriving at an accident scene may provide one or more tools for entering vehicles. The following tools are usually found near an accident scene:

* Spare tires - Use these to prevent heavy vehicles from slipping and trapping persons. They can also be used to hold electrical wires in place to reduce the hazard of being hurt. Spare tires make excellent flotation devices in a water accident (Figure 15-9).

* Lug wrench - Use this wrench to open windows and doors. Use this wrench to remove additional spare wheels and tires if needed (Figure 15-10).

* Vehicle jacks - Use these jacks to pull, pry, and lift heavy objects (Figure 15-11).

* Hand tools (Figure 15-12).
    Pliers - You can use pliers to pull glass, lift chrome, or remove plastic covers, and to help cutting tools work easier.
    Screwdrivers - You can use screwdrivers to pry, lift objects, and prevent injury by wedging heavy objects.
    Hacksaws - You can use hacksaws to cut light metal.
    Hammers - You can use hammers to break glass, wedge and lift heavy objects, or as cutting tools for sheet metal.
    Axes or hatchets - Use these for both cutting and prying tools.
    Pocket knives - Use these to cut seat belts, rubber gaskets, and clothes to use as bandages.

* Rope - Use rope as a safety line to keep heavy objects from moving. Rope can also be helpful in pulling and spreading operations.

* Wreckers - Use wreckers to lift, pull, or pry weights equal to their own weight. Some wreckers come equipped with special rescue tools like air bags or cutters.

* Gloves prevent minor injuries to the hands of the First Responder.

* Eye glasses will protect the eyes from flying objects. If available, use safety glasses; they are more effective.

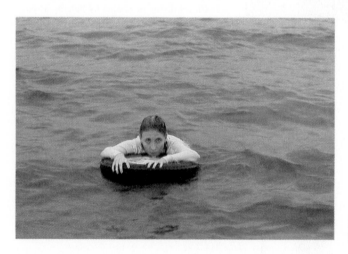

Figure 15-9. A spare tire makes an excellent flotation device.

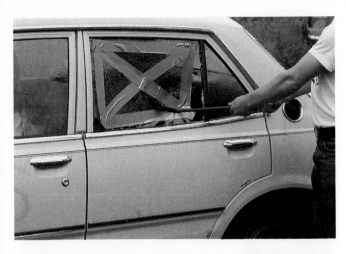

Figure 15-10. A lug wrench may be used to open windows and doors.

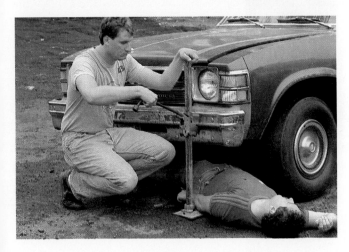

Figure 15-11. A vehicle jack may be used to pull, pry or lift heavy objects.

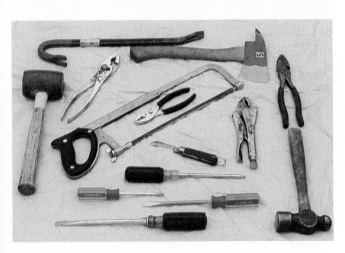

Figure 15-12. These hand tools are very useful to gain access to a vehicle.

Gaining Access

The primary responsibility for the First Responder is to gain access to an accident scene to prevent further harm. If this goal cannot be accomplished safely, for both the responders and the injured, do not attempt access. Before forcing entry, always try to open all vehicle doors by using their handles. If all doors and windows are jammed closed, enter the vehicle through the easiest point. Secure the vehicle before applying any cutting, prying, or pulling tools (Figure 15-13). The steps to secure a vehicle include:

✳ Preventing ignition from all controllable sources. Turn off ignitions, cut battery ground cables, and do not smoke.

✳ Using cribbing to prevent the vehicle from falling over on you or others (Figure 15-14).

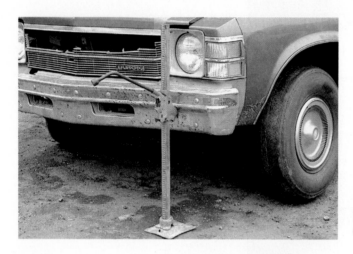

Figure 15-13. Secure the vehicle before using cutting, prying, or pulling tools.

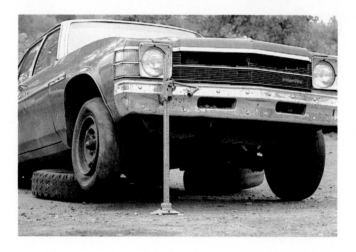

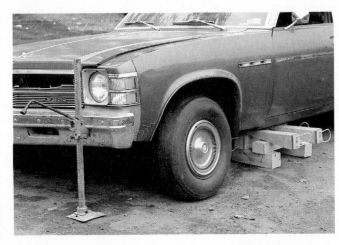

Figure 15-14. Use cribbing to prevent the vehicle from falling over on you.

Windows and Doors

Windows are usually the most effective way to enter a wrecked vehicle. Once a window is opened or removed, the doors can usually be opened. Select a window away from the patient(s). Use as little force as necessary to break the window. Enter windows using one of the following methods:

✳ Side windows - Force any vent windows open with a hammer, screwdriver, or pliers. Strike the very corner of the window with a hammer, lug wrench, or screwdriver and hammer (Figure 15-15). Clear all glass away and enter the vehicle. The doors do not have to be open for you to begin patient care.

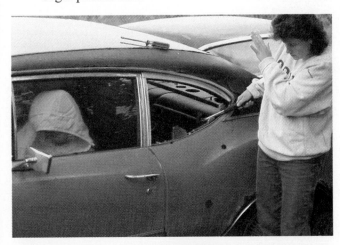

Figure 15-15. Breaking the side window.

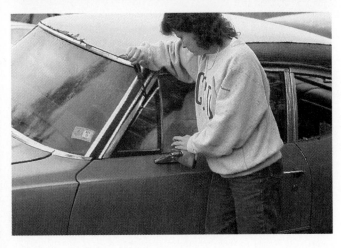

✳ Front or rear windows - Remove all rubber mounted windshields and rear windows by cutting the rubber seals away. The chrome protectors may have to be removed as shown in Figures 15-16. Many of the newer cars have both front and rear windows that are glued in place. Cut these windows away using an axe, hatchet, or hammer.

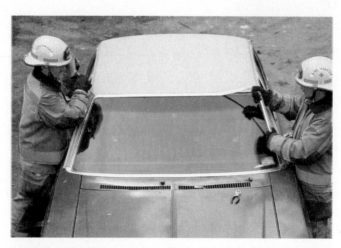

Figure 15-16. Removing the chrome protectors on a window.

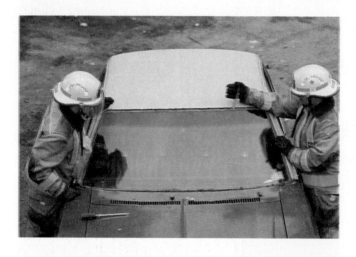

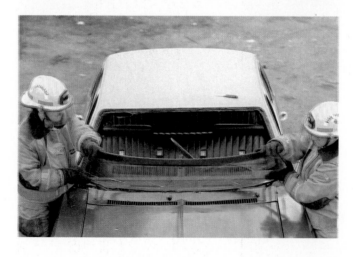

One of the important differences found between the construction of the side glass, which is tempered, and the windshield or back window is the safety protection found in some front and rear windows. When struck, the side glass will break into many small pieces; windshield and back window glass will often be protected by a strong plastic innershield. Many back windows are constructed like side windows. Try to remove them. Search for windows that can be opened quickly.

The tints applied to the inside of car windows are an asset to the First Responder. If this tint is properly applied, the window will remain firm when broken and can be lifted out intact (Figure 15-17).

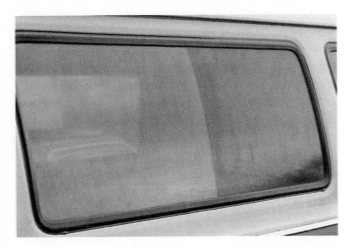

Figure 15-17. Tinted windows.

Overturned Vehicles

Most overturned vehicles can be entered through the windows or doors. *Do not* attempt to right an overturned vehicle before removing the patients. Use one of the following methods to stabilize the vehicle while access is being attempted:

❋ Place a jack strategically under the vehicle to prevent rocking motion (Figure 15-18a).

❋ Use a spare tire with a rope and jack to stabilize the vehicle (Figure 15-18b).

❋ Use a spare tire with a rope and jack to stabilize the vehicle (Figure 15-19).

If you cannot gain access to the vehicle through a window, cut through the floor with an axe, hatchet, or even a hammer. You can rapidly expand the size of the hole using a hacksaw. It is usually safer to cut floor holes in the rear of the vehicle. One can easily cut out the floorwell and have excellent access to the injured. Vans can be cut almost anywhere. They are usually composed of a single layer of thin metal on all sides. You do not have to be as selective when looking for a spot to open a van. The most important concern during this procedure is not to further injure anyone that may be in the van.

Never enter an unstable vehicle. Always secure the vehicle using one of the methods discussed. Any openings like metal flaps or doors should be tied off to prevent them from falling into and injuring you or one of the patients.

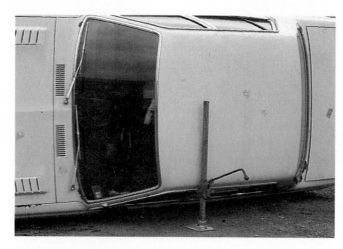

Figure 15-18a. A jack may be used to prevent a rocking motion.

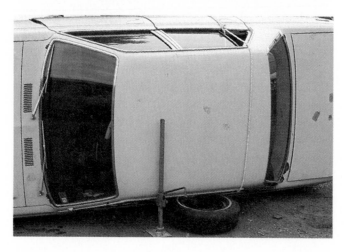

Figure 15-18b. A spare tire used with a rope and jack may be used to stabilize and lift a vehicle.

Electrical Hazards

If a vehicle involved in an accident comes in contact with electrical wires, assume they are energized until proven otherwise. *Do not* touch the vehicle. All conscious persons trapped in the vehicle should be instructed to provide needed care; bleeding control, fracture immobilization, and other care. Try to access or remove them *only* after the power company has secured the electrical current and makes sure the area is safe. Unless absolutely necessary, have entrapped persons remain in the vehlicle.

If other factors require removing the patient from the vehicle, take extreme care to protect them. Potential fires, explosive, or toxic hazards may require removing the injured from the vehicle. Tell the victim to leap from the vehicle without making contact with the ground and the car at the same time. Tell the victim to land on one foot and proceed to hop out of the energized area (Figure 15-19). This helps prevent the victim from closing the circuit and being shocked while in the accident area. An area around the vehicle, especially in sandy soil, may be energized with electricity. Small children may be tossed out of the energized area to the arms of First Responders. *Do not* rush in to danger and be patient. This is a risky procedure and should not be attempted unless danger to life is imminent.

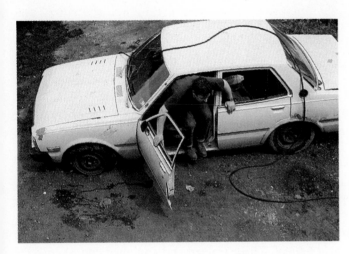

Figure 15-19. Hop on one foot out of the energized area.

Trapped Persons

Use a jack or a fulcrum process to lift a heavy object or a vehicle off a trapped person. An object, like a spare tire, may be used for wedging cribbage. Make sure the object used for lifting has enough strength to allow you to safely lift the object trapping the person. Never place a part of your body under the object being lifted (Figure 15-20). A slip may cause the object to fall trapping you and further injuring both you and the person. Be careful when using people to lift. The lifted object may slide creating further injury to the patient.

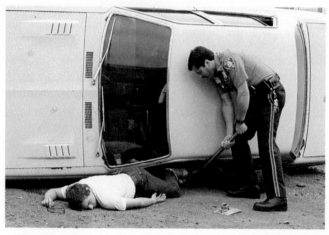

Figure 15-20. Never place a part of your body under the object being lifted.

The First Responder will seldom be required to extricate an entrapped person. This job should be left for the team having the tools, expertise, and personnel to quickly, safely, and effectively remove objects from around patients.

If a portion of a patient's body, such as their head, arm or leg, has been extruded through a window or other opening in the vehicle, pad the part with protective dressings. Try to remove the torn metal or glass away from the injured part. This can often be accomplished by using pliers, hacksaws, or other pulling and cutting tools.

The First Responder will rarely need to do more than move the front seat back or remove the back seat (Figure 15-21) to make room to treat a patient. Those trained and equipped can remove the injured from the vehicle. Splint all suspected broken bones before moving persons in or out of vehicles.

Do not disengage seat belts until full spinal immobilization has been accomplished. The only reason for moving a patient is when a life-threatening danger exists. Most belts may be released using the release button. If this is not successful, a knife will cut the nylon strap and allow the belt to be removed. Never cut a seat belt when the patient is strapped in and the vehicle is upside down. Make sure enough personnel are available to properly support and secure the injured patient.

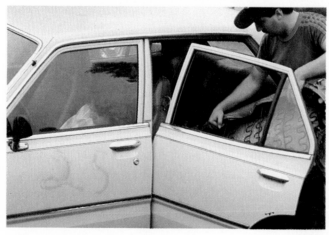

Figure 15-21. Removing the back seat.

MOVING INJURED PATIENTS

The First Responder should *never* attempt to move anyone unless the patient is in imminent danger. Many persons have sustained greater injury from being improperly moved. Most conditions allow time for stabilizing injured body parts before moving.

The only reasons to move an injured patient are:

* Serious contamination by hazardous materials.

* A real danger of fire or explosion.

* Need to gain access to other severely injured patients. This should only be accomplished when others are in danger of dying.

* It is impossible to provide protection of the accident scene.

Ask yourself this question before moving an accident victim. Is there sufficient cause to suspect signal injury? If you answer "yes" to this question, quickly splint the spine before moving the injured patient. Flexion, extension, and lateral movements of the spine must be minimized. You can often use the patient's clothing to temporarily splint the spine. An example of good neck immobilization is to use the vehicle's sun visor. Remove the visor and place one end down the patient's shirt or jacket. Secure the collar to hold the visor in place. Pull a sock or stocking over the patient's head and the other end of the sun visor (Figure 15-22). This holds the head and neck in a secure position. Use any of the methods to secure the spine or other bones discussed in the previous chapters for this purpose.

Always pull the patient by the long axis of the body. Follow this rule even when proper equipment for immobilization is used (Figure 15-23).

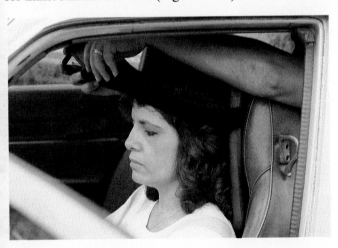

Figure 15-22. A belt and sun visor may be used to hold the head and neck in a secure position.

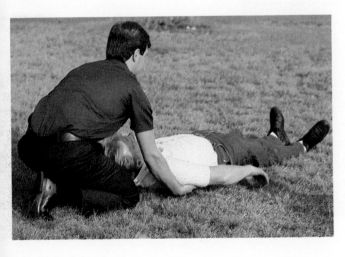

Figure 15-23. Always pull the patient by the long axis of the body.

Use the following techniques to move the patient in imminent danger:

❋ Collar drag (Figure 15-24)

❋ Fireman's drag (Figure 15-25)

❋ Blanket drag (Figure 15-26)

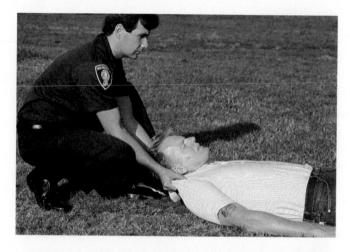

Figure 15-24. The collar drag.

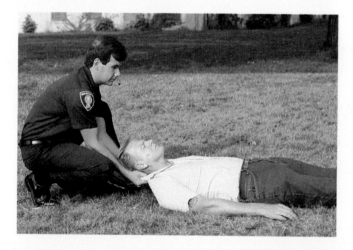

Figure 15-25. The fireman's drag.

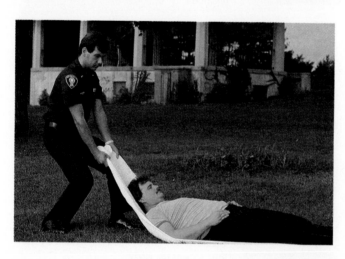

Figure 15-26. The blanket drag.

Nonemergency Moves

The First Responder should wait for help from the responsible agency before moving patients unnecessarily. Communicate with those responsible and follow their directions. The following are a few single-person lifts and carries that are used to move patients:

✳ Walking assist (Figure 15-27). The patient must be conscious and capable of helping. To perform this move:

> Place that patient's arm around your shoulders and grasp his or her wrist.
> Place you other arm around the patient's waist.

✳ Fireman's carry (Figure 15-28). This carry allows you to lift and carry any patient equal to, or smaller than the lifter. The patient must be conscious for this lift to be effective. This lift frees one of your arms to open doors and push other harmful objects out of the way. To perform this, use the following method:

> Roll the patient on his or her back.
> Flex the patient's knees and block his or her toes with yours to prevent sliding.
> Grasp the patient's wrist, your right to the patient's right and left to the patient's left. Cross your arms at the wrists.
> Drag the person up on your shoulder with a smooth pulling and lifting motion.
> Stand carefully.
> Grasp one of the patient's hands and one of his feet with one of your hands.

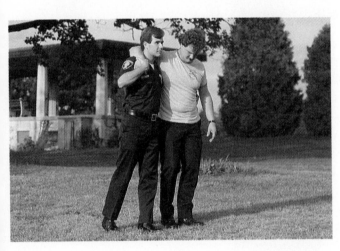

Figure 15-27. The walking assist.

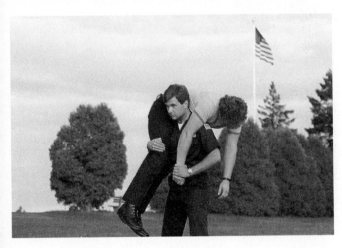

Figure 15-28. The fireman's carry.

❋ Use the packstrap carry (Figure 15-29) when the patient is larger than the First Responder.

Place your body parallel to the injured person.
Pull the patient's arm around your neck.
Roll face down and rise to your hand and knees.
Stand using leg muscles only.

❋ Use the blanket drag (Figure 15-30) when a blanket is present and can be easily placed beneath the injured person. The number of lifters may indicate the lifting and carrying method.

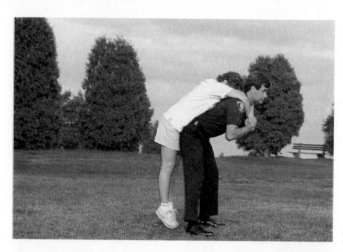

Figure 15-29. The packstrap carry.

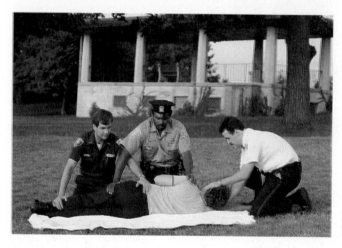

Figure 15-30. Positioning the blanket for the blanket drag.

Multiperson Lifts

Learn the multiperson lifts from your local EMS personnel. Variations of these lifts exist in many areas of the country. The most effective patient moves require teamwork. This teamwork must be developed among those persons working together. Take advantage of the expertise of those around your community and form a working team to allow you to help them more easily perform their jobs.

WATER ACCIDENTS

Due to the popularity of water related sports in our country, everyone should know how to secure a near-drowned person. Many people drown in shallow water. As stated earlier, First Responders should never enter a situation for which they are neither equipped or trained. Water rescue is no exception. The First Responder should only enter the water as a last resort. Many objects found around the scene will float. A few of these include:

* Rope - Don't forget to hold on to one end.

* Spare tire and wheel - A standard spare tire and wheel is capable of floating up to 20 persons at the same time (Figure 15-31).

* Plastic jug - Put a little water inside and tie a rope to the handle. Milk jugs work very well for this purpose.

* Gas can - Gas weighs less than water so the can will float.

* An ice cooler - Tape the lid on and tie a rope to the handle.

* Plastic garbage bags - Place a little water inside the bag and tie a rope to the open end to seal it.

* Other objects - Wood, chairs and other similar objects will float.

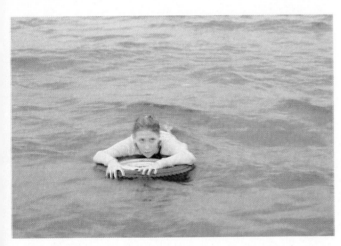

Figure 15-31. A spare tire makes an excellent flotation device.

Most human bodies will float. Learn to float in a safe place. Fill your lungs with air, hold this air in and breathe only when necessary. Hold your head back and you will float face up. Prove you can, it may save your life someday. If you find yourself in unknown water:

Check the depth; you may not be over your head

You can bob out if the water is less than 12-15 feet deep. Bounce down to the bottom, push up to the surface, take a breath, go to the bottom again and repeat the steps while bouncing toward shore.

If you are in water that is too deep, float.

Do not attempt to move a person from a pool until their spine is immobile if you suspect spinal injury. Float the person onto the ledge at the side of the pool and work with them there.

The basic rules of saving a person from drowning are:

* THROW them an object to grasp that floats.

* TOW them to shallow water.

* GO in the water only if equipped and trained to do so.

SUMMARY

First Responders should remember all the steps required to gain access to injured patients. The initial steps include:

❋ Survey the scene for dangers, including:
   Hazards.
   Protect the scene and others arriving.
   Secure hazards if possible.
   Gain access.
   Secure the injured persons.

❋ Call for needed help.

The First Responder will seldom need to move a patient before additional help arrives. The only reasons to move a patient involve life or death situations. No injured person should be moved unless absolutely necessary. *Do not* attempt any procedure or rescue you are untrained or unequipped to do.

THE MEDICOLEGAL ASPECTS OF EMERGENCY CARE

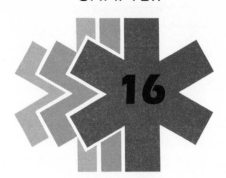

16

KEY CONCEPTS AND SKILLS

By the end of this chapter, you will be able to:

✱ Discuss the medical and legal (medicolegal) aspects of emergency care, including:

What constitutes an emergency.
Your duty to act.
Standard of care to provide the patients.
Consent: actual, implied, minors, and mind-altered patients.
Forcible restraint.
Good Samaritan laws.
Certification.

✱ Sort patients using triage for ordinary and mass casualty purposes.

✱ Describe the general considerations for communication, interface, and working with other units in a mass casualty situation.

✱ Describe the general rules of communication in emergency medical care.

✱ Describe the basics of report writing and the importance of the written report in the Emergency Medical Services System (EMSS).

KEY WORDS

Abandonment – The unilateral termination of care by the EMS provider without the patient's consent and without making provision for continuing care at the same level or higher.

Certification – A process in which a person, an institution, or program is evaluated and recognized as meeting certain predetermined standards. The purpose of certification is to assure that the standards met are those necessary for safe and ethical care.

Consent – In medicolegal terms, granting permission to another to render care.

Duty to Act – A medicolegal term relating to certain personnel who either by statute or function have a responsibility to provide care.

Emergency – A serious situation that arises suddenly and threatens the life or welfare of a person or a group of people.

Forcible Restraint – The process of confining an individual from any action, mental or physical.

Good Samaritan Laws – Statutory provisions enacted by many states to protect citizens from civil and criminal liability in rendering gratuitous emergency medical care, unless there is willful, wrong, or gross negligence.

Mass Casualty Triage – Sorting of patients into priority categories for care and transport, usually in emergencies involving more than five patients.

Medicolegal – A term relating to medical jurisprudence or forensic medicine.

Ordinary Triage – Sorting patients into priority categories for care and transport, usually in emergencies involving less than five patients.

Standard of Care – Written, accepted levels of emergency care expected by reason of training and profession.

Rendering emergency medical care in an organized system is a recent phenomenon. As the scope and nature of emergency medical care becomes more sophisticated and available, litigation involving participants in the Emergency Medical Services System (EMSS) will no doubt increase. For this reason, First Responders must understand the various legal aspects of emergency care.

A basic principle of emergency care is to do no further harm. Any health care provider acting in good faith and according to an appropriate standard of care may avoid legal exposure.

DEFINITIONS

What is an Emergency? – An emergency is a serious situation that arises suddenly and threatens the life or welfare of a person or group of people. First Responders usually deal with traumatic events that may be an accident or illness requiring immediate intervention.

Emergency Medical Assistance – Emergency medical assistance is defined as immediate care or treatment. The First Responder is often the first link in the chain of prehospital care.

Negligence – Negligence is the omission to do something that a reasonable person would do acting under the same or similar circumstances. It may be defined as deviation from accepted standards of care (Figure 16-1).

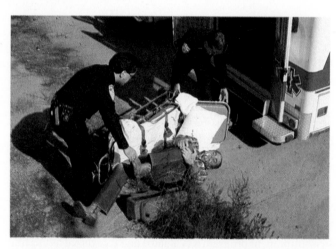

Figure 16-1. An example of negligence.

Standards of care are written by law or professional organizations for the purpose of not exposing others to unreasonable risk or harm. Negligence is the failure to provide the same care that a person of similar training would provide.

Determining negligence is based on the following factors:

* Duty: It is the responsibility of the First Responder to act reasonably. Conduct is measured by standards of care based upon training. How would a person with similar training act under the same circumstances?

* Breach of duty: Not acting within an expected and reasonable standard of care.

* Damages: The patient is harmed in some noticeable way.

* Proximate cause: There must be a reasonable cause and effect, e.g., you drop the stretcher and the patient falls off and fractures a leg.

Standards of Care

Many standards of care may be imposed on the First Responder. State health department regulations usually govern the scope and level of training. Court decisions have resulted in case law defining standards of care. Professional standards are also imposed. An example is the American Heart Association standard for BLS-CPR.

Ordinary Care

Ordinary care is a minimum standard. In general, it is expected that anyone who offers assistance will exercise reasonable care and act prudently. If you act reasonably, according to the accepted standard, the risk of civil suit is small. By applying standard practices you have been trained to use, liability is likely to be avoided. Various organizations have defined standards for CPR. Deviating from these standards may cause the First Responder to be liable.

STANDARDS IMPOSED BY LAW

Medical Practices Act

Most states exempt emergency medical services personnel from the licensure requirements of medical practices acts. The First Responder is regarded as a nonmedical professional. The practice of medicine is defined as the diagnosis and treatment of disease or illness. An unlicensed person who engages in such activities can be liable for both civil and criminal action. There is little question that First Responders and others in the prehospital care chain assess the need for life support and start care. The standard of care must be maintained within the scope of your state's provisions and licensing requirements.

Certification

Some states provide for either certification or licensure of persons who perform emergency medical care. These certifications obligate you to conform to these standards. The standards are generally recognized nationally by various registry groups and provide an important link in the nationwide EMSS. In order to be protected, certification or licensure must remain current; skill levels must be kept up to date (Figure 16-2).

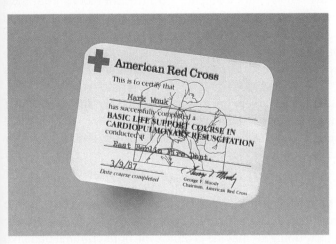

Figure 16-2. A CPR card.

Many associations have recently changed their concept. The American Heart Association, for example, now only acknowledges one's successful completion of a BLS-CPR course. Certification has specific legal meaning and is generally restricted to licensing agencies.

MEDICOLEGAL CONSIDERATIONS

Duty to Act

A bystander is under no obligation to assist a stranger in distress; there is no duty to act. However, there may be a duty to act in certain instances, including:

* ✳ If the person is charged with emergency medical response.
* ✳ If assisting in any emergency is the stated policy of your service or department.

If a person has a duty and abuses it, and harms another individual, the First Responder and/or the agency may be sued for negligence.

Abandonment

Abandonment, in terms for the First Responder, means the unilateral termination of care without the patient's consent, and without making any provisions for continuing care at the same or a higher level. In terms for the First Responder, once care is started, it must not stop until an equally competent person assumes responsibility. When care is started, the First Responder has assumed a duty. Not performing that duty exposes the patient to harm and is a basis for a negligence suit.

Consider the following set of circumstances. You arrive at the scene of a single-car accident with two injured persons and begin care. A passerby stops and tells you that there is a two-car accident down the road with five injured people. You turn care over to the passerby and leave to go to the other accident.

What problems may develop from the above actions?

* ✳ Did you neglect your duty to the persons in the first accident?
* ✳ What was the level of training of the passerby?
* ✳ Did you abandon the person you were helping?
* ✳ Did you violate a standard of care?
* ✳ Did you act prudently?

An abandonment of duty is reflected in the case of *Pettee versus Elk Grove Village* involving the volunteer fire department. June Pettee, who was pregnant, began having an acute respiratory problem. Her husband called the Elk Grove Village Fire Company, located five blocks from their home. The ambulance was dispatched, but when the chief of the department realized that the family had not paid the required fee for service, he cancelled the response. He then notified the EMS in the district where the family lived. The chief failed to notify the family that a transfer had been made. The second ambulance took 20 minutes to respond to the call. The patient was dead upon arrival; the fetus died 40 minutes after delivery.

The jury awarded $355,000 to the estate based largely on the premise that the fire department receiving the first call had made a voluntary assumption and terminated aid without notifying the caller. The fire department thereby breached its duty, increased the patient's danger, and deprived her of the help she rightfully had an expectation to receive.

Consent

Under most circumstances, consent is required before care can be started. A person receiving care must give permission for treatment. If a person is in control of his or her actions, even though injured, and refuses care, you may not assist. In fact, doing so may be grounds for both criminal and civil action such as unlawful battery.

Consent can be actual or implied, and can involve the care of a minor or a mind-altered patient.

Actual Consent

Actual consent must be informed consent. The person being cared for must not only give permission for treatment, but also must understand the nature of the assistance to be rendered. The legal basis for this doctrine rests on the assumption that the patient has a right to determine what is to be done with his or her body.

A patient might agree to certain emergency medical care but not to other care. For example, a patient might agree to have you remove him from a car, but refuse further care. An injured person might agree to emergency care in her home, but refuse to be transported to a medical facility. Informed consent is valid if given orally. Merely signing a consent form does not eliminate the requirement to tell that patient what is involved.

Implied Consent

When a person is unconscious and unable to give consent or when a serious threat to life exists, the law holds that the patient has consented. However, many things may be unclear about what represents a "serious threat." Legal action would likely revolve around that question. This becomes a medicolegal judgment, which should be supported by maximum efforts of the First Responder to obtain consent. Refusal or your intention to render emergency care also may be implied. For example, a patient's action in pulling his arm from your splint may be an indication of nonconsent (Figure 16-3).

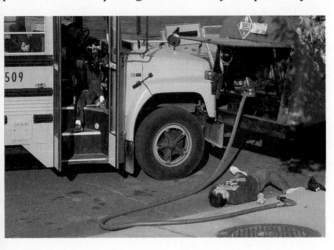

Figure 16-3. Implied consent is represented by this example.

Consent For Minors

The right of consent involving care of a minor belongs to the parent or guardian. If possible, make an effort to contact the parent or guardian, but in serious cases consent is implied.

REMEMBER: Never withhold lifesaving care.

Mind-Altered Patients

Assisting patients who are mentally ill, in behavioral (psychologic) crisis, under the influence of drugs or alcohol, or retarded is complicated. Medicolegally, it is similar to situations involving minors. The approval to render emergency care should be obtained from those legally responsible. In many cases, however, such permission will not be readily obtainable. Many states have protective custody statutes allowing such a person to be taken, under law enforcement authority, to a medical facility. Know the provisions in your area.

Forcible Restraint

Before emergency care can be rendered, forcible restraint of the mind-altered individual may be required. In most states only a law enforcement officer may forcibly restrain an individual. The First Responder should be clearly informed about local laws. Restraint without authority exposes you to both litigation and possible personal danger. Restraint may only be used in circumstances of risk to yourself or others.

If forcible restraint is required, law enforcement officers must be called. Your service should have clearly defined protocols to deal with this aspect. After restraints are applied, they must not be removed enroute even if the patient promises to behave.

> **REMEMBER:** If the patient is conscious and the situation is not urgent, consent is required. Adults who appear to be in control of their senses cannot be forced to submit to either care or transportation.

Good Samaritan Laws

Most states have adopted Good Samaritan laws. These provisions are based on the common law principle. This principle holds that when you reasonably help another person, you should not be liable for ordinary negligence. However, Good Samaritan laws do not protect you from a law suit. Only a few statutory provisions provide immunity from a law suit and those usually are reserved to governments.

The Good Samaritan law provides an affirmative defense if you are sued for rendering care. It does not protect you from liability or for failure to provide proper care, nor does it pertain to acts outside the scope of care. The law does not protect anyone from wanton, gross, or willful negligence, e.g., the failure to exercise due care.

Consider these circumstances. You are a member of a volunteer squad. You respond to a pool-side accident in which a person, under the influence of alcohol, dove into the shallow end of the pool. His friends pull the victim out, who is still breathing. You place the patient on a stretcher but do not provide for cervical spine stabilization because the patient is belligerent. Enroute to the medical facility, the patient sits up and complains of pain in the neck and has great difficulty in breathing. Upon examination in the emergency room, the patient is found to have a fracture of the cervical spine and is quadriplegic.

What are some of the issues in this case?

* Are the squad members exempt from civil damages because they were volunteers and covered under the Good Samaritan act?
* Did they act in accordance with a standard of care?
* Were the patient's subsequent injuries related to the care not rendered?
* In a similar case *(Rose versus Foothill Ambulance Service, California, 1976)*, a man under the influence of alcohol dove into a pool and struck his head. He was lifted out by a bystander. Care was rendered by bystanders, but the EMS responder failed to properly protect the patient's spine. The jury awarded $500,000 in damages in favor of Mr. Rosa. The basis for the decision rested on the assumption that the EMTs should have understood that an intoxicated person has a diminished capacity to reason. In spite of Mr. Rosa's drunken actions, the EMS responder must extend more care to him than to a sober person. This case illustrates an increased standard of care required when treating inebriated persons.

TRIAGE

Triage was first used as a system to sort various commodities. In France, during World War I, the concept of triage was used to sort battlefield casualties. In ordinary triage you deal with a small number of patients, generally no more than five. In mass casualty triage some of the priorities change due to a large number of patients.

Triage follows the ABCs:

* Maintain an airway with spine control.

* Maintain breathing.

* Control breathing.

The First Responder must determine which patients require lifesaving care. In ordinary triage, the goal is to establish a priority of care for those most critically injured. In mass casualty triage, the goal is to determine priority of those seriously injured who have the best chance of survival.

> **REMEMBER:** An important principle is to do no harm. Be conscious of your own safety by not placing your own life in danger. The most immediate concerns are lack of breathing and extensive bleeding (hemorrhage).

Ordinary Triage

As discussed in Chapter 3, triage is divided into three categories (Figure 16-4). *First priority* (immediate care) patients require immediate stabilization and transportation to a medical facility. The priorities are:

* Acute respiratory insufficiency.

* Cardiac arrest.

* Massive, uncontrollable bleeding (hemorrhage).

* Open chest or abdominal trauma.

* Severe laceration involving open fractures of the major bones.

* Severe burns of the face or upper respiratory tract.

* Burns covering 40% of the Body Surface Area (BSA).

* Severe medical problems such as poisoning or diabetic emergencies.

* Severe head injury.

* Shock.

Second priority (urgent care) patients show the following conditions and should be transported to a medical facility as soon as possible:

* Rapidly correctable mechanical respiratory defects (obstructions).

* Controllable bleeding (hemorrhage) from an easily accessible site.

* Severe crushing wounds of the extremities.

* Burns on 15-40% of BSA.

* Major multiple fractures.

* Injuries to the spine.

* Severe eye injuries.

* Penetrating abdominal wounds (perforating wounds as well).

Third priority (delayed care) patients show the following conditions and should be transported to a medical facility as soon as it becomes practical:

* Obviously or imminently dead.
* Minor injuries.
* Closed fractures (simple).
* Lacerations without severe bleeding.
* Burns on less than 15% of BSA (except of the respiratory tract).
* Emotionally distressed but not severely injured.

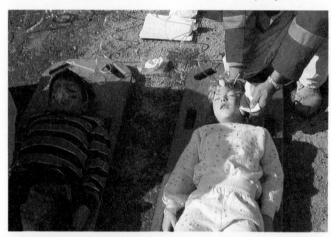

Figure 16-4. Examples of triage. **A,** First priority (immediate care).

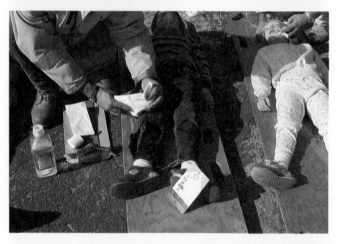

B, Second priority (urgent care).

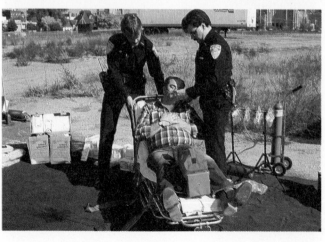

C, Third priority (delayed care).

Mass Casualty Triage

In a mass casualty, it is not always the severity of the injuries that determine priority. Rather, it is how quickly and efficiently you can do what is required. While you must pay attention to urgent needs, overall care is based on a determination of who has the best prognosis for recovery at the time of assessment (Figure 16-5).

> **REMEMBER:** It is important to recognize that no triage, whether ordinary or mass, is final. The process must be constantly updated to meet changing conditions. Also, the changes in resources in the field and at the receiving hospitals must be considered. Generally those stabilized first should be the first to leave the scene. Recognize that if an insufficient number of vehicles is available, a different order may have to be arranged, so transport patients using these guidelines:

IMMEDIATE: Approximately 20% of casualties. Conditions are:

* Rapidly correctable mechanical respiratory defect, e.g., opening the airway by using the chin-lift/head-tilt.
* Controllable bleeding from an easily accessible site.
* Severe crushing wounds of the extremities.
* Incomplete amputation.
* Severe lacerations involving open fracture of the large bones.
* Severe burns of the upper respiratory tract.
* Second- or third-degree burns of 15-40% of BSA.
* Major medical complications such as heart attack or severe bleeding disorders.

DELAYED: Approximately 20% of casualties. The conditions are:

* Closed fracture wounds.
* Moderate lacerations without bleeding.
* Severe eye injury.
* Noncritical central nervous system injury.
* Penetrating or perforating abdominal injury.

MINIMAL: Approximately 40% of casualties. The conditions are:

* Small lacerations with controllable bleeding.
* Closed fracture wounds of the small bones.
* Second-degree burns of less than 15% BSA, not including burns of the hand and/or face.
* Moderate mental health problems.
* Minor short-term whole body ionizing radiation.

EXPECTANT DEAD: Approximately 20% of casualties. The conditions are:

* Critical injuries to the central nervous system and respiratory systems.
* Multiple critical injuries.
* Burns of more than 40% BSA.
* Established lethal dose of total body radiation.

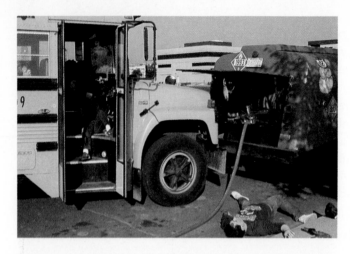

Figure 16-5. **A,** A mass casualty scene.

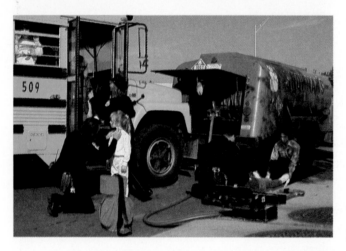

B, Initial care.

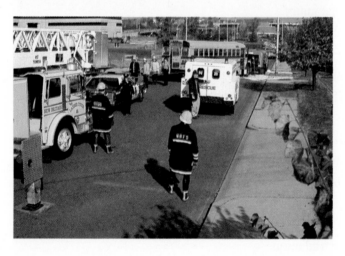

C, Fire suppression.

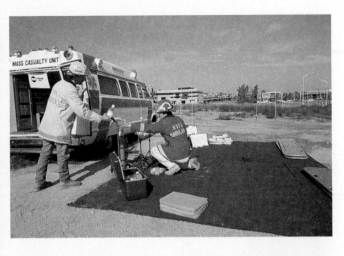

D, Setting up the mass casualty area.

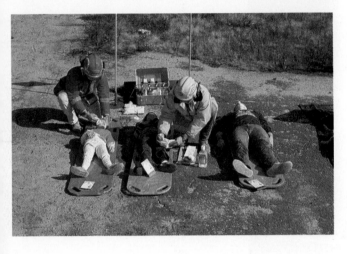

E, Emergency care and triage tagging.

Assessment of the Scene

The First Responder may be the first person on the scene to assess a disaster and activate the mass disaster plan. This means alerting your department to the type of disaster and number of casualties. This will allow preplanned notifications to be made. Notification includes the hospital, other public safety agencies, county and statewide EMS resources, and other units, e.g., civil preparedness and the Red Cross (Figure 16-6).

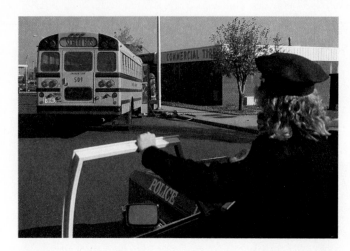

Figure 16-6. **A,** Police arriving at the scene.

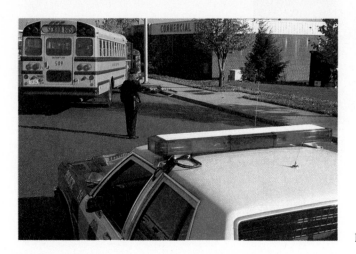

B, Scene assessment.

Classifying a Disaster

A disaster can be classified according to the number of casualties known or expected. The following classification is used by many states:

✳ Class 1: 3-15 casualties.

✳ Class 2: 16-150 casualties.

✳ Class 3: 150 or more casualties.

This system of classification is not the only one used; however, First Responders should use the method dictated by local guidelines and protocols.

Psychological Aspects

The behavior of those involved in a mass disaster may be severely affected. The general carnage, different sights and smells perceived can be overwhelming.

> **REMEMBER:** Staying calm, cool, and collected at the scene goes a long way to assure the injured as well as other emergency personnel. A First Responder with past experience and training should be able to handle the situation until additional help arrives. Bystanders and others with little or no previous experience may respond with great emotional distress. Preparing for such an occurrence may make management of the scene easier. Teams prepared to deal with psychological stress can be called on to help all responders and other persons involved in the disaster. However, the total impact may not be felt until hours, days, or months after the incident.

COMMUNICATIONS

One of the important responsibilities of the First Responder is using the communications system (Figure 16-7). Such a system may require:

✳ Transmitting information about the number of patients to central communications agencies.

✳ Knowledge of major problems and conditions.

✳ Kinds of assistance needed.

✳ Estimated times of arrival of patients to substations or area hospitals.

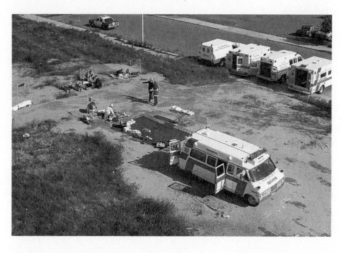

Figure 16-7. Triage area showing command center.

Many agencies will respond during a mass disaster (Figure 16-8). This may present communications and leadership problems. First Responders should follow the directions of the person or agency in charge. This will vary with the type of emergency services most urgently needed at the moment.

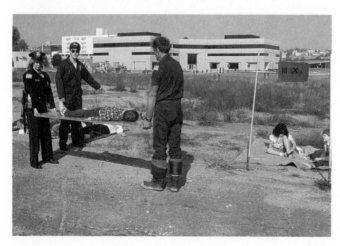

Figure 16-8. Multiple public safety service response.

Each agency should have a predefined communications plan. In the transmission of emergency data, it may be necessary to establish new guidelines. The rules of communication of any data, however, are not difficult to grasp:

✳ Be clear.

✳ Be concise.

✳ Remain calm; do not shout into microphone units.

✳ Be careful about transmitting the names of patients over radio frequencies because of possible violation of patient confidentiality. This is now more of a concern because of the widespread use of scanners.

In any communication, it is important that the sender is certain that the receiver has fully understood the data transmitted. This may be done by simply asking for assurance. If necessary, a brief repetition of the data may be requested, particularly when vital signs or other medical information is relayed.

In the presence of patients or family members, be careful about how much information is relayed over the radio. This helps avoid increased levels of anxiety, fear, or even worsening the patient's condition. Some information may best be relayed to the receiving agency or public safety department by some means other than radio.

Report Writing

Many individuals consider writing reports as a bothersome and time-consuming administrative duty. Reports of an emergency medical incident are of great significance. The report is important:

* To a First Responder.
* For medicolegal reasons.
* For follow-up data in reviewing patient care.

A report begins with the First Responder's observations of the incident, including:

* Response.
* Nature of the presenting situation.
* Care rendered.
* Notes of the accident.

The function of a report is to answer questions. Usually those questions will be provided on forms developed by your agency. In some states the data you provide is considered privileged information. Such data may not be released without the patient's permission, authorized by the hospital, or ordered by an appropriate legal authority.

> **REMEMBER:** The data collected becomes part of the patient's record and may be used in a variety of situations. Accuracy is important. Note every aspect of the care rendered and the surrounding circumstances.

If the incident was unusual, it is recommended that you write an "incident report." Such a report documents and records special impressions about any unusual activity; it is filed with the primary report. This is important because of the delays between the actual incident and later administrative or court reviews. Such notes will provide documentation.

The facts and activities of a medical emergency are significant because they contain important and vital information. This information will be used by other health care providers. The First Responder is often the "entry point" in the chain of events that may have resulted in lifesaving care. Everything reported is important to the health care providers who provide final responsibility.

SUMMARY

Never fail to provide lifesaving care because of fear of legal recourse. The Good Samaritan concept should prevail. Do those things necessary to preserve life, prevent further harm, reduce pain, reduce shock, and shorten the victim's hospital stay.

Know and understand the laws of your area. There is no greater reward than saving a life.

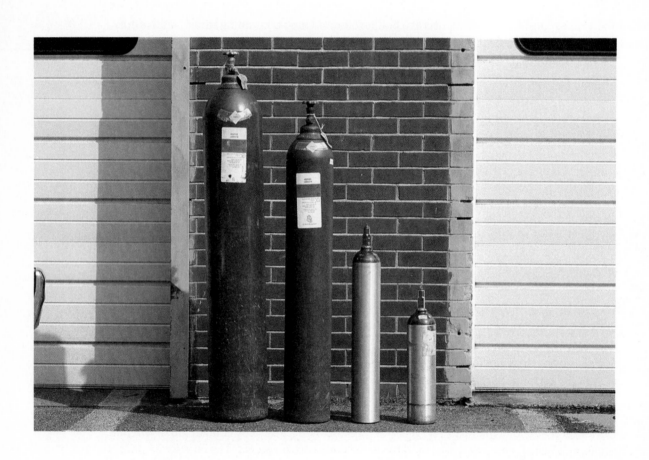

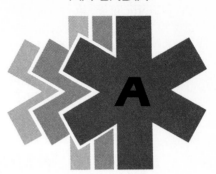

OXYGEN ADMINISTRATION

KEY WORDS

Bag-Valve Mask – A manual breathing device used for nonbreathing patients to exchange air.

Liter – A metric measure that equals approximately one quart.

Manually-Controlled Oxygen Powered Resuscitator – A device provided with a manual button to allow controlled air administration on command.

Pressure-Cycled Resuscitator – A back pressure controlled device that allows air exchange in relationship to the compliance of the lungs.

OXYGEN ADMINISTRATION

Oxygen is an odorless, colorless gas found in the atmosphere. The air in which we live contains approximately 21% oxygen with the remainder being primarily nitrogen. Medical (pure) oxygen can be fractionally distilled from the air of the atmosphere. The result of this process is liquid oxygen. Oxygen is not used in a liquid state by prehospital providers due to the extreme danger of injury if the holding container is damaged. However it is routinely used in some aircraft for oxygen systems.

Oxygen can be converted from a liquid to a gaseous form by placing it under extreme pressure. When a medical oxygen cylinder is full, the oxygen within generates approximately 2200 lbs. of pressure/square inch (PSI). These cylinders are made of steel or aluminum. Have all cylinders tested to assure they can withstand the pressure they are required to contain. The steel cylinders will feel heavier than the aluminum ones, but this does not change the amount of oxygen they hold. You cannot tell if a container is full by its weight.

To protect against placing the wrong breathing appliance on any cylinder, the cylinders are both color coded and have either a pin index system (Figure A-1) or a thread compatibility factor to make it

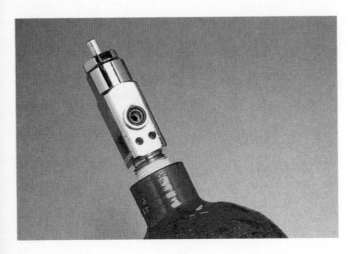

Figure A-1. The pin index system.

difficult to attach any control head other than an oxygen regulator to an oxygen container. Most medical oxygen cylinders are painted green for identification.

Oxygen cylinders come in many sizes but all hold approximately 2200 PSI. They are given letter designations to denote their size. The highest letters of the alphabet denote oxygen bottles with a larger capacity. For example, a "D" bottle holds less oxygen than an "E" bottle and an "E" bottle holds less than an "M" bottle (Figure A-2). You can tell how full a bottle is by the pressure it generates. The more oxygen present, the higher the pressure. A bottle that is half full should generate approximately 1100 PSI.

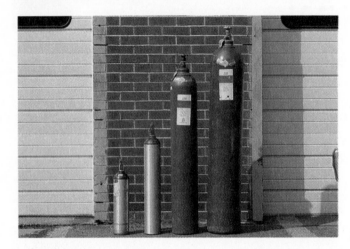

Figure A-2. Bottle sizes.

Gas flow from a cylinder is controlled by a regulator. The regulator is responsible for reducing the bottle pressure. Most oxygen appliances operate between 40-70 PSI. Some regulators are single stage and include liter flow devices (Figure A-3) while others simply work as pressure reducers. Liter flow devices work at pressures between 40-70 PSI and provide a flow rate between 1-15 liters of oxygen/min.

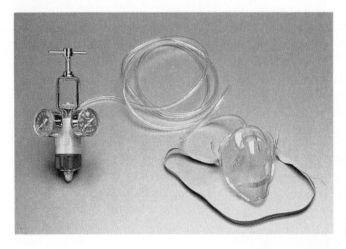

Figure A-3. The liter flow device.

Precautions must be observed when storing, handling, or using oxygen cylinders. These precautions include:

✳ Oxygen cylinders must be stored in an atmospheric temperature of less than 125 °F (50 °C).

✳ Never allow smoking in an area where oxygen is stored or in use.

✳ Oil, grease, or other combustibles must not be allowed to come in contact with oxygen cylinders, valves, or fittings.

✳ All oxygen bottles, whether stored or in use, must be securely protected from falling over since any damage to a valve may allow rapid release of the stored oxygen. In such an event the tank may become a deadly missile. Strap all stored bottles, secure all bottles upright in a vehicle, and protect all bottles with safety stands when oxygen is being used.

✳ Never use an oxygen bottle unless it is attached to an approved, properly fitted regulator. Have each regulator tested regularly to assure compliance.

✳ Be careful when working around oxygen bottles. Do not drop them or place any part of your body over the valve stem when they are in use.

OXYGEN ADMINISTRATION APPLIANCES

Oxygen Administrators

Remember that the atmosphere contains approximately 21% oxygen so use this appliance when 2 atmospheres are required to support the patient. Later in this chapter we will discuss how to help determine which patients need more oxygen. The following table shows the flow rate of oxygen in comparison to the percentage of oxygen provided.

Oxygen Flow Rate	Percent of Oxygen Provided (in percent)
1 liter/minute	24%
2 liter/minute	28%
3 liter/minute	32%
4 liter/minute	36%
5 liter/minute	40%
6 liter/minute	44%

Liter flow devices reduce the line pressure from 40-70 PSI to a flow pressure that is usable for the patient. They all have a dial that allows the First Responder to control the rate of flow from 1-15 liters/min. A liter is approximately equal to 1 quart of oxygen.

APPLIANCES FOR ADMINISTRATION

Oxygen can be administered using the following devices:

✳ Nasal cannulas.

✳ Simple face masks.

✳ Pocket masks.

✳ Pressure cycled resuscitators.

✳ Manually controlled oxygen-powered resuscitators.

✳ Bag valve mask resuscitators.

Nasal Cannula

One method of administering oxygen to a patient who is exchanging a sufficient air volume is to use a nasal cannula (prongs) as shown in Figure A-4. The two small prongs fit into the patient's nose and provide increased amounts of oxygen as the liter flow is increased. They should be used when no more than a 44% concentration of oxygen is required for the patient. If the liter flow device is set for 5-8 liters/min., an inspired oxygen concentration of 35-50% is possible.

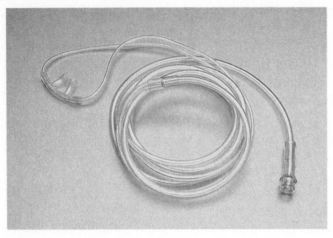

Figure A-4. The nasal cannula.

The nasal cannula is the most common appliance used for oxygen administration for patients needing minor support. Whenever they are used, the patient must be able to breathe a sufficient amount to support their functions. Remember, if a patient is a mouth breather or has obstructions involving the nasal passages, he or she will receive little oxygen flow from this device. *Do not* use them for patients who are not breathing or are moving insufficient amounts of air to support consciousness.

Simple face Masks

Simple face masks are used when greater amounts of oxygen are required for the patient. There are different sizes for adults, children, and infants. They are clear and fit over the patient's mouth and nose (Figure A-5). These masks are attached firmly to the patient's face with a strap to prevent oxygen from leaking around the mask. Some people are unable to wear masks due to feelings of claustrophobia. Some masks have reservoirs attached to allow an increased amount of oxygen to be given to the patient.

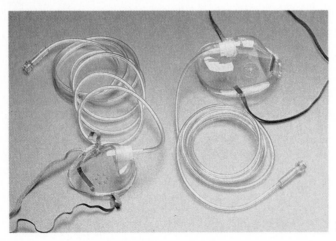

Figure A-5. Simple face masks.

With a flow rate of 6-10 liters/min., these masks will provide approximately 35-60% of inspired oxygen if firmly attached to the face. Most masks have ports on the side of the face piece that will increase the exhalation of carbon dioxide and increase the amount of oxygen inhaled. Some of these masks have port covers that can be easily removed, which reduce the amount of oxygen given to the patient. They should only be used on breathing patients in marked respiratory distress. The First Responder should never use a standard mask on a nonbreathing patient.

Pocket Masks

Pocket masks (Figure A-6) can be used for the nonbreathing patient. They provide a sufficient flow of oxygen if attached to a liter flow device set at a flow rate of 15 liters/min. The pocket mask can also be used without oxygen. Use the mask in conjunction with rescue breathing. The use of a pocket mask with a one-way valve is strongly recommended for use by First Responders. This device may serve as a preventive measure against certain communicable diseases. See Appendix B for more information. It is the best overall oxygen appliance for the First Responder's kit.

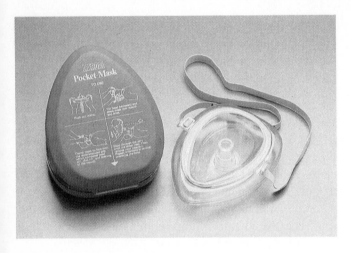

Figure A-6. Pocket mask.

Pressure Cycled Resuscitators

Pressure cycled resuscitators, such as the old Emerson, E & J, and Stephenson, are still in use. Never use the resuscitators to ventilate a patient since they are controlled by back pressure and do not provide a sufficient amount of oxygen to support life. These devices should not be used by prehospital EMS personnel, especially when performing CPR. Compressions of the chest will stop the inhalation cycle. The result is an inadequate supply of inspired oxygen. Contact your local EMS agency for information on updating this equipment.

Manually Controlled Oxygen Powered Resuscitators

Manually controlled oxygen powered resuscitators (Figure A-7) are simple to operate and quite effective when properly used. The First Responder needs to press the button on the resuscitator quickly and watch to see the chest rise. These devices are also called demand valves. Some of the commercial names are Robert Shaw, Elder, and Hare. The DOT regulations require ambulances to use manually controlled or demand type resuscitators.

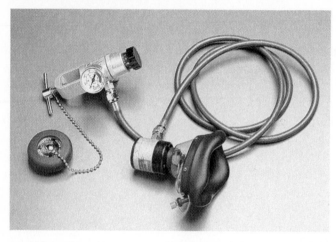

Figure A-7. Manually controlled oxygen powered resuscitator.

Demand type resuscitators have high flow rates that allow their use in rescue breathing as well as when performing CPR. When used in the demand mode, the patient will simply inhale through the firmly fitted mask attached to the valve. Oxygen at 100% will come out at varying flow rates until a pre-set pressure is achieved or the patient's lungs have been sufficiently expanded. The unit then stops delivering oxygen and the patient breathes out (exhales). These units will provide a flow rate of 40 liters/min. The First Responder must be alert for gastric distention caused by overinflation. This will increase the likelihood of vomiting. Malposition of the head and airway is also possible. In addition, the high flow rate may also hamper ventilation. The use of demand units requires much practice and training. The use of demand units is best suited for full-time EMS personnel.

Bag Valve Masks

Bag valve masks (Figure A-8) will hold approximately 1500 cc's of oxygen. They may have an oxygen reservoir to increase the amount of oxygen they can provide. The mask must be firmly attached to the patient's face and a sufficient amount of air squeezed from the bag for each breath. These masks should only be used for nonbreathing patients. A great amount of training and constant refresher courses are required to properly use this mask.

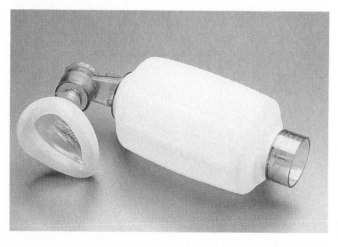

Figure A-8. Bag valve mask.

USING MASKS AND RESUSCITATORS

Always assure that no ignition source, such as matches, are present when oxygen is being used. Before using any device, explain to the patient what you are doing and how it will help them breathe. Learn how to properly use oxygen equipment before administering oxygen.

The following information summarizes how to properly use each oxygen administration device. For the cannula:

✳ Explain what you are going to do.

✳ Place a prong gently in each nostril.

✳ Attach the tube to the liter flow device.

✳ Turn the oxygen on and set the flow from 1-6 liters/min.

✳ Watch the patient closely to assure proper air exchange.

For the simple face mask:

✳ Explain what you are going to do.

✳ Remove the rubber ports from the side of the face piece as necessary to reduce the percentage flow of oxygen. The more a mask allows air to escape, the lower the percentage of oxygen that can be given. If both ports are left covered, approximately 90% oxygen by volume can be administered. When one port cover is removed, approximately 75-86% can be given. When 60-75% is required, remove both ports. Masks without reservoirs can only produce 50-60%. The liter flow setting should provide 6-10 liters/min. Remember that 10 liters of oxygen/min. will provide the patient with inspired air of approximately 50% oxygen.

For the pocket masks:

✳ Explain what you are going to do.

✳ Attach the tube to a liter flow device and set the flow at 15 liters/min.

✳ Seat the mask firmly around the patient's mouth and nose.

✳ Give 1 breath every 5 seconds.

NOTE: These appliances should only be used for nonbreathing patients.

This appliance will provide the best breath volumes and the highest volume of oxygen possible, and is the best appliance for use by the First Responder. For manually controlled oxygen-powered resuscitators:

✳ These appliances can provide air exchange for the nonbreathing patient but may blow air into the stomach and reduce blood flow and air exchange. Use of the resuscitators requires extensive training and practice.

For bag valve masks:

✳ Some people do not have hands that are large enough to fully deflate the bag. The volume of oxygen produced is related to the user's ability to stroke the bag. This appliance should only be used by well-trained and experienced First Responders.

SECRETION CONTROL

Most people experiencing breathing difficulty produce large amounts of mucous. There is really no appliance that will sufficiently remove this fluid outside a prehospital or hospital setting. The prehospital team may have a sufficient suction unit on board the ambulance but no portable unit has proven to be fully effective.

The only successful method to remove secretions may be to turn the patient over or to lift the patient upside down and drain the fluid. Unless fluids are removed they may be aspirated into the lungs of the patient. A bulb respirator, such as that used to suction an infant, may be of some minor help.

WHO NEEDS OXYGEN?

The following table provides an overview of which patients need a given amount of oxygen.

Oxygen Given (in percent)	Cause of Breathing Difficulty
1-20%	Emphysema
24-44%	Mild breathing problems
	Asthma
	Pneumonia
	Minor trauma
50-60%	Acute heart attack
	Major trauma
	Stroke
	Head Injury
more than 60%	Near drownings
	Major trauma
	Nonbreathing persons
	Pulmonary edema

REMEMBER: Never withhold oxygen from a nonbreathing patient or when a patient is in respiratory distress.

AIRWAYS:

Airways are devices that are helpful when assistance is needed to hold the tongue from the back of the throat. They can be effective when extra help is needed and no help is available. The airway (Figure A-9) should be inserted in a manner that keeps the airway open without the First Responder having to use both hands. Insert airways using the following procedure:

✳ Select an airway that is not too small, so that it will reach from the mouth to the curve of the jaw (Figure A-9a).

✳ Lift the patient's jaw (Figure A-9b).

✳ Insert the airway alongside the cheek (in a 90 ° position) and slide it along the inside of the cheek (Figure A-9c). When the airway is in the posterior portion of the throat, rotate the airway 45 °. Retract the tongue. Position the flange of the airway in front of the teeth and lips. Check the airway to see that it is in the correct position. Do this by either rescue breathing or listening for air exchange.

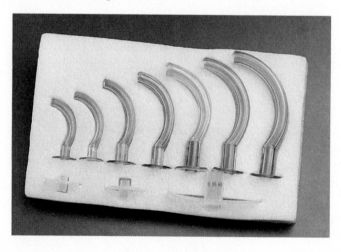

Figure A-9. Airways.

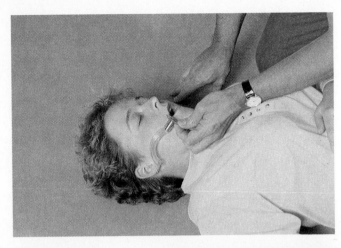

Figure A-9a. Select the correct size.

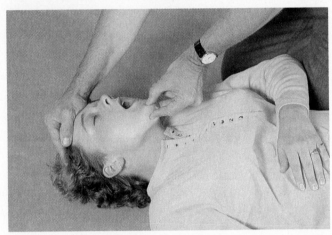

Figure A-9b. Lift the patient's jaw.

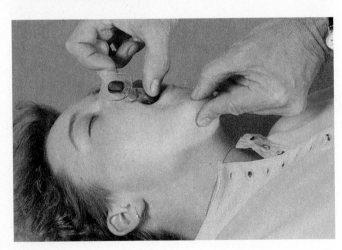

Figure A-9c. Insert the airway.

SUMMARY:

Airway management is one of the most important skills required of the First Responder. You should become familiar with the appliances used in your area since local protocol may vary. Respiratory support is one of the most urgent skills that must be provided by the First Responder.

The function of respiration is to remove carbon dioxide and provide oxygen to the body tissue. The respiratory system must have a clear route of air exchange, sufficient breath volume, and enough oxygen to support life. The appliances listed in this appendix will help you support patients more effectively.

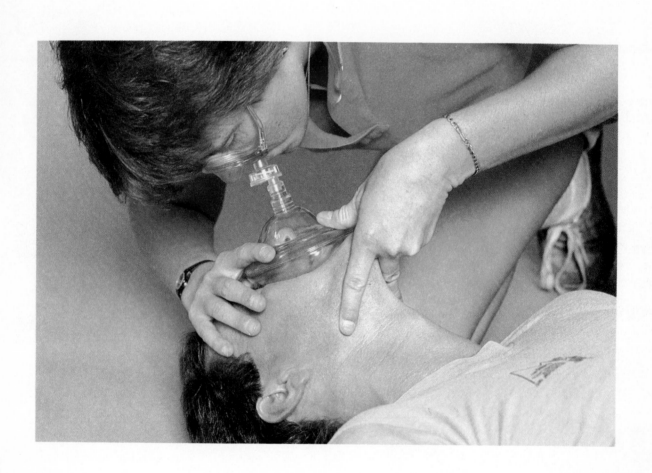

COMMUNICABLE DISEASES AND THE FIRST RESPONDER

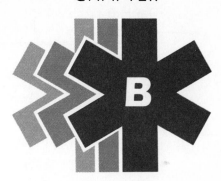

Communicable diseases (also called contagious or infectious diseases) are those diseases that can be transmitted from one individual to another. There are many ways that these diseases can be transmitted:

❋ Direct - from the infected person.

❋ Indirect - from dressings, linens, or surfaces.

❋ Airborne - from the patient through sneezing or coughing.

❋ Vehicle - via ingestion of contaminated food, water, or by contaminated drugs, fluids, or blood.

❋ Vector - via animals, e.g., ticks.

Communicable diseases have always existed but only a small number of these should concern the prehospital emergency medical care providers. The First Responder is no exception, especially since he or she is often at the scene of an incident first.

This appendix covers three communicable diseases: AIDS, hepatitis, and meningitis. Table B-1 outlines common childhood and adult diseases.

Table B-1 Common Childhood Diseases

Disease	Signs and Symptoms	Mode of Transmission	Infective Material	Protective Measures
Bacterial Meningitis	fever, severe headache, stiff neck, sore throat	direct contact	oral, nasal secretions	mask
Chicken Pox (Vaicella)	fever, rash, cutaneous vesicles	airborne, direct contact with drainage	respiratory secretions, drainage from vesicles	mask good hand washing
German Measles (Rubella)	fever, rash	airborne, direct contact with oral secretions	oral secretions	mask
Hepatitis A	fever, loss of appetite, jaundice, fatigue	direct contact oral ingestion of virus	urine, stool	mask

*Reprinted and adapted with permission from Heckman, James D. *Emergency Care and the Transportation of the Sick and Injured*. ed. 4 Park Ridge, Il American Academy of Orthopedic Surgeons, pp 361-362.

Table B-1 *(continued)*

Adult Diseases

Disease	Signs and Symptoms	Mode of Transmission	Infective Material	Protective Measures
Measles (Rubeola)	fever, rash bronchitis	airborne, direct contact with secretions	oral secretions	gloves, hand washing
Mumps	fever, swelling of salivary glands (parotid)	airborne, direct contact	saliva	mask
Whooping Cough (Pertussis)	violent cough at night, whooping sound when cough subsides	airborne, direct contact	oral secretions	mask
Scarlet Fever	fever, headache, nausea, vomiting	airborne, direct contact	oral secretions	mask
AIDS	fever, night sweats, weight loss, cough	sexual contact, blood, needles	blood, semen, possibly saliva	gloves, hand washing
Gonorrhea	discharge from urethra or vagina lower abdominal pain, fever	sexual contact secretions	genital-urinary secretions	gloves if in contact with secretions sexual protection
Hepatitis B	fever, fatigue, loss of appetite, nausea, headache, jaundice	blood, oral secretions, sexual contact	blood, saliva, semen	gloves, hand washing
Hepatitis Non A Non B	fever, headache fatigue, jaundice	blood	blood	gloves, hand washing
Malaria	cyclic fever, chills, fever	blood-mosquito vector	blood	hand washing
Mononucleosis	fever, sore throat, fatigue	mouth-to-mouth kiss	oral	none
Pneumonia	fever, cough	airborne	sputum	mask
Syphilis	genital and cutaneous lesions nerve degeneration (late)	sexual contact, blood	drainage from genital lesions, blood	gloves, hand washing sexual protection
Tuberculosis	fever, night sweats, weight loss, cough	airborne	sputum	mask

*Reprinted and adapted with permission from Heckman, James D. *Emergency Care and the Transportation of the Sick and Injured.* ed. 4 Park Ridge, Il American Academy of Orthopedic Surgeons, pp 361-362.

ACQUIRED IMMUNE DEFICIENCY SYNDROME (AIDS)

AIDS is caused by a virus that attacks the immune system of the body and damages a person's ability to fight other diseases, and ultimately causes death. There is presently no cure for AIDS, and there is no vaccine to prevent this condition.

Risk Groups

Ninety-eight percent of the reported cases of AIDS in the United States fall into the following categories:

* Homosexual or bisexual men with multiple sex partners.
* Intravenous drug abusers.
* Recent immigrants from Haiti or Central Africa.
* Sex partners of person in these groups.
* Children born to infected mothers.

AIDS is believed to be transmitted mainly by blood or sexual contact. Although the AIDS virus is found in several body fluids, e.g., saliva and tears, the usual route of transmission of the AIDS virus in the affected risk groups occurs during sexual contact with an infected person's semen, blood, and possibly an infected person's vaginal secretions.

The virus then usually enters a person's bloodstream through the rectum, vagina, or penis. Small lacerations invisible to the eye in the surface lining of the vagina or rectum may occur during insertion of the penis, finger, or other objects, thus providing an avenue for the virus to directly enter the bloodstream.

In the case of intravenous drug abusers, transmission of the AIDS virus occurs through the use of contaminated needles and syringes. The AIDS virus is carried into contaminated blood left in the needle, syringe, or other drug-related implements. The virus is injected into the new victim by using these dirty syringes or needles.

Incidents of transmission of the virus via secondary transfer of blood or other body fluids have been reported in several areas of the United States. These cases have involved medical personnel.

Emergency medical care workers, like the First Responder, are often involved in critical illness and trauma situations that may expose them to AIDS. These situations may involve direct person-to-person contact when CPR is being performed or by coming into contact with an infected person's blood during rescue attempts. It is important for the First Responder to take precautions to prevent or reduce the likelihood transmission of AIDS.

The Signs and Symptoms of AIDS

Some people remain apparently healthy after becoming infected with AIDS. There may be no physical symptoms of the illness. Many people are carriers of the virus and remain without symptoms for an extended period of time.

Persons with AIDS-Related Complex (ARC) have a condition caused by the AIDS virus in which the person tests positive for AIDS and has specific clinical signs and symptoms (of at least 1 month's duration), including:

* Loss of appetite.
* Weight loss.
* Fever.
* Night sweats.
* Skin rashes.
* Diarrhea.
* Tiredness, extreme and constant.
* Lack of resistance to infection.
* Swollen lymph nodes.

Persons in which the AIDS virus has destroyed the body's immune system are exposed to additional diseases. These diseases, called opportunistic diseases, may eventually cause death. Some of the signs and symptoms of these opportunistic diseases may include:

* Pneumonia (Pneumocystis carinii).

    Persistent cough.
    Fever.
    Shortness of breath or difficulty in breathing.

* Kaposi's syndrome.

    Multiple purplish blotches and bumps on the skin.

* Central nervous system damage (usually a long-term development; these symptoms may occur alone or with the other signs and symptoms listed above).

    Memory loss.
    Indifference.
    Loss of coordination.
    Partial paralysis.
    Mental disorders.

Precautions

Precautions to be observed in treating AIDS patients have been recommended by the Centers Disease Control (CDC) and other health agencies. These precautions include:

1. Know the facts about AIDS, including its nature, persons affected by the disease, and the routes of transmission.

2. Prevent accidental injury from needles or other sharp instruments used by these patients, e.g., knives or damaged sharp metal pieces of a motor vehicle that may have been contaminated with blood, serum, or other body fluids. The body fluids of concern are:

   * Blood.
   * Respiratory secretions.
   * Feces.
   * Urine.
   * Vomitus.
   * Semen.
   * Vaginal secretions; amniotic fluid may also carry the virus.
   * Cerebrospinal fluid (CSF).
   * Saliva (possibly).

3. Wear latex rubber gloves if hand contact with body fluids may occur. Rubber gloves should be worn when involved in any incident in which contact with body fluids may be anticipated.

4. In addition to gloves and masks, if the patient's environment involves high risk or a high blood profile, additional protective measures may be necessary. The use of eye goggles, face masks, and gowns may be prudent protective steps. This is particularly true for police/fire department first responders who often have a higher risk exposure. Disposable kits are available from medical supply houses. OSHA has included AIDS as an occupationally-related hazard. Therefore, employees are advised to consult with their local/state labor offices.

5. If rescue breathing is necessary, use a face mask with a one-way valve. Any airway equipment used should be disposable. Avoid mouth-to-mouth contact.

6. Hands or other affected skin areas of the First Responder should be thoroughly washed with soap and running water for approximately 10 seconds. Use paper towels to dry the hands.

7. Any equipment, including vehicle surface, clothing, or other material that may have come into contact with any body fluids of a suspected or confirmed AIDS patient must be thoroughly cleaned and disinfected. Recommended cleaning and disinfection procedures include the following:*

   ❋ Use an immediate-level disinfectant to clean surfaces contaminated with body fluids. These disinfectants will kill vegetative bacteria, fungi, tubercle bacillus, and viruses. The disinfectant should be registered by the United States Environmental Protection Agency (EPA) for use as a disinfectant in medical facilities and hospitals.

   ❋ Various classes of disinfectants are listed below. Hypochlorite solution (bleach) is preferred for objects that may be put in the mouth. The disinfectants include:

   Ethyl or isopropyl alcohol (70%).
   Phenolic germicidal detergent in a 1% aqueous solution (e.g., Lysol®).
   Sodium hypochlorite with at least 100 parts per million (ppm) in available chlorine (½ cup of household bleach in 1 gallon of water, which needs to be freshly prepared each time it is used).
   Quaternary ammonium germicidal detergent in a 2% aqueous solution (e.g., Tri-quat®, Mytar®, or Sage®).
   Iodophor germicidal detergent with 500 ppm available (e.g., Wescodyne®).

   All body fluids should be removed and any equipment used thoroughly washed with one of these disinfectants. Special cleaning and disinfection methods of equipment may be required (consult the manufacturer's guidelines).

   ❋ Clothing - The most important consideration in laundering contaminated clothing is to eliminate potentially infectious agents by using soap and water. Adding bleach will further reduce the number of potentially infectious agents, Wash clothing contaminated with body fluids separately. Presoaking may be required for heavily soiled clothing. Otherwise, wash and dry clothing in a normal fashion. If the material is not colorfast, add ½ cup of nonchlorox bleach (e.g., Clorox II®, or Borateem®) to the wash cycle.

   It is recommended that you consult your local hospital or health department for specific recommendations. Special cleaning and disinfection may be required depending on the equipment used. In these cases, follow the manufacturer's instructions carefully.

8. If you have had exposure to the blood or other body fluids of a suspected AIDS patient, for example, blood that has entered a cut on your finger, or a splash of another body fluid into you mouth, contact your local hospital for further guidance and testing.

*Courtesy of the State of Connecticut Office of Emergency Medical Services.

Sources of Additional Information

The CDC as well as most state and local health departments and your local American Red Cross maintain AIDS hotlines. You may call these toll-free hotlines for further information:

✳ United States Centers for Disease Control
   1-800-342-AIDS - recorded information.
   1-800-447-AIDS - specific questions.

You may write or call these agencies for information:

✳ United States Centers for Disease Control
   Atlanta, GA
   Phone:1-404-329-3543 for printed material.

✳ United States Public Health Office
   Public Affairs Office
   Hubert H. Humphrey Building
   Room 725H
   200 Independence Ave. SW
   Washington, DC 20201
   Phone: 1-202-245-6867

✳ Local Red Cross chapter or American Red Cross
   AIDS Education Office
   1730 D St. NW
   Washington, DC 20006
   Phone:1-202-737-8300

✳ Local or state health agency AIDS department

HEPATITIS

Hepatitis is an inflammatory disease of the liver, the major causes of which are Type A, B, and non-A, non-B viruses; alcohol; and drugs. The following sections describe the various types of hepatitis.

Type A Hepatitis

Type A hepatitis is caused by an RNA virus. It is spread primarily via the fecal-oral route and is responsible for localized outbreaks of hepatitis due to contaminated food, water, or shellfish. Blood and possibly other body secretions are also infectious. Type A hepatitis is also seen in children, most of whom do not show any symptoms. Children pass the disease onto their parents during close contact, for example, when diapers are changed. Type A hepatitis is generally mild in severity, except when found in the elderly, and has an excellent prognosis.

Type B Hepatitis

Type B hepatitis is caused by a DNA virus. It is usually transmitted by injection and sexual contact. The injected route may involve transmission of contaminated blood or blood products, the sharing of needles of drug abusers, or intravenous equipment used in renal dialysis treatment. The type B virus is present in the blood, saliva, semen, and urine of infected persons. Sexual partners of Type B hepatitis patients are at risk for infection.

Among the at-risk population are intravenous drug abusers, homosexual or bisexual males, medical personnel, and hemodialysis patients. First Responders can become infected from the blood or saliva of an accident victim, from contact with body fluids that enter the First Responder's body, accidental needle punctures from a drug abuser, or from contaminated or soiled bedding or dressings. Type B hepatitis is a serious illness and is often life-threatening.

Type Non-A, Non-B Hepatitis

Type non-A, non-B hepatitis is caused by at least two difference viruses that are unlike those involved with either types A or B. Transmission of this type of hepatitis is usually related to a transfusion or contaminated needle puncture.

The Signs and Symptoms of Hepatitis

Hepatitis may vary from a minor flu-like illness to fatal liver failure. The usual signs and symptoms are:

* Loss of appetite
* Weakness, exhaustion
* Nausea
* Vomiting
* Fever
* Skin rash
* Dark urine
* Jaundice

Precautions

Precautions in treating hepatitis patients, especially those with Type B, are similar to those identified for suspected or identified AIDS patients. If you are a First Responder exposed to Type B hepatitis or work in a high-risk environment, consider being vaccinated. Vaccination will provide you with active immunity against Type B hepatitis infection. Your physician or local hospital can give you appropriate medical advice on this vaccination.

MENINGITIS

Meningitis is an inflammation of the membrane (meninges) of the brain and spinal cord. Meningitis is caused by either bacteria or viruses. Both viral and bacterial meningitis are discussed here.

Viral Meningitis

Most viral meningitis cases occur as a complication of viral infection. Some of these complications occur following measles, chickenpox, smallpox vaccination, and other viral infections. Viral meningitis does not present a high risk to the First Responder. It is usually transmitted via food or water or by an insect bite.

The Signs and Symptoms of Viral Meningitis

The signs and symptoms of viral meningitis include:

* Fever (usually low grade, less than 100° F, 37.8° C).
* Headache.
* Photophobia (light avoidance).
* Stiffness in the neck and back.
* Malaise.

In cases involving the brain, other signs and symptoms may include:

* Alteration in the level of consciousness.
* Personality change.
* Seizures.
* Paralysis.

Bacterial Meningitis

Bacterial meningitis is caused by several types of bacteria, some of which are influenza, meningococci, and pneumococci. Bacterial meningitis presents a risk to the First Responder, especially if there is direct contact with respiratory secretions during rescue breathing, or from an infected patient coughing or spitting in a First Responder's face. Be careful with suspected meningitis patients who have skull fractures or fluid coming from the nose or ears. Be very careful with patients whose rashes appear to be hemorrhagic; these may appear as tiny purple dots on the skin.

Also be careful of the elderly, people whose immune systems may be depressed, and alcoholics who may have some or all of the listed signs and symptoms. These persons are more susceptible to bacterial meningitis.

The Signs and Symptoms of Bacterial Meningitis

The signs and symptoms of bacterial meningitis include:

* Sore throat (often precedes the other symptoms).
* Fever (temperature is usually higher than 104 °F, 40 °C).
* Headache.
* Vomiting.
* Stiff neck.
* Skin rash.

As bacterial meningitis progresses, more serious signs and symptoms usually develop, including

* Changes in the level of consciousness.
* Confusion.
* Stupor.
* Coma.

Precautions in Treating Meningitis

Precautions in treating meningitis are similar to those of the other infectious diseases discussed in this appendix. Avoid direct contact with body fluids and secretions. In the presence of a coughing meningitis patient, use a protective face mask and eye goggles. If rescue breathing is required, use a pocket mask with a one-way valve rather than using mouth-to-mouth resuscitation.

If you have been exposed to a meningitis patient, contact your physician or local hospital and follow their recommendations.

PREVENTION

First Responders may be exposed to a wide variety of communicable diseases so you should have an annual health examination. In addition, and with the advise of your agency and personal physician, consider immunizations for:

* German measles (Rubella).
* Tetanus and diptheria boosters.
* Influenza.
* Hepatitis Type B.

SUMMARY

Communicable diseases expose the First Responder to certain risks. These risks can be minimized by taking certain precautions when confronted with an infected person, and obtaining medical advice in the handling of these patients.

Questions worth considering are:

* Does this person have a communicable disease?
* Am I protected from this communicable disease?
* Have I decontaminated myself, equipment, and vehicle, if used, following exposure to an infected person?
* Did I receive, from appropriate medical officials, e.g., the hospital emergency department, information regarding the final diagnosis of this patient?

Remember that most communicable diseases generally produce systematic signs and symptoms that usually involve fever and increased pulse rate. A fever is generally a sign of infection. In these circumstances the First Responder should employ appropriate self-protective measures.